Communication
DISORDERS
SOURCEBOOK

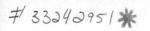

Health Reference Series

Volume Eleven

Communication
DISORDERS
SOURCEBOOK

*Basic Information about Deafness and
Hearing Loss, Speech and Language
Disorders, Voice Disorders, Balance and
Vestibular Disorders, and Disorders of
Smell, Taste, and Touch*

Edited by
Linda M. Ross

Omnigraphics, Inc.

Penobscot Building / Detroit, MI 48226

BIBLIOGRAPHIC NOTE

This volume contains individual publications issued by subagencies of the National Institutes of Health, including the National Institute for Deafness and Other Communication Disorders (NIDCD) and the National Institutes on Aging; the Department of Health and Human Services; and selected articles from the Food and Drug Administration's *FDA Consumer*. Copyrighted documents produced by the the the National Information Center on Deafness; Gallaudet University; The National Association of the Deaf; The American Speech-Language-Hearing Association; Communication Skill Builder; The American Academy of Otolaryngology—Head and Neck Surgery; The Cleft Palate Foundation; and The National Center for Voice and Speech are also included along with selected copyrighted articles from *Indiana Medicine, The Journal of the American Board of Family Practice, SHHH Journal, Tinnitus Today, Audecibel, The American Journal of Audiology,* and the House Ear Institute's *Review*. All copyrighted docments are used with the permission of the copyright holder. Docu:nent numbers, where applicable, and specific source citations are listed on the first page of each publication.

Edited by
Linda M. Ross

Peter D. Dresser, Managing Editor, *Health Reference Series*
Karen Bellenir, Series Editor, *Health Reference Series*

Omnigraphics, Inc.

Matthew P. Barbour, *Production Manager*
Laurie Lanzen Harris, *Vice President, Editorial*
Peter E. Ruffner, *Vice President, Administration*
James A. Sellgren, *Vice President, Operations and Finance*
Jane J. Steele, *Vice President, Research*

Frederick G. Ruffner, Jr., *Publisher*

Copyright © 1996, Omnigraphics, Inc.

Library of Congress Cataloging-in-Publication Data

Communication disorders sourcebook : basic information about deafness
  and hearing loss, speech and language disorders, voice disorders,
  balance and vestibular disorders, and disorders of smell, taste, and
  touch / edited by Linda M. Ross.
     p.   cm. — (Health reference series ;)
  Includes bibliographical references and index.
  ISBN 0-7808-0077-X (lib. bdg. acid-free paper)
     1. Communicative disorders.   I. Ross, Linda M. (Linda Michelle)
  II. Series.
  RC423.C644   1995
  616.8'55—dc20   95-42157
                                                                       CIP

∞

This book is printed on acid-free paper meeting the ANSI Z39.48 Standard. The infinity symbol that appears above indicates that the paper in this book meets that standard.

Printed in the United States.

Table of Contents

Preface

Part I: Deafness and Hearing Loss

Section 1: General Information

Section 2: Childhood Hearing Problems

Part II: Speech and Language Disorders

Section 1: General Information

Section 2: Adult Aphasia

Section 3: Stuttering and Spasmodic Dysphonia

Section 4: Craniofacial Anomalies

Part III: Voice Disorders

Part IV: Other Sensory Communication Disorders Including Balance, Vestibular, Smell, and Taste Disorders

Preface

About This Book

Each year, thousands of people struggle with communication disorders that affect hearing, speech and language, voice, balance, smell, taste, or touch. This book contains information compiled from a variety of sources to help those impacted by communication disorders. Many of the articles are from government agencies, including the Food and Drug Administration, the National Institute on Deafness and Other Communication Disorders (NIDCD) and other divisions of the National Institutes of Health. The material that appears in this publication was selected because it offers basic medical information to the layperson, patient, and concerned family and friends.

How to Use This Book

The NIDCD has arranged communication disorders into several categories in its National Strategic Research Plan, a research report updated regularly. The editor has followed the NIDCDs categories to organize the information presented in this book.

Part I: Deafness and Hearing Loss provides information on what is arguably the most widespread communication disorder. It is divided into seven sections, each addressing a separate area of concern. Section 1 offers general information on deafness and hearing loss. Section

2 addresses Childhood Hearing Problems including chronic ear aches, otitis media, genetics, and hereditary deafness. Noise-induced hearing loss is the subject of Section 3, while Section 4 explores Tinnitus in depth. Section 5 relates specifically to the problems of aging and hearing loss. Section 6 looks at other causes of deafness including cholesteatoma, barotrauma, otosclerosis, and the perforated ear drum. Lastly, Section 7 provides information about Cochlear Implants.

Part II: Speech and Language Disorders is organized into sections that cover general information, adult aphasia, stuttering, spasmodic dysphonia, and cleft palate and other craniofacial anomalies.

Part III: Voice Disorders gives general information on voice disorders, rehabilitation, therapy and training.

Part IV: Other Sensory Communication Disorders Including Balance, Vestibular, Smell, and Taste Disorders are often associated with the inner ear and can involve hearing loss. This section covers general information about balance and vestibular disorders, dizziness, acoustic neuroma, and Ménière's Disease. Although smell and taste disorders represent a relatively unexplored field at the present time, Part IV provides the most recent information available from the NIDCD.

Acknowledgements

The editor would like to thank Margaret Mary Missar whose expert research skills resulted in the substance of this book; Bruce the Scanman for his fantastic scanning abilities; and last, but not least, Peter and Karen for their guidance and encouragement on this project.

Note from the Editor

This book is part of Omnigraphics' *Health Reference Series*. The series provides basic information about a broad range of medical concerns. It is not intended to serve as a tool for diagnosing illness, in prescribing treatments, or as a substitute for the physician/patient relationship. All persons concerned about medical symptoms or the possibility of disease are encouraged to seek professional care from an appropriate health care provider.

Part One

Deafness and Hearing Loss

Chapter 1

Hearing and Hearing Impairment

Overview

Prevalence, Incidence and Cost of Hearing Impairment

More than 28 million Americans are believed to have impaired hearing. Levels of hearing impairment vary from a mild but important loss of sensitivity to a total loss of hearing. Approximately one of every 1000 infants is born with a hearing impairment that is severe enough to prevent the spontaneous development of spoken language. Many more infants have a less severe but substantial impairment or will acquire one by age three or four. Over 50 percent of these impairments are believed to be of genetic origin. These impairments have serious and far-reaching implications for all aspects of development, and the costs of treatment and education for these children are enormous.

The most common cause of hearing loss in children is otitis media, an infection in the middle ear. Otitis media is predominantly a disease of infants and young children. Recent studies show that about 75 percent of all American children have an episode of otitis media by the time they are three years of age. This disease is estimated to account for over 10 million visits to the offices of physicians per year and

This document is a portion of the National Strategic Research Plan for Hearing and Hearing Impairment and Voice and Voice Disorders, compiled by the National Institute on Deafness and Other Communication Disorders, a division of the National Institutes of Health.

to have a total annual cost of over $3.5 billion. The cost of managing otitis media is enormous, but it pales in comparison to the developmental and educational sequelae of otitis media.

The number of hearing-impaired people in the United States is expected to increase substantially in the next few decades due to increasing longevity and the consequent overall aging of the population. By far, the largest group of Americans suffering from hearing loss are the elderly. Thirty to 35 percent of the United States population between the ages 65 to 75 years have a hearing loss severe enough to require a hearing aid. The percentage increases with age, and 40 percent over the age of 75 years would benefit from amplification with a hearing aid. The costs of managing hearing impairments in the elderly are enormous and growing, but they are overshadowed by the costs in terms of quality of life. There are many and obvious benefits of eliminating or alleviating hearing impairments in the elderly. Recent advances in drug therapy suggest that it may be possible to replace neurotransmitters of the auditory system that are diminished in the aging process.

Hearing impairment includes auditory disorders that are not necessarily accompanied by a loss of sensitivity. Auditory processing disorders occur in learning disabled children. A substantial number of hearing impairments are caused by exposure to noise, either in the workplace or as a result of leisure activities. Strategies need to be developed to educate the public on the importance of preventing noise-induced hearing impairment. The costs associated with prevention are minimal compared to the enormous costs of rehabilitating individuals once affected.

At least 15 percent of the population are affected by tinnitus, many so severely that it disrupts their lives. The socioeconomic impact of this form of hearing disorder is great but has not been fully quantified.

Historical Background

Research on hearing impairment has not progressed as well as on other disorders. Research on the ear and the processes associated with hearing and its disorders was inhibited for many years by the fact that the tiny sensory organ for hearing, the organ of Corti, is encased by the bony cochlea (shaped like a snail shell) and was inaccessible to direct observation and experimental manipulation. The cochlea was, in fact, a "black box," which could be investigated in the living state only by indirect methods. Studies of pathology were also difficult, since the preservation and histologic preparation of the delicate structures of the inner ear were complicated by the presence of the surrounding bone.

There is insufficient public appreciation of the vital importance of good hearing to overall health and employment opportunities. All societies depend upon the mutual abilities of their citizens to understand and produce speech and language. Hearing is essential to everyday human communication, and yet it is taken for granted much more than other areas of health. Furthermore, hearing is widely and thoughtlessly abused.

Some individuals who do not hear are members of a cultural community with its own language, American Sign Language. There is great interest about the nature and acquisition of signed language and about visual processing of language by deaf people within the 1991 update of the Language and Language Impairments section of the National Strategic Research Plan.

Recent research on deafness and hearing impairment has benefited greatly from major advances in biomedical research as a whole, such as molecular biology. Rapid advances in the molecular genetics of hereditary hearing impairment are at hand.

Hearing

Transduction and Homeostasis

The sensory cells of the auditory system are located in the organ of Corti (hearing organ) and are in contact with the fibers of the auditory nerve. The sensory cells in the organ of Corti consist of inner and outer hair cells. In the auditory system, transduction is the process in which acoustic energy is converted to electrical energy, resulting in the propagation of nerve impulses in the auditory nerve. Homeostasis is the process of maintaining a tendency of stability in the internal environment. Cochlearhomeostasis is essential for the maintenance of normal hearing. Intracellular recordings from inner and outer hair cells have revealed important functional differences between the two hair cell populations. Sound energy is transduced by inner hair cells, which are now understood as mechanoreceptors. The transduction is mediated by ion channels that are directly gated by mechanical force. The hair cell's transduction channels thus differ importantly from previously characterized channels responsive to membrane potential or ligand binding.

The inner ear not only receives but also produces acoustic energy. The signals resulting from this energy are called otoacoustic emissions which can be detected with sensitive microphones in the external auditory canal. This finding has opened a new era of investigation. The source of the otoacoustic emissions is thought to be the outer hair cells. The isolation and maintenance of outer hair cells *in vitro* has led to the discovery that outer hair cells move in response to acoustical and electrical stimulation and changes in their chemical environment. Furthermore, the outer hair cell motility is influenced by nerves from the central nervous system to the inner ear. It is believed that the motility of the outer hair cells results in mechanical changes in the organ of Corti which make the inner hair cells more sensitive and capable of detecting fine frequency differences.

The origin of the unique fluid environment within the cochlea and details of intracochlear blood flow have been established, and the understanding of the biochemical mechanisms involved in transmembrane signaling is increasing.

Sound Processing in the Brain

When presented with the complex sounds of speech, the normally hearing listener is able to extract many different features of speech such as its frequencies, intensities, rhythm, location and identity of the speaker and the meaning of the words. The brain extracts these stimulus features by processing patterns of neural activity along different pathways to different subregions of the brain. Each pathway may be specialized to analyze only certain aspects of the sound. These parallel pathways are constructed from a complex network of nerve cells interconnected by excitatory and inhibitory synapses.

At present, our understanding of the neuronal processes underlying sound analysis is incomplete. Nevertheless, important progress has been made in some areas, such as understanding how sources of sounds are located in space and how speech and other complex sounds are coded at lower levels of the auditory central nervous system.

To understand how complex sounds such as speech are processed, a variety of anatomic and physiologic techniques are being used to measure and analyze responses to sounds from neurons located in different subregions of the brain. Neuronal activity patterns are associated with different cell types within each region and with the chemicals (transmitters) they use for interneuronal communication.

The aim is to describe, for each subsystem, the chain of neurons involved in the analysis and how the relevant information is represented in patterns of neural activity. Knowledge of the subsystems' transmitters can be critical in selectively stimulating or blocking elements of the neural circuits and thereby dissecting their functional roles or treating their disorders. This knowledge also can be used in mapping the location of different cell types by the application of immunologic or molecular probes.

In view of the complexity of the inner ear and the brain, small disturbances in normal function can produce substantial hearing impairments. To provide successful treatment strategies for hearing disorders or to design neural prostheses and therapeutic agents, there must be an understanding of the normal anatomy, physiology and biochemistry of the auditory system. Progress already made in these areas is being applied to the periphery in the design of cochlear prostheses and hearing aids and has led to great improvements in the ability to overcome the disabling consequences of many types of hearing impairments. Identification of transmitters could ultimately lead to the development of drug therapies for a variety of auditory system disorders including hearing impairment and tinnitus.

Auditory Perception

The study of auditory perception is concerned with how sound patterns are converted by the auditory system to experiences by the listener. Auditory perceptual research extends and relates work on physiologic aspects of sound coding to the resulting experience of sound.

Research on auditory perception also determines the relation between physical properties of complex sounds (such as environmental sounds and speech) and the experiences arising from them. Work on determining how listeners recognize the source of sounds or individual speakers and how they separate and locate inputs from several different sound sources is in progress. The benefits to be derived from increasing our understanding of how normal and impaired auditory systems mediate the perception of sound are many, and they include: (1) innovative designs for auditory prostheses, (2) greatly improved behavioral tests for diagnosis of specific auditory disorders and (3) improved methods for training and rehabilitation of hearing-impaired individuals.

Regeneration of Sensory Cells

Sensory cells in the ear of coldblooded animals can be regenerated. Even in species such as birds, in which the production of sensory cells normally ceases in early embryonic development, regeneration can occur in young and adult birds. Furthermore, the regeneration of sensory cells has been shown to contribute to recovery of hearing. Recent investigations have shown that the regenerated hair cells originate from cells produced by the proliferation of supporting cells that survive at sites of damage in the inner ear. Efforts are now under way to identify the molecular events that stimulate the proliferation of those cells, so that those events or their analogs may be tested for their potential to induce sensory cell regeneration in mammalian ears where it does not appear to occur spontaneously. Investigations of sensory cell regeneration must utilize a combination of conventional methods and methods that originate from the cutting edge of biotechnology. The questions are formidable, but the potential payoff from this research may be the long-hoped-for regeneration of auditory hair cells in humans.

Hearing Impairment

Hereditary Hearing Impairment

Hereditary hearing impairment accounts for at least 60 percent of congenital deafness. Syndromes in which there is some other finding associated with the hearing impairment account for 30 percent while nonsyndromic forms (hearing impairment alone) account for 70 percent of congenital hereditary hearing impairment. Of the nonsyndromic forms, 70 to 85 percent are transmitted as autosomal recessive, 12 to 27 percent are autosomal dominant and approximately three percent are sex-linked. A large percentage of hearing impairment with onset in childhood and adulthood also has a genetic basis, and an underlying genetic susceptibility probably contributes to many forms of hearing loss attributed to environmental factors such as noise-induced hearing loss and presbycusis.

8

The mapping of genes involved in hearing impairment will continue to provide important information and depends on the identification of families with the gene and their participation in molecular genetic studies. Location of the gene in a specific chromosomal region provides more precise information for genetic counseling and is an important first step towards isolating the gene, determining its protein product and understanding the cause of the hearing impairment.

Advances in comparative mapping of the human and mouse genomes promise to be valuable for identifying human genes responsible for hearing impairment. The insertion of genetic material into cells to prevent or ameliorate hereditary hearing impairment may soon become a possible treatment option.

Acquired Sensorineural Hearing Loss

There are a great variety of causes of acquired sensorineural hearing loss. These include: noise exposure, infections, neoplasms, trauma, degeneration and aging and immune-mediated disorders as well as unknown causes. Although the term "acquired" sensorineural hearing loss implies a nongenetic cause, there may be a genetic predisposition for the development of hearing loss from these causes.

It has been estimated that as many as 38,250 new cases of Meniere's disease are diagnosed each year in the United States. This condition results in hearing impairment and balance disturbances that wax and wane, yet continue in a progressive fashion. Despite the vexing nature of this illness, studies have led to a better understanding of the fluid homeostasis within the inner ear and the anatomical sites responsible for its maintenance. Studies of temporal bone pathology have suggested possible viral, immunologic, allergic, hormonal and environmental causes for this disease. While animal models have been developed which show some of the histologic features seen in the human condition, no model has been found which simulates recurrent attacks described in this patient population. A number of longitudinal, controlled studies on the medical and surgical treatment for this condition have been reported, however, no treatment has been shown to improve or stabilize the hearing in these patients. Furthermore, there is a disturbing tendency for this disease to become bilateral (20 to 40 percent). Therefore, there is a critical need to discover the cause of this condition and to develop treatment strategies to prevent the late sequelae of this relentless illness.

Bacterial, fungal or viral infections including acquired immuno-deficiency syndrome (AIDS) can cause sensorineural hearing loss. Bacterial and viral infections may cause sensorineural hearing loss by spreading from the middle ear or mastoid cavity into the inner ear or may spread into the inner ear from the subarachnoid space as in meningitis.

Viruses have also been implicated in sudden deafness. Patients with AIDS may have hearing loss from the AIDS virus itself or from other pathogens, including viral and fungal agents that cause opportunistic infections.

The immune system is not only an important factor in the defense of the ear against infections, but it also may be involved in hearing loss in autoimmune diseases and other types of immune-mediated hearing loss. These include systemic diseases such as polyarteritis nodosa, Cogan's syndrome and lupus erythematosus, in which the inner ear may become the target organ of antibodies or become damaged by the resultant inflammatory process. Research is needed in the diagnosis and the treatment of these disorders. Special opportunities exist to study these problems because of new technology derived from molecular biology and immunology. The role that allergic processes play in the cause of hearing impairment has been suggested but requires further study to establish its relationship.

A variety of tumors may result in a sensorineural hearing loss. One of the most frequent tumors is acoustic neurinoma (vestibular Schwannoma), the most common tumor in the posterior cranial fossa. Both benign tumors and malignant tumors, such as squamous cell carcinoma and chemodectomas, may affect the temporal bone. Further studies of the natural history, genetics, factors controlling growth and treatment, including chemotherapy, radiation therapy and surgery, are needed. For example, the recent application of the gamma knife and laser surgery to the removal of acoustic neurinomas should be studied to evaluate the efficacy of these new therapeutic approaches. During the last decade, important progress has been made in understanding how hearing loss may be caused by environmental factors such as noise, drugs and toxins. For the first time, rational hypotheses have been advanced for the mechanisms underlying hearing loss induced by aminoglycoside antibiotics, leading the way to the design of protective measures and drug modification. The understanding of inner-ear damage by diuretics has allowed the development of preventive pharmacologic strategies to be successful in animal models.

The mechanisms by which intense noise affects the inner ear are better understood. Advances include novel and important information about the effects of noise on the cochlear microcirculation, fluid homeostasis and mechanical properties of the sensory cells. These advances provide an excellent basis for future research to elucidate the molecular mechanisms underlying environmentally induced hearing deficits and strengthen the hope of finding means to prevent or ameliorate these forms of hearing impairment.

Inner ear, auditory nerve and brain stem degeneration probably contribute to the hearing disorders seen in aging persons. In most cases, no discrete cause can be found. In these instances, the term presbycusis is used. Noise exposure, both occupational and nonoccupational, is often partially responsible for the inner-ear damage observed. Some people are genetically predisposed to premature loss of hearing. Systemic illnesses such as atherosclerosis and diabetes are poorly assessed as risk factors for hearing loss in aging.

The prevalence of presbycusis has been reasonably well documented, but future population-based studies are needed to identify more clearly risk factors, including moderate (especially nonoccupational) noise exposure, smoking, diet and systemic disease. These studies should go beyond pure-tone audiometry to include measures of speech perception performance and other high-level auditory processes. Family studies can help elucidate the genetic component. Finally, epidemiologic studies should explore the impact of presbycusis on affected persons and on society.

Unfortunately, there are many disorders of the inner ear for which the cause is unknown. These include disorders as perilymphatic fistula, noises in the ear or head (tinnitus) and Meniere's disease. There is a critical need to elucidate the pathogenesis and develop treatments for these puzzling disorders.

Otitis Media, Otosclerosis and Other Middle-Ear Disorders

Otitis Media. Otitis media is the most common treatable disease of infants and young children and the most frequent cause of fluctuating hearing loss. Three-fourths of the children born each year experience at least one episode of otitis media by their third birthday, and one-third have repeated bouts of otitis media. The disease necessitates frequent health care visits for the child and parents, with an enormous impact on family lifestyle and parent work productivity. The economic impact of this disorder for families with young children is extraordinary; estimated annual health care costs for otitis media in the United States are $3.5 billion. Furthermore, some of the children who experience frequent otitis media during early childhood experience difficulty in speech and language development and some have lifelong hearing impairment. These sequelae compound the economic and societal costs of otitis media.

Remarkable advances have occurred in improving the understanding of the epidemiology, natural history and pathophysiology of otitis media. This progress is being translated into improved methods of prevention, diagnosis and treatment. New techniques of molecular and cellular biology and genetics are being applied to elucidate underlying mechanisms that predispose children to the entire spectrum of middle-ear inflammatory disorders grouped within otitis media.

Otosclerosis and Other Middle-Ear Disorders. Otosclerosis is one of the most common causes of progressive, adult-onset hearing loss, affecting one in 100 persons. It is a localized disorder of bone remodeling within the middle and inner ears. Recent advances in genetics, molecular biology and ultrastructure have improved the understanding of this disease, however, its exact cause is still unknown.

Middle-ear structures collect environmental sound and transmit it to the inner ear. An understanding of middle-ear micromechanics is essential to the development of improved middle-ear implants and implantable hearing aids.

Assessment, Diagnosis, Treatment and Rehabilitation. The identification and assessment of hearing impairment and the diagnosis of specific disorders involve collaboration among primary care physicians, otolaryngologists, audiologists and geneticists. The procedures in current use include measurement of auditory thresholds, determination of the acoustic properties of the external and middle ears, measurement of speech recognition thresholds, quantification of the acoustic reflex threshold, measurements of otoacoustic emissions and recording of the electrical activity of the brain in response to sound. Assessment and diagnosis are precursors to treatment and essential to the determination of treatment efficacy.

During the past decades, major progress has been made in the medical and surgical treatment of some hearing impairments. For the hearing impairments that cannot be alleviated by medical or surgical treatment, there is a rich array of rehabilitative intervention. This intervention has two basic components: prosthetic management and auditory rehabilitation. Prosthetic management seeks to provide access to sound patterns by means of hearing aids, cochlear implants, tactile aids, visual speech training aids and other sensory aids. Auditory rehabilitation involves training to accelerate adaptation to novel sensory inputs; develop auditory (and nonauditory) perceptual skills; enhance the integration of inputs from different modalities, such as vision and hearing; and create an emotional state that is optimally conducive for communicating.

For children with hearing impairment of sufficient severity to prevent or impair the spontaneous development of spoken language, intervention and management go well beyond prosthetics and auditory rehabilitation. The development of the basic cognitive and language skills on which subsequent development and education depend is addressed in depth in the 1991 update of the Language and Language Impairments section of the National Strategic Research Plan.

Recent Accomplishments

Basic and clinical investigators in hearing and hearing impairment are undertaking research in many new directions. They are exploiting past accomplishments and taking advantage of the tools and insights offered by recent progress in neuroscience, cellular biology, immunology, molecular biology, genetics and computer technology. Progress in understanding the mechanisms of normal hearing is accelerating. However, transferring new knowledge into clinical applications is not occurring at a comparable rate.

The relatively slow rate of applying new knowledge to the problems of patients is due to many factors: the difficulty of the problems, the incomplete state of knowledge in the basic sciences, the lack of appropriate tools and models and the shortage of investigators bridging basic and applied areas. There is a severe shortage of clinical investigators who are conversant with the state-of-the-art research methods and their applicability to relevant clinical issues.

Hearing

Transduction and Homeostasis

Many insights into the function of the cochlea have been derived recently from *in vivo* and *in vitro* studies. Considerable progress is being reported in the measurement of cochlear blood flow and the study of its regulation. Studies of the composition, production, circulation and absorption of endolymph (the fluid in the membranous inner ear) are providing insights into the regulation of the properties of this unique fluid as well as the effects of these properties on transduction. Immuno-histologic techniques have been employed and allow for an in-depth characterization of the inner ear. New research has shown that changes in hearing are associated with the loss of outer hair cells. Scientists have learned more about stereocilia and how they are physically linked at their tips and participate in frequency selectivity or tuning.

In vitro studies of isolated hair cells have led to a greater understanding of the biophysics of mechanoelectrical transduction and of ion channels in hair cell membranes. Progress has been made in the molecular and functional characterization of the structural and contractile proteins of stereocilia, hair cells and the cuticular plate. This knowledge contributes to a better understanding of how stereociliary stiffness and hair-cell micromechanics are modulated.

Important progress has been made in understanding fast and slow motility of the outer hair cell. Stimulus and response characteristics have been detailed and provide clues about the function of these mechanisms *in vivo*. Biochemical studies have revealed the presence of second messenger molecules in outer hair cells, which may play a role in their slow motile mechanisms. Modern immunohistochemical techniques have shown the presence of more than one neurotransmitter at hair-cell synapses and are being used to identify the proteins associated with ion channels. Characterization of the membrane properties of sensory and neuronal elements using *in vitro* biophysical approaches is beginning to provide an understanding of the molecular basis of auditory function. For example, the ion-channel basis of electrical resonance has been elucidated in hair-cell membranes of several species. Ultrastructural studies have revealed details about the contact zones between outer hair cells and efferent nerve fibers. In addition, cells and tissues from the inner ear can be grown in tissue culture and hence are available for *in vitro* studies.

Recent studies of basilar-membrane motion and receptor potentials in the intact animal have led to a finer appreciation of the active process responsible for cochlear frequency selectivity. In certain species, including the human, the hearing organ generates sound spontaneously or in response to acoustic stimulation. In humans, these otoacoustic emissions are produced by outer hair cells and have great promise for practical diagnostic use to identify hearing loss.

Sound Processing in the Brain

Auditory nerve fibers connecting hair cells to the cochlear nucleus in the brain stem have been identified with intracellular marking techniques. New information is also available concerning the transformation of auditory nerve input in the cochlear nucleus. The membrane properties of some of these cochlear nucleus cells have been analyzed with *in vitro* techniques that allow the manipulation of the electrical and chemical environment and subsequent intracellular staining to elucidate cell morphology, including the arborization of the entire axon. There has been substantial additional progress in understanding the encoding of complex signals transmitted from the auditory nerve to the cochlear nuclei. The relationship between the neural code for sound intensity, frequency and temporal characteristics and the perception of these stimulus variables has been further clarified. Chemical neuroanatomical studies have successfully used immunocytochemical, neurochemical, neuro-pharmacologic and molecular techniques to identify many of the neurotransmitters and receptors involved at specific synapses in structures throughout the auditory neural axis, especially with respect to the cochlear nuclei and the efferent feedback to the inner ear. The mapping of transmitter-receptor subtypes in the central auditory system has been initiated.

Research conducted in the central nervous system has produced exciting new findings. Progress has been made in understanding the structure and function of efferent feedback pathways to the inner and middle ears. There is now good evidence that both systems aid in the detection of signals in noisy environments, and there is the possibility that both may serve to protect the ear from acoustic injury. Changes in the central nervous system have been described in response to enriched and deprived acoustic environments. New insights have been generated with respect to how the brain performs complex computations to create maps of auditory space and how these maps interact with visual space.

Auditory Perception

Recent research in auditory psycho-physics has produced a set of working models of auditory perception that far exceed the bounds of the simple "energy detector" models of hearing in general use. Research underway in a variety of areas is providing remarkable advances in the understanding of how human and non-human listeners make sense of the auditory world around them; that is, how they assign identities and sources to the sounds they perceive and how they recognize the communication sounds of single and multiple speakers. This research provides the essential link that will enable the application of advances at the molecular, anatomic and physiologic levels to the design of improved auditory prosthetic devices.

There have been a number of exciting recent advances in the linking of psychoacoustical and physiological research. Behavioral measures of frequency selectivity have been developed that allow comparison with electrophysiologic measures of auditory tuning. These measures can now be used to characterize normal and impaired hearing, and the potential exists for the diagnostic application of such measures. Perceptual evidence of the role of various populations of auditory nerve fibers in coding sound intensity has recently been obtained. The influences of adaptation and active cochlear processes on perception have been elucidated in psychophysical tasks.

Increased understanding of the perception of spectral shapes and the ability of the ear to distinguish changes in shape from changes in intensity have been achieved. Spectral shape cues are used to distinguish many classes of speech sounds and contribute to auditory localization. Studies on the role of across-frequency band enhancement and interference effects on the detection and localization of sounds are providing improved understanding of complex "real-world" auditory perception.

New approaches are being used to characterize auditory localization by humans. Sounds presented over headphones can now provide the perceptions found in real auditory space, particularly when head movements are accounted for. These results provide new possibilities for presenting sounds in simulated situations and through prosthetic devices.

Increased study of the role of perceptual learning, selective attention, auditory memory and streaming in the formation of auditory percepts has contributed to the understanding of how we attend to multiple sound sources in complex acoustic environments.

Regeneration of Sensory Cells

Decades ago, it was shown that production of sensory cells in the ears of mammals ceases before birth. This finding confirmed that sensory cells are produced only during embryonic development and meant that damage to sensory cells later in life was irreparable. This fact is the basis for considering sensory hearing impairment as a permanent and irreversible condition.

It is now known that sensory cells are continually being added to the functional populations of cells in the ears of cold-blooded animals. Even more recently, it was shown that sensory cells can be regenerated in damaged cochlear epithelia in juvenile birds in which the production of these cells normally ceases early in embryonic development. This regenerative potential has been confirmed in several species and is not limited to immature animals. The results have provided an opening to understanding and perhaps manipulating the growth of human sensory cells.

Hearing Impairment

Hereditary Hearing Impairment

The genes causing a number of syndromes that involve hearing impairment have now been mapped. Recent accomplishments include the mapping of an Usher syndrome (deafness, vestibular loss and blindness due to retinitis pigmentosa) type 2 gene to the long arm of chromosome 1 and a gene for Waardenburg syndrome (deafness and pigmentary and integumentary changes) type 1 (WS1) to the long arm of chromosome 2. More than one gene is involved in both of these syndromes. At the same time, considerable effort is being expended to isolate the two genes that have been mapped. Comparative mapping suggests that WS1 is homologous to the Splotch gene in the deaf mouse.

Analyses of a large Costa Rican family in which many members have progressive low frequency hearing loss recently allowed the mapping of a gene for an autosomal dominant nonsyndromic form of hearing impairment to the long arm of chromosome 5. Other families with similar audiometric findings can now be tested to determine whether the same gene causes their impairment.

At least 28 X-linked (sex-linked) disorders involve hearing loss. Recent accomplishments include precise location of the gene causing albinism-deafness and tentative evidence of more than one X-linked gene for clinically identical forms of progressive mixed deafness. The gene for Alport syndrome has been located to the same region as one of the collagen genes (COL4A6). Further studies of several individuals with Alport syndrome suggest that mutations in the collagen gene cause this syndrome. It is of interest to note that hearing loss is associated with other syndromes caused by collagen defects, such as Stickler syndrome (COL2A1) and one form of osteogenesis imperfecta (COLlA1).

The development of human and animal cochlea-specific cDNA libraries is proceeding rapidly.

Acquired Sensorineural Hearing Loss

The role of genetic factors in disease processes that would otherwise be considered acquired has been underscored by the recent demonstration of a genetically controlled mitochondria defect which predisposes to aminoglycoside ototoxicity.

Similarly, mouse models of genetically induced sensorineural hearing loss of late onset may provide a better understanding of the genetic predisposition to presbycusis. The recent elucidation of the nature of a variety of afferent and efferent neurotransmitters will provide better understanding and possible therapy for sensorineural hearing loss. For example, the discovery of a variety of oncogenes associated with various tumors holds promise for better understanding of the development and growth of acoustic neurinomas and other tumors of the temporal bone. New insights into the prevention and treatment of ototoxicity may result from studies of pharmacologic blocking of ototoxic actions of various drugs. A better understanding of how ototoxic metabolites may cause damage to the cochlea may provide new insights into prevention and treatment of this problem.

Application of new immunobiologic techniques will provide an understanding to the normal and disrupted immune mechanisms responsible for damage to the inner ear in immune-mediated disorders. Recent evidence suggests that some individuals with progressive deafness have autoantibodies directed against inner-ear proteins. These studies open up avenues for the diagnosis of treatable forms of sensorineural hearing loss. Better techniques to diagnose perilymphatic fistulae might emerge from the findings of recent studies, suggesting a specific inner-ear protein may be detectable in perilymph that is not found in serum, cerebrospinal fluid or middle-ear fluid.

Recent developments of animal models for bacterial and viral infections, such as bacterial labyrinthitis, congenital cytomegalovirus infection and other viral infections holds promise for the development of new diagnostic and treatment modalities for sensorineural hearing loss caused by infections. In particular, recent developments in antiviral therapy hold promise for the treatment of inner-ear viral infection. Studies of biochemical factors including enzymes and the susceptibility of developing animals to ototoxic drugs will help clarify the unique susceptibility of the immature human to ototoxic drugs.

Otitis Media, Otosclerosis and Other Middle-Ear Disorders

Otitis Media. The most common cause of hearing loss in children is otitis media. Primarily a disease of infants and children, otitis media produces sequelae that may affect hearing later in life.

During the past three years, there has been important progress in understanding the epidemiology and pathophysiology of otitis media, and this progress has led to advances in prevention and treatment. This research has led to new questions and has revealed pathways for more detailed investigation.

Research in epidemiology and natural history indicates that otitis media forms a continuum of clinical and pathologic entities from acute, self-limited disease to chronic forms with destruction of middle-ear structures. Many persons affected with otitis media do not display clinical symptoms and ordinarily would go undetected. Several risk factors for acute otitis media and otitis media with effusion have been identified using multivariate models, and a genetic basis for otitis media has been suggested.

Research on eustachian-tube and middle-ear physiology and pathophysiology has provided new information on a surfactant-like substance, mucociliary clearance, neural connections between the middle ear and brain stem, tubal muscles, tubal compliance and effects of pharmacologic agents and adenoidectomy on tubal function. Anatomic, pathologic and cellular biologic research has revealed the importance of cellular regulation and differentiation and receptor expression in the pathogenesis of otitis media. Developmental changes in tubotympanic anatomy have been recorded, and ultrastructural changes of the tubotympanum have been studied in normal and several pathological

19

conditions. The application of immunocytochemistry to the study of the pathogenesis of otitis media has led to characterization of filament proteins, neuropeptides, oxidative enzymes, immunocompetent cells and inflammatory mediators. In addition, cellular patterns of middle-ear alteration, including epithelial metaplasia and migration and bone-cell activation, have been identified.

Microbiological, immunological and biochemical research has yielded additional evidence that upper-respiratory viral infections contribute to a high proportion of acute episodes of otitis media. The importance of the interaction between respiratory viruses and bacterial infection in the pathogenesis of otitis media has been revealed by human and animal studies. Research at molecular and cellular levels has begun to characterize cell-membrane receptors for bacteria causing otitis media and to reveal the contribution of bacterial cell-envelope products in middle-ear inflammation. Evidence suggests that the middle-ear immune response can be manipulated by donor T-lymphocytes from animals presensitized by oral antigen. Research has suggested that the presence or absence of an impaired immune response to certain bacterial antigens may allow differentiation between otitis media-prone and normal children.

Improving the immunogenecity of pneumococcal polysaccharide antigens and identification of common nontypable *Haemophilus influenzae* antigens have been primary goals in vaccine development for prevention of otitis media. The development, licensing and widespread use of *Haemophilus influenzae* type b polysaccharide-protein conjugate vaccines beginning in infancy is causing a major reduction in bacterial meningitis, which is an important cause of acquired sensorineural deafness.

Important progress has been made in the biochemical and molecular characterization of middle-ear inflammation including the role of bacterial products and host responses. Molecular studies have explored the bacterial genome that is related to adherence and antibiotic resistance.

Clinical research has yielded important progress in the screening and diagnosis of otitis media and has improved the medical and surgical management of otitis media. Advances in tympanometry have resulted in improved terminology and objective parameters. Bacterial surveillance has revealed changing patterns of bacterial resistance among the microorganisms that cause otitis media. The pharmacology of antibiotics used in the treatment of otitis media and their distribution into and out of the middle ear have become the subjects of intense investigation. Surgical prophylaxis and chemoprophylaxis of recurrent acute otitis media have been explored in several recent studies.

Otosclerosis and Other Middle-Ear Disorders. The understanding of otosclerosis and other types of conductive hearing losses due to infection or trauma has advanced in recent years. Using immunohistochemical and ultrastructural techniques, viral antigens of rubella and rubeola have been identified in otosclerotic tissues. These findings suggest that childhood viral infections may play a role in the genesis of otosclerosis. Recent ultrastructural studies have further elucidated this unique disorder of localized bone remodeling.

Advances have occurred in the development of biocompatible implants for the replacement of middle-ear ossicles. Additionally, there has been progress in the development of implantable or partially implantable hearing aids.

Assessment, Diagnosis, Treatment and Rehabilitation

Considerable progress has been made in the technology of hearing aids and auditory prostheses. Digital and programmable hearing aids with vastly increased potential for signal processing are being developed and fitted clinically. Programmable hearing aids permit much more precise fitting of hearing aid characteristics on the basis of individual needs than is possible with nonprogrammable hearing aids. In addition, a variety of noise-reduction schemes are being incorporated into hearing aids, ranging from those that vary the frequency response as the background noise spectrum and level change to those that process the outputs of arrays of microphones.

The multichannel cochlear implant has become a widely accepted auditory prosthesis for both adults and children. The vast majority of adult implant recipients derive substantial benefit in conjunction with speechreading, and many can communicate effectively without speechreading. Some implanted children, including the prelingually deaf, derive substantial benefit, particularly with continued use. New sound processing techniques based on high-rate, nonsimultaneous (interleaved), pulsatile stimulation have been shown to improve the effectiveness of cochlear implants. A neural prostheses for insertion into the cochlear nucleus of the brain stem has provided encouraging levels of speech reception in individuals who have had bilateral

21

destruction of the nerves of hearing caused by bilateral acoustic neurinomas or head trauma.

Studies of methods of tactual communication used by deaf and blind persons demonstrate the capacity of the skin and the proprioceptive system to provide a secure basis for the development of tactile aids. Such aids could serve as effective alternatives to powerful hearing aids and auditory prostheses.

Recent accomplishments in the area of auditory rehabilitation include use of computer-controlled video and audio laser disc systems for fully or semi-automated instruction, development of connected discourse tracking procedures for speechreading instruction, efficient enhancement of speech perception and increased understanding of the contributions of context and prior knowledge to the perception of spoken language from impoverished sensory input.

The areas of assessment and diagnosis have benefited from numerous developments in recent years, including development of noninvasive methods for measurement of the acoustical properties of the external and middle ears (acoustic immittance), that permit precise assessment and diagnosis of middle-ear disorders and disorders of discrete portions of the central auditory pathways, computer-based techniques for assessment of sound-evoked electrical activity in the cochlea (electrocochleography) and in the brain (auditory brain stem and cortical responses) and discovery and exploitation of spontaneous and induced emissions of sound from the inner ear (otoacoustic emissions). Measurements of otoacoustic emissions holds great promise for precise evaluation of defects within the inner ear and early identification of hearing impairments in infants.

Chapter 2

National Information Center on Deafness

A Provider of Information that Can Make a Difference

More than 22 million Americans have some degree of hearing loss. Young or old, deaf or hard of hearing, these people are our relatives, friends, neighbors, and co-workers.

Deaf and hard of hearing people and people who live or work with them have questions and concerns. The National Information Center on Deafness answers these questions and provides helpful information to people who need it.

NICD: A Unique Resource

The National Information Center on Deafness (NICD) is a centralized resource of accurate, up-to-date, and objective information on all aspects of hearing loss and deafness. Staff members of NICD keep in touch with experts in the field of deafness, collect information on programs, services, and a wide array of topics related to deaf and hard of hearing people, and develop publications that are highly respected.

The NICD staff and dedicated volunteers use a systematic process to ensure that all inquiries are answered efficiently and accurately. Whether it arrives by letter, telephone, or TDD, or involves a personal visit, each request for information is given the utmost care

This document was produced by the National Information Center on Deafness.

23

and answered through selected materials, personalized letters, and/or referrals to experts and supporting agencies.

Access to Resources and Experts in the Field of Deafness

Located in Washington, D.C., at Gallaudet University, the world's only liberal arts university for deaf students, NICD has access to experts knowledgeable in the field of deafness and to other resources not available anywhere else in the world.

The Gallaudet University Library, for example, contains materials on deafness dating back to 1546. The Gallaudet Research Institute is internationally recognized as a leader in deafness-related research, and the National Center for Law and the Deaf serves as a national clearinghouse on legal issues and deafness. In addition, other Gallaudet offices provide NICD with invaluable information and resources.

NICD also maintains contact with offices and commissions on deafness and countless other programs, people, resource centers, associations, and organizations across the country.

The NICD Resource Room houses more than 500 brochures and pamphlets from organizations and agencies working in deafness and related fields. Its files contain literature on almost 700 different topic areas related to deafness and hearing loss, and a database identifies programs and services for deaf and hard of hearing people throughout the United States.

NICD Publications: Objective, Up-to-date, and Easy to Read

The National Information Center on Deafness has developed more than 85 publications that answer many questions people have about hearing loss and deafness. These publications are non-technical, easy to read, and inexpensive. All NICD publications are reviewed by experts in the field for accuracy and by consumers for readability. Selected complimentary copies of publications are used frequently to respond to information requests. The NICD publications list entitled Publications from the National Information Center on Deafness is available at no charge and identifies NICD's most popular publications.

The National Information Center on Deafness
Gallaudet University
800 Florida Ave. NE
Washington, DC 20002-3695
(202) 651-5051 Voice
(202) 651-5052 TDD
(202) 651-5054 Fax

Chapter 3

Deafness: A Fact Sheet

Introduction

An estimated 21 million Americans have some degree of hearing impairment. Hearing impairments affect individuals of all ages, and may occur at any time from infancy through old age. The degree of loss may range from mild to severe. This variability in age at onset and degree of loss plus the fact that each individual adjusts differently to a loss of hearing makes it impossible to define uniformly the consequences of a loss.

Although the National Center for Health Statistics through its Health Interview Survey has been able to estimate the number of people with hearing impairments, there have been no recent national surveys which can be used to estimate the number of people who are deaf. As a result, estimates for the number of deaf people range anywhere from 350,000 to two million.

Audiological/Medical Information

There are four types of hearing loss, each of which can result in different problems and different possibilities for medical and nonmedical remediation.

This fact sheet was written cooperatively by the National Information Center of Deafness and the National Association of the Deaf.

27

Conductive hearing losses are caused by diseases or obstructions in the outer or middle ear (the conduction pathways for sound to reach the inner ear). Conductive hearing losses usually affect evenly all frequencies of hearing and do not result in severe losses. A person with a conductive hearing loss usually is able to use a hearing aid well, or can be helped medically or surgically.

Sensorineural hearing losses result from damage to the delicate sensory hair cells of the inner ear or the nerves which supply it. These hearing losses can range from mild to profound. They often affect certain frequencies more than others. Thus, even with amplification to increase the sound level, the hearing impaired person perceives distorted sounds. This distortion accompanying some forms of sensorineural hearing loss is so severe that successful use of a hearing aid is impossible.

Mixed hearing losses are those in which the problem occurs both in the outer or middle and the inner ear.

A **central** hearing loss results from damage or impairment to the nerves or nuclei of the central nervous system, either in the pathways to the brain or in the brain itself.

Among the causes of deafness are heredity, accident, and illness. An unborn child can inherit hearing loss from its parents. In about 50 percent of all cases of deafness, genetic factors are a probable cause of deafness. Environmental factors (accident, illness, ototoxic drugs, etc.) are responsible for deafness in the remaining cases. Rubella or other viral infections contracted by the pregnant mother may deafen an unborn child. Hazards associated with the birth process (for example, a cut-off in the oxygen supply) may affect hearing. Illness or infection may cause deafness in young children. Constant high noise levels can cause progressive and eventually severe sensorineural hearing loss, as can tumors, exposure to explosive sounds, heavy medication, injury to the skull or ear, or a combination of these factors.

Central hearing loss may result from congenital brain abnormalities, tumors or lesions of the central nervous system, strokes, or some medications that specifically harm the ear.

The detection and diagnosis of hearing impairment have come a long way in the last few years. It is now possible to detect the presence of hearing loss and evaluate its severity in a newborn child. While medical and surgical techniques of correcting conductive hearing losses have also improved, medical correction for sensorineural hearing loss has been more elusive. Current research on a cochlear implant which provides electrical stimulation to the inner ear may lead to important improvements in the ability to medically correct profound sensorineural hearing loss.

Educational Implications

Deafness itself does not affect a person's intellectual capacity or ability to learn. Yet, deaf children generally require some form of special schooling in order to gain an adequate education.

Deaf children have unique communication needs. Unable to hear the continuous, repeated flow of language interchange around them, deaf children are not automatically exposed to the enormous amounts of language stimulation experienced by hearing children during their early years. For deaf children, early, consistent, and conscious use of visible communication modes (such as sign language, fingerspelling, and Cued Speech) and/or amplification and aural/oral training can help reduce this language delay. Without such assistance from infancy, problems in the use of English typically persist throughout the deaf child's school years. With such assistance, the language learning task is easier but by no means easy.

This problem of English language acquisition affects content areas as well. While the academic lag may be small during the primary grades, it tends to be cumulative. A deaf adolescent may be a number of grade levels behind hearing peers. However, the extent to which hearing impairment affects school achievement depends on many factors—the degree and type of hearing loss, the age at which it occurred, the presence of additional handicaps, the quality of the child's schooling, and the support available both at home and at school.

Many deaf children now begin their education between ages one to three years in a clinical program with heavy parental involvement. Since the great majority of deaf children—over 90 percent—are born to hearing parents, these programs provide instruction for parents on implications of deafness within the family. By age four or five, most deaf children are enrolled in school on a full-day basis. Approximately one-third of school-age deaf children attend private or public residential schools. Some attend as day students and the rest usually travel home on weekends. Two-thirds attend day programs in schools for the deaf or special day classes located in regular schools, or are mainstreamed into regular school programs. Some mainstreamed deaf children do most or all of their schoolwork in regular classes, occasionally with the help of an interpreter, while others are mainstreamed only for special activities or for one or two classes.

In addition to regular school subjects, most programs do special work on communication and language development. Class size is often limited to approximately eight children to give more attention to the children's language and communication needs.

At the secondary school level, students may work toward a vocational objective or follow a more academic course of study aimed at postsecondary education at a regular college, a special college program for deaf students (such as Gallaudet University or the National Technical Institute for the Deaf) or one of the 100 or more community colleges and technical schools that have special provisions for deaf students.

Communication: Some Choices

Communication is an important component of everyone's life. The possible choices for communication involve a variety of symbol systems. For example, you may communicate in English through speaking and writing. Despite your skills, you probably cannot communicate with someone whose only language is Chinese, even though that person also speaks, reads, and writes quite fluently.

In the United States, deaf people also use a variety of communication systems. They may choose among speaking, speechreading, writing, and manual communication. Manual communication is a generic term referring to the use of manual signs and fingerspelling.

American Sign Language

American Sign Language (ASL) is a language whose medium is visible rather than aural. Like any other language, ASL has its own vocabulary, idioms, grammar, and syntax—different from English. The elements of this language (the individual signs) consist of the handshape, position, movement, and orientation of the hands to the body and each other. ASL also uses space, direction and speed of movements, and facial expression to help convey meaning.

Fingerspelling

When you spell with your fingers, you are in effect "writing in the air." Instead of using an alphabet written on paper, you are using a manual alphabet, that is, one with handshapes and positions corresponding to each of the letters of the written alphabet.

Conversations can be entirely fingerspelled. Among deaf people, however, fingerspelling is more typically used to augment American Sign Language. Proper names and terms for which there are no signs are usually fingerspelled. In the educational setting, the use of fingerspelling as the primary mode of communication in combination with spoken English is known as the Rochester method.

Manual English

When the vocabulary of the American Sign Language and fingerspelled words are presented in English word order, a "pidgin" results. Pidgin Sign English (PSE) is neither strictly English nor ASL, but combines elements of both.

A number of systems have recently been devised to assist deaf children in learning English. These systems supplement some ASL signs with invented signs that correspond to elements of English words (plurals, prefixes, and suffixes, for example). There is usually a set of rules for word (sign) formation within the particular system. These systems are generically known as manually coded English or manual English systems. The two most commonly used today are Signing Exact English and Signed English. While each of these systems was devised primarily for use by parents and teachers in the educational setting, many of the invented and initialized signs from their lexicons are filtering into the vocabulary of the general deaf community.

Oral Communication

This term denotes the use of speech, residual hearing, and speechreading as the primary means of communication for deaf people.

The application of research findings and technological advances through the years has led to refinements in the rationale for and approach to teaching speech to deaf children. Several findings are pertinent here. Deaf children may actually have functional residual hearing. The speech signal is redundant. Since it carries excess information, it is not necessary to hear every sound to understand a message. For language learning to be successful with deaf children (no

matter what the educational approach), programs of early intervention must take place during the critical language-learning years of
birth through six years of age. Hearing screening procedures that accurately detect hearing impairments in very young children make it
possible to fit hearing aids and other amplification devices and to introduce auditory and language training programs as soon as the problem is detected.

Almost all auditory approaches today rely heavily on the training
of residual hearing. The traditional auditory/oral approach trains the
hearing impaired child to acquire language through speechreading
(lipreading), augmented by the use of residual hearing, and sometimes
vibro-tactile cues. The auditory/verbal approach (also called
unisensory or acoupedic method) teaches children to process language
through amplified residual hearing, so that language is learned
through auditory channels.

Speechreading

Recognizing spoken words by watching the speaker's lips, face,
and gestures is a daily challenge for all deaf people. Speechreading is
the least consistently visible of the communication choices available to
deaf people; only about 30 percent of English sounds are visible on the
lips, and 60 percent are homophonous, that is, they look like something else. Try it for yourself. Look in a mirror and "say" without voice
the words "kite," "height," "night." You'll see almost no changes on your
lips to distinguish among those three words. Then say the following
three words—"maybe," "baby," "pay me." They look exactly alike on the
lips.

Some deaf people become skilled speechreaders, especially if they
can supplement what they see with some hearing. Many do not develop great skill at speechreading, but most deaf people do speechread
to some extent. Because speechreading requires guesswork, very few
deaf people rely on speechreading alone for exchanges of important information.

Cued Speech

Cued Speech is a system of communication in which eight hand
shapes in four possible positions supplement the information visible
on the lips. The hand "cue" signals a visual difference between sounds

that look alike on the lips—such as /p/, /b/, /m/. These cues enable the hearing impaired person to see the phonetic equivalent of what others hear. It is a speech-based method of communication aimed at taking the guesswork out of speechreading.

Simultaneous Communication

This term denotes the combined use of speech, signs, and fingerspelling. Simultaneous communication offers the benefit of seeing two forms of a message at the same time. The deaf individual speechreads what is being spoken and simultaneously reads the signs and fingerspelling of the speaker.

Total Communication

Total Communication is a philosophy which implies acceptance and use of all possible methods of communication to assist the deaf child in acquiring language and the deaf person in understanding.

Historically, proponents of particular systems have often been at odds with proponents of other systems or modes. There is increasing consensus that whatever system or systems work best for the individual should be used to allow the hearing impaired person access to clear and understandable communication.

Deaf Adults in Today's Society

The deaf adult population in the United States is composed both of individuals deaf since early childhood and individuals who lost their hearing later in life. People who were deafened as adults, or after the age of 18, are sometimes called post-vocationally deaf. Having already embarked on their careers, these people may have serious problems both personally and professionally adjusting to their hearing loss. People who were deafened prior to age 18 may have problems not only with English language skills, but also, because of fewer opportunities for interaction with hearing people in pre-work settings, they may be less well prepared for interpersonal relationships they encounter in the job market. Discrimination is a common problem for minority groups. Deaf people as members of a minority group experience their share of discrimination. Deaf people as a group are underemployed. Together with members of other minority and disabled groups, deaf people are working to change attitudes which have given them jobs but inadequate advancement opportunities.

In the United States, deaf people work in almost every occupational field. Some have become doctors, dentists, lawyers, and members of the clergy. A number of deaf people enter careers within the field of deafness. Thirteen-hundred teachers of deaf students in the United States are themselves hearing impaired individuals. In addition, there are deaf administrators, psychologists, social workers, counselors, and vocational rehabilitation specialists. Deaf people drive cars and hold noncommercial pilot's licenses and pursue the same leisure time interests as everyone else.

Many deaf young people have attended school with deaf classmates. This educational pattern, coupled with ease of communication and compatibility encouraged by shared experiences as deaf individuals, leads to socializing with other deaf individuals in maturity. Many deaf people (80 percent) tend to marry other deaf people; most of their children (approximately 90 percent) are hearing.

The Deaf Community

Because the problem in dealing with the hearing world is one of communication, deaf people tend to socialize together more than do people with other disabilities. However, members of the deaf community have contacts with other people, too. Some are active members of organizations of hearing people. Some deaf people move freely between hearing and deaf groups, while other deaf people may have almost no social contact with hearing people. A few deaf people may choose to socialize only with hearing people.

While it is possible to find deaf individuals in every section of the United States, there are major concentrations of deaf people in the larger metropolitan areas of the East and West coasts.

Organizations of and for Deaf People

Clubs and organizations of deaf people range in purpose from those with social motives (watching captioned films, for example) to those with charitable aims. Organizations offer deaf people the opportunity to pursue a hobby (athletics, drama) or civic commitment (political action) on the local, regional or national level. Local or state associations of deaf people may be affiliated with the National Association of the

Deaf. The Oral Deaf Adults Section of the Alexander Graham Bell Association for the Deaf has local chapters that provide social opportunities for deaf people who favor oral communication. The National Fraternal Society of the Deaf provides insurance and supports social and charitable functions. It has 120 divisions throughout the United States and Canada.

A few of the more than 20 national organizations of and for deaf people in the United States are briefly described in the following list. Many of these organizations publish newsletters, magazines, or journals. Add to these the publications developed by clubs and schools for the deaf (for students and alumni) and it is possible to identify 400 publications aimed at a readership within the deaf community.

Alexander Graham Bell Association for the Deaf
3417 Volta Place, NW
Washington, DC 20007
(202) 337-5220 (V/TDD)

A private, nonprofit organization serving as an information resource, advocate, publisher, and conference organizer, the Alexander Graham Bell Association is committed to finding more effective ways of teaching deaf and hard of hearing people to communicate orally. Sections within the organization focus on the needs of deaf adults (Oral Deaf Adults Section) and parents (International Parent Organization).

American Deafness and Rehabilitation Association (ADARA)
P.O. Box 21554
Little Rock, AR 72225
(501) 663-7074 (V/TDD)

An interdisciplinary organization for professional and lay persons concerned with services to adult deaf people, ADARA sponsors workshops for state rehabilitation coordinators.

American Society for Deaf Children
814 Thayer Avenue
Silver Spring, MD 20910
(301) 585-5400 (V/TDD)

Composed of parents and concerned professionals, ASDC provides information, organizes conventions, and offers training to parents and families with children who are hearing impaired.

National Association of the Deaf
814 Thayer Avenue
Silver Spring, MD 20910
(301) 587-1788 (V/TDD)

With 50 state association affiliates and an aggregate membership exceeding 20,000, the NAD is a consumer advocate organization concerned about and involved with every area of interest affecting life opportunities for deaf people. It serves as a clearinghouse of information on deafness, offers for sale over 200 books on various aspects of deafness, and works cooperatively with other organizations representing both deafness and other disabilities on matters of common concern.

Educational Institutions

Schools for deaf students have traditionally played an important role in advancing the welfare of deaf people through education of deaf students and public information efforts about the capabilities and accomplishments of deaf people. Two national institutions each have enrollments of over 1,000 deaf students.

Gallaudet University
800 Florida Ave. NE
Washington, DC 20002-3695

National Technical Institute for the Deaf
Rochester Institute of Technology
1 Lomb Memorial Drive
Rochester, NY 14623

For descriptions of the more than 100 postsecondary programs for deaf students at community colleges and technical schools around the country, order a copy of *College and Career Programs for Deaf Students*. For price information, contact:

College and Career Guide
c/o Gallaudet Research Institute
Center for Assessment and Demographic Studies
800 Florida Ave. NE
Washington, DC 20002-3695

Special Devices for Deaf People

Technology and inventiveness have lead to a number of devices which aid deaf people and increase convenience in their daily lives. Many of these devices are commercially available under different trade names.

Telecommunications Devices for Deaf People (TDDs) are mechanical/electronic devices which enable people to type phone messages over the telephone network. The term TDD is generic and replaces the earlier term TTY which refers specifically to teletypewriter machines. Telecaption adapters, sometimes called decoders, are devices which are either added to existing television sets or built into certain new sets to enable viewers to read dialogue and narrative as captions (subtitles) on the TV screen. These captions are not visible without such adapters.

Signalling Devices which add a flashing and/or vibrating signal to the existing auditory signal are popular with hearing impaired users. Among devices using flashing light signals are door "bells," telephone ring signallers, baby-cry signals (which alert the parent that the baby is crying), and smoke alarm systems. Alarm clocks may feature either the flashing light or vibrating signal.

Some Special Services

Numerous social service agencies extend their program services to deaf clients. In addition, various agencies and organizations—either related to deafness or to disability in general—provide specific services to deaf people. Among these special services are the following:

Captioned Films for the Deaf

A loan service of theatrical and educational films captioned for deaf viewers. Captioned Films for the Deaf is one of the projects funded by the Captioning and Adaptations Branch of the U.S. Department of Education to promote the education and welfare of deaf people through the use of media. This branch also provides funds for closed-captioned television programs, including the live-captioned ABC-TV news.

Registry of Interpreters for the Deaf, Inc. (RID)

A professional organization, RID maintains a national listing of individuals skilled in the use of American Sign Language and other sign systems and provides information on interpreting and evaluation and certification of interpreters for deaf people.

State Departments of Vocational Rehabilitation

Each state has specific provisions for the type and extent of vocational rehabilitation service, but all provide vocational evaluation, financial assistance for education and training, and job placement help.

Telecommunications for the Deaf, Inc.

TDI publishes an international telephone directory of individuals and organizations who own and maintain TDDs (telecommunications devices for deaf people) for personal or business use.

Contributors to the original fact sheet:

Roger Beach, Ph.D., Asst. Professor, Department of Counseling, Gallaudet University.

Bernadette Kappen, Ph.D., Asst. Principal, Overbrook School for the Blind, Philadelphia, PA.

William McFarland, Ph.D., Director of Audiology, Otologic Medical Group, Los Angeles, CA.

Philip Schmitt, Ph.D., Professor, Department of Education, Gallaudet University.

Ben M. Schowe, Jr., Ph.D., Learning Resources Center, MSSD, Gallaudet University.

Leticia Taubena-Bogatz, M.A., Teacher, KDES, Gallaudet University.

Revised by Loraine DiPietro, Director, National Information Center on Deafness, Gallaudet University.

Suggested Readings

Davis, H. and R. S. Silverman. *Hearing and Deafness*. 4th ed. New York: Holt, Rinehart and Winston, 1978.

Freeman, R., C. F. Carbin, and R. Boese. *Can't Your Child Hear? A Guide for Those Who Care About Deaf Children*. Baltimore: University Park Press, 1981.

Gannon, J. *Deaf Heritage*. Silver Spring, MD; National Association of the Deaf, 1981.

Katz, L., S. Mathis, and E. C. Merrill, Jr. *The Deaf Child in the Public Schools: A Handbook for Parents of Deaf Children*. 2nd ed. Danville, IL: Interstate Printers and Publishers, 1978.

Mindel, E. and M. Vernon. *They Grow in Silence: The Deaf Child and His Family*. Silver Spring, MD: National Association of the Deaf, 1971.

Moores, D. *Educating the Deaf: Psychology, Principles, and Practices*. 3rd. ed. Boston: Houghton Mifflin Co., 1987.

Ogden, P. and S. Lipsett. *The Silent Garden: Understanding the Hearing Impaired Child*. New York City: St. Martin's Press, 1982.

Schlesinger, H. and K. Meadow. (1974). *Sound and Sign: Childhood Deafness and Mental Health*. Berkeley University of California, 1974.

Spradley, T. S. and J. P. Spradley. *Deaf Like Me*. Washington, DC: Gallaudet University Press, 1978.

Directory of Services

The April issue of the American Annals of the Deaf is a directory of the various programs and services for deaf persons in the United States. Copies of this reference may be purchased from:

American Annals of the Deaf
Gallaudet University
KDES, PAS 6
800 Florida Ave. NE Washington, DC 20002-3695

Additional Information

If you have specific questions that were not answered by this fact sheet, please contact either the National Information Center on Deafness, Gallaudet University, Washington, DC 20002, or the National Association of the Deaf, 814 Thayer Avenue, Silver Spring, MD 20910.

The National Information Center on Deafness (NICD) is a centralized source of information on all aspects of deafness and hearing loss, including education of deaf children, hearing loss and aging, careers in the field of deafness, assistive devices and communication with hearing impaired people.

Chapter 4

Treatment of Sensorineural Hearing Loss

Abstract

Of the 25 million people who are hearing impaired, 85% suffer from sensorineural hearing loss (SNL). In the past decade, the identification and treatment of SNL have evolved from futile efforts to active intervention. This paper identifies nine forms of inner ear disorders causing SNL for which medical/surgical treatment is available. Physicians must realize that, with appropriate diagnosis and treatment, hearing nerve loss can have a satisfactory outcome.

During the past decade, otologists have focused their attention on identifying and treating sensorineural hearing loss (SNL). Before this time, a loss of hearing due to decreased hearing nerve function was untreatable, except by amplification.

The conquest of middle ear deafness by replacing ossicles, restoring the tympanic membrane or removing diseased tissue using microsurgical techniques has become an accomplished fact. The success in conductive deafness treatment has overshadowed recent progress in hearing improvement in the larger population of sensorineurally deaf patients. Conductive deafness affects only 15% of the 25 million people who are hearing-impaired.

This excerpt was originally published in *Indiana Medicine*, August 1991. Used by permission.

There are nine forms of inner ear disorders causing SNL for which medical/surgical treatment is available. Although responses to treatment vary, any relief is appreciated by the afflicted patient.

This article will review the progress in managing sensorineural deafness and outline nine forms of SNL for which treatment should be instituted (Table 4.1).

Ménière's Disease

Ménière's disease is a clear-cut clinical entity characterized by hearing loss, vertigo, ear fullness and tinnitus. Substantial benefit is obtained from dietary, medical and/or surgical treatments. The major spells can be stopped in more than 90% of patients, and hearing can be improved or stabilized in two-thirds of patients.

All patients are placed on a salt- and caffeine-restricted diet and advised to stop smoking. Other medications such as diuretics, vasodilators and vestibular suppressants can be used.

Diazepam frequently is used and is beneficial in the latter category. Meclizine is seldom beneficial.

Surgery is offered to patients who do not improve with medical and dietary therapies. If hearing is salvageable, an endolymphatic sac-mastoid shunt is usually the first choice. The shunt is an outpatient surgical procedure offering more than an 80% chance of controlling dizziness and, especially in the early stages of the disease, about a 60% chance of stabilizing or reversing sensorineural hearing loss. If this procedure fails to control the vertigo and there is reasonably good hearing, a retro-sigmoid or suboccipital vestibular nerve section is performed to save auditory nerve function.

Intraoperative surgical monitoring is recommended to minimize risk to the facial and auditory nerves. This procedure does nothing to alter the basic disease process in the cochlea and, after a period of time, hearing can deteriorate severely. If no useable hearing is present and tinnitus is severe, total VIIIth nerve section is done to provide relief of tinnitus and vertigo. If tinnitus is not a primary complaint, labyrinthectomy usually is curative.

The goals of therapy today are not only to relieve dizzy spells but also to improve and stabilize hearing.

Table 4.1. Treatment of Sensorineural Hearing Loss (SNL)

TYPE	CHARACTERISTICS	*SPECIFIC DIAGNOSTIC TESTS	MEDICAL TREATMENT	SURGICAL Rx	SUCCESS WITH EARLY INTERVENTION
MENIERE'S DISEASE	Fluctuating hearing loss, fullness, tinnitus, episodic vertigo	ECoG Audiogram ENG	Salt, caffeine restriction, cessation smoking, diuretic, vasodilators, vestibular suppressants.	Endolymphatic sac-mastoid shunt; Vestibular nerve section; Cochleo-vestibular nerve section; Labyrinthectomy	80% vertigo control, hearing stabilization; 95% vertigo control; hearing preservation; 95% vertigo control; no hearing; 90% vertigo control; no hearing
AUTOIMMUNE SNL	Rapid hearing loss Possible vestibular sx	Immune screen	Steroids Cyclophosphamide Plasmaphoresis	None	95% control
SYPHILITIC DEAFNESS	Variable; Meniere's-like Sx	FTA-ABS	Steroids Antibiotics	None	Good
COCHLEAR OTOSCLEROSIS	Flat hearing loss Usual family history	CT Scan	Flouride, calcium, Vit. D	None	Good degree of stabilization
SUDDEN DEAFNESS	Rapid (< 72 hrs) loss of hearing; possible vertigo		Steroids Carbogen I.V. contrast media	None	20-80%
TOXIC DEAFNESS	Hearing loss, tinnitus Imbalance on medication	Posturography Serial Audiometry and ENG	Cessation or reduction of offending medication	None	Variable; depends on particular ototoxic medication
PROFOUND SNL	No hearing; no benefit from amplification	Complete test battery Psychological profile	None	Cochlear Implant	Improved
NOISE INDUCED SNL	Tinnitus; hearing loss after noise exposure	Serial Audiology	Ear protection Possible steroids Hearing Aids	None	Good to excellent with early intervention
PERILYMPH FISTULA	Hearing loss, dizziness	ECoG ENG - Impedence test	Bedrest, stool softeners, cough suppressants	Tympanotomy and fistula grafting	95% dizziness control 50-80% hearing control

*Although all patients receive other diagnostic tests, these tests have great diagnostic specificity.

Perilymph Fistula

Perilymph fistula is a leakage of fluid (perilymph) from the inner ear (labyrinth) into the middle ear through the round and/or oval windows. A history of exertion, barotrauma or an audible "pop" in the ear at the time of the hearing loss suggests this entity. A fistula within the cochlea also can develop, causing a mixing of the inner ear fluids (endolymph and perilymph). This condition disrupts the delicate balance of electrolytes within the inner ear compartment. Although symptoms characteristically are fluctuating hearing loss alone (15%) or vestibular symptoms alone (12%), both symptoms commonly are present. Developmental anomalies, such as a widely patent cochlear aqueduct or cochlear modiolar defects, may predispose the involved ear to this condition.

Historical features suggesting fistula of the inner ear include compressive/decompressive episodes, heavy lifting or straining, head injury or stapedectomy. Conservative treatment consists of bed rest, stool softeners and avoiding heavy lifting, coughing or straining. Sensorineural hearing loss that continues to progress, with or without positional vertigo and ataxia while walking, indicates the need for surgery. A tympanotomy with tissue sealing of the oval and round windows will eliminate dizzy symptoms in 95% of patients and improve or stabilize hearing in 50% of patients.

Autoimmune Sensorineural Deafness

Autoimmune sensorineural deafness is a treatable form of severe hearing loss when the body's immune system attacks and progressively destroys the inner ear. Reports indicate that it may involve patients of any age. It may take the form of sudden or fluctuating hearing losses. Any patient with a bilateral or asymmetric sensorineural deafness for which the cause is not readily apparent is suspect for this disease. It is important to recognize it since there is no treatment other than immunosuppression that may salvage or restore hearing. Without treatment, all hearing is lost.

Any patient suspected of having this disease should have an immune screen (sedimentation rate, rheumoid factor, anti-nuclear antibody with and without culture cells and quantitative IgA and IgG). If any two of these are positive, treatment should be started.

Our treatment is dexamethasone, 16 mg daily in divided doses for a period of approximately three months before tapering the medication begins. Twice-weekly audiograms are used to monitor the patient. In severe bilateral cases, some investigators have used cyclophosphamide infusion. We have not needed to use this medication. Patients who cannot tolerate steroid therapy are candidates for plasmapheresis.

Identifying this cause of sensorineural deafness is of paramount importance since it can be reversed totally.

Syphilitic Deafness

Sensorineural hearing loss due to syphilis has been around for years. The benefits of steroid therapy after appropriate antibiotic treatment are well-documented. This form of deafness and vertigo may mimic Ménière's disease; thus, all patients suspected of Ménière's must have appropriate testing for tertiary syphilis. A fluorescent treponemal antibody/absorbed is suggested.

Steroid therapy eliminates vertigo and allows patients to hear for up to 10 years. Steroid therapy every other day can provide relief without significant side effects.

Medications with Toxic Effects on Hearing

The medications listed below have toxic effects on the hearing or balance function of the inner ear. The prescribing physician should consult the *Physicians' Desk Reference,* a pharmacist or similar source before prescribing these medications.

This list is not exhaustive but provides guidance in using some common medications. Hearing and balance function monitoring is recommended when potentially ototoxic medications are used. [Medications are listed in this format: chemical name; trade name.]

Aminoglycoside Antibiotics

Streptomycin; —
Neomycin; Mycifradin, Neobiotic
Kanamycin; Dantrex, Klebcil
Tobramycin; Nebcin

Paromomycin; Humatin
Gentamicin; Garamycin
Sisomycin; Sispetin
Amikacin; Amikin
Netilmicin; Netromycin

Chemotherapeutic

Cisplatin; Platinol

Salicylic Acid Derivatives

Aspirin; Various (effects reversible)

Other Antibiotics

Vancomycin; Vancocin
Erythromycin; Various (rarely ototoxic)
Capreomycin; Capastat (rarely ototoxic)

Metal Antagonist

Deferoxamine; Desferal (usually reversible)

Loop Diuretics

Ethacrynic acid; Edecrin
Furosemide; Lasix
Bumetanide; Bumex

Drug Combination

Neomycin; Aminoglycoside
Polymyxin B; Loop Diuretics
Dexamethasone

Cochlear Otosclerosis

Cochlear otosclerosis is characterized by a flat audiometric loss and good to excellent speech understanding and starts in the third or fourth decade of life. Although a positive family history of proven stapedial otosclerosis is usually present, this is not necessary. This type of hearing nerve loss can be arrested (85%) or even reversed (15% of the 85%) with appropriate doses of daily fluoride, Vitamin D and calcium. Since fluoride therapy can prematurely close the epiphyseal plate in developing bones, it must be used with caution in children or pregnant women.

Sudden Deafness

Sudden hearing loss is defined as a loss of at least 30 dB in three contiguous frequencies in less than 72 hours and occurs in about 10 people per 100,000 per year. Both men and women are affected, with an average age of 43 years at onset. In most cases, the etiology cannot be determined. Most commonly, the sudden loss is attributed to either viral infection or compromised circulation to the inner ear.

Our treatment for this idiopathic loss is primarily steroid therapy. The prognosis for recovery depends upon: 1) the hearing loss configuration; 2) the patient's age; 3) the degree of vestibular injury defined by the electronystagmogram; 4) the presence or absence of vertigo; and 5) the duration of the loss. Patients with a mild mid-frequency hearing loss often recover all of the lost hearing. Patients with a moderate sensorineural hearing loss will have a partial recovery rate, ranging from 40% to 80%. Patients with severe to profound loss have a 20% chance of recovery.

Administering intravenous iodinated contrast media is another treatment that we have used for sudden idiopathic hearing nerve deafness. Inhaling carbogen (95% O_2 and 5% CO_2), which has a strong vasodilating effect, also has been useful.

Toxic Deafness

Physicians must be aware of the potentially toxic effects of medications on the hearing and balance nerves of the inner ear.

Aminoglycosides and loop diuretics are especially hazardous, especially when used in combination. Chemotherapeutic agents, such as cisplatin, are capable of producing a devastating effect on the auditory/vestibular apparatus.

Preoperative audiometric and vestibular testing with close monitoring during treatment is strongly advised. Potentially dangerous medications are listed in [the section titled, "Medications with Toxic Effects on Hearing"].

Profound Sensorineural Deafness: Cochlear Electrode Implant

Total bilateral hearing nerve deafness is untreatable with the most powerful means of hearing aid amplification but can be treated with cochlear electrode implants. Although there are not many suitable candidates, selected centers can provide this treatment for adults and children with total deafness.

Noise-Induced Hearing Loss

Sensorineural hearing loss due to loud noise exposure can be arrested in its early stages and reversed with appropriate sound protection devices and, occasionally, with medication. The early warning signs after noise exposure include fullness in the ear, tinnitus and a temporary decrease in hearing and should be seriously addressed.

Evaluation

As with all medical disorders, a thorough history forms the basis for diagnosis and treatment. Particular attention is paid to antecedent ear disease or surgery, trauma, activity at the time of onset and symptoms of hearing fluctuation, tinnitus, vertigo and ear pressure. Physical examination should include microscopic ear examination and neurological examination. Audiologic evaluation should include measuring the air and bone conduction with speech discrimination. Auditory brain stem responses will show the status of eighth nerve and brain stem structures if hearing is not too depressed.

Electrocochleography (ECoG) measures the electrical activity within the cochlea in response to sound stimuli. It can distinguish between nerve loss originating in the cochlea versus the eighth nerve or higher structures. Ménière's disease often gives a distinctive signature on ECoG. Vestibular evaluation consists of electronystagmography (ENG) and a fistula test with ENG-impedance testing if fistula is suspected. Posturography often is helpful in cases of confusing balance findings. Radiologic studies include magnetic resonance imaging (MRI) and computed tomography (CT). MRI is used when a tumor is suspected, and CT may be helpful if a fracture or other bony abnormality is suspected. Laboratory work consists of an FTA/ABS, complete blood count and erythrocyte sedimentation rate, unless a specific clinical entity is suspected.

Summary

Sudden or rapid progressive sensorineural hearing loss is an otologic emergency demanding expeditious evaluation and initiation of therapy if the patient's hearing is to be preserved. Nine distinct entities have been identified in which a patient's hearing can be preserved, stabilized or restored to normal. Early intervention is of great importance.

The authors are with The Ear Institute of Indiana in Indianapolis.

Correspondence and reprints: George W. Hicks, M.D., Ear Institute of Indiana, 8103 Clearvista Parkway, Indianapolis, IN 46256.

References

1. Nagahara K, Fisch U, Dillier N: Experimental Study on the Perilymphatic Pressure. *Am J Otolaryngol*, 3:1-8, 1981.

2. Coats AC: The Summating Potential and Ménière's Disease. *Arch Otolaryngol*, 107:199-208, 1981.

3. Maddox HE 111: Endolymphatic Sac Surgery. *Laryngoscope*, 88:1676-1679, 1977.

4. Gibson WPR: A Study of Endolymphatic Sac Surgery. *Otolaryngol Clin North Am*, 16(1):181-188, 1983.

5. Anderson RG, Meyerhoff WL: Sudden Sensorineural Hearing Loss. *Otolaryngol Clin North Am*, 16(1):189-195, 1983.

6. Daspit CP, Churchill D, Linthicum FH: Diagnosis of Perilymph Fistula Using ENG and Impedance. *Laryngoscope*, 90:217223, 1980.

7. Hicks GW, Wright III JW: Delayed Endolymphatic Hydrops. *Laryngoscope*, 98(8): 840-845, 1988.

8. Wright Jr JW, Wright III JW, Hicks GW: Valve Implants: Comparative Analysis of the First Year's Experience with Results in Other Sac Operations. *Otolaryngol Clin North Am*, 16(1):175-179, 1983.

9. Silverstein H, Norrell H, Rosenberg S: The Resurrection of Vestibular Neurectomy: A 10-year Experience with 115 Cases. *J Neurosurg*, 72:533-539, 1990.

10. McCabe B: Autoimmune Sensorineural Hearing Loss. *Ann Otol Rhinol Laryngol*, 88:585-589, 1979.

11. Guzya AJ: Sudden Sensorineural Hearing Loss. *The Hearing Journal*, 40(2):2331, 1987.

12. Schuknecht HF, Donovan ED: The Pathology of Idiopathic Sudden Sensorineural Hearing Loss. *Arch Otolaryngol*, 243:1-15, 1986.

13. Sismanis A, Hughes GB, Butts F: Bilateral Spontaneous Perilymph Fistula: A Diagnostic and Management Dilemma. *Otolaryngol Head Neck Surg*, 103(3):436-438, 1990.

14. Wilson WR, Byl FM, Laird N: The Efficacy of Steroids in the Treatment of Idiopathic Sudden Hearing Loss: A Double-Blind Study. *Arch Otolaryngol*, 106:772-776, 1980.

—by George W. Hicks, M.D. and
J. William Wright III, M.D.,
Indianapolis.

Chapter 5

Early Identification of Hearing Impairment in Infants and Young Children

Approximately one of every 1,000 infants is born deaf. Many more children develop some degree of hearing impairment later in childhood. Any degree of hearing impairment during infancy and early childhood can have devastating effects on speech and language development, affecting learning and social/emotional growth. Furthermore, reduced ability to hear at a young age adversely affects the person's vocational and economic potential.

Despite the consequences of hearing impairment in infants and young children, the average age of identification in the United States is close to three years, well past the critical period for speech and language development. To evaluate current research and provide recommendations regarding hearing assessments from birth through five years of age, the National Institute on Deafness and Other Communication Disorders and the NIH Office of Medical Applications of Research sponsored a Consensus Development Conference on the Early Identification of Hearing Impairment in Infants and Young Children, March 1-3, 1993. Following 1 1/2 days of presentations from experts in relevant fields and audience discussion, a 15-member non-Federal panel weighed the information and developed a consensus statement.

The consensus panel concluded that all infants should be screened for hearing impairment. The panel was able to make this recommendation since recent advances in technology have led to

Summary of the NIH Consensus Statement; March 1-3, 1993.

improved screening methods that provide the capability to identify hearing impairments in infants soon after birth.

Currently, the only infants screened are those identified with one or more high risk factors associated with hearing impairment, including low birth weight or a family history or hearing impairment. These criteria, however, fail to identify 50 to 70 percent of children born with hearing impairment.

The screening procedure recommended by the panel would involve first screening the hearing of all infants with a test that measures otoacoustic emissions (OAE's). OAE's are low-intensity sounds produced by the inner ear that can be measured with a sensitive microphone placed in the ear canal. Measurement of OAE's was selected as the first test of the recommended screening procedure since it is a quick, inexpensive, accurate test of hearing sensitivity.

The panel further recommended that infants who fail the OAE screening have additional testing for auditory brain stem responses (ABR) which can confirm the validity of the OAE failure. Those infants who fail ASR should have a comprehensive hearing evaluation no later than 6 months of age.

Because infants admitted to neonatal intensive care units (NICUI) have an increased risk of hearing impairment, the panel recommended that these infants' hearing should be screened just before discharge from the hospital. The panel also suggested that infants in the well-baby nursery with a family history of hearing impairment or diagnoses of craniofacial anomalies or intra-uterine infections should have their hearing screened prior to discharge from the hospital.

Furthermore, the panel recommended that the hearing of all other infants be screened within the first three months of life, but added that this will be achieved most efficiently by screening prior to discharge from the well-baby nursery since the infants are more accessible for testing at that time.

However, the panel cautioned that 20 to 30 percent of hearing impairment in children occurs during infancy and early childhood. Therefore, the panel strongly urged that hearing screening be continued at intervals throughout early childhood. Parental concern should be elicited during well-baby visits to physicians, and speech and language development should be evaluated during those visits using formal assessment tools. Failure to reach appropriate language milestones should result in prompt referral for hearing evaluation.

Parental concern expressed about the hearing of their child should be sufficient reason to initiate prompt formal hearing evaluation.

The panel also recommended that children recovering from bacterial meningitis as well as those with a history of significant head trauma, viral encephalitis or labyrinthitis, excessive noise exposure, exposure to ototoxic drugs, congenital-perinatal cytomegalovirus infection, familial hearing impairment, chronic lung disease or diuretic therapy, and children with repeated episodes of otitis media with persistent middle ear effusion have their hearing tested. School entry screening at both public and private schools should continue in order to provide another opportunity for universal identification of children with hearing impairments.

The panel urged future research to evaluate the validity and reliability of screening instruments and to compare various screening procedures for time and cost. The cost effectiveness of universal screening for infant hearing impairment also needs to be investigated. The panel identified the need to develop innovative behavioral audiometry tests that are applicable for screening programs. Furthermore, the panel felt that large-scale studies should be conducted to evaluate the efficacy of early identification and intervention.

Free, single copies of the complete NIH Consensus Statement on the Early Identification of Hearing Impairment in Infants and Young Children may be obtained from the Office of Medical Applications of Research, NIH, Federal Building, Room 618, Bethesda, Maryland 20892, phone 301-496-1143.

Chapter 6

Hearing Tests for Infants and Young Children

Assessing hearing in infants and children is complicated by differences in children's development and the need to use different tests to assess various aspects of hearing. These tests, along with observations by parents or caregivers are used to obtain an accurate measure of a child's hearing.

The various tests used to evaluate hearing function in children can be classified into two major types: 1) behavioral assessment techniques and 2) physiological assessment techniques.

Behavioral Assessment Techniques

Informal observation. This method of hearing assessment involves observing how the child responds to everyday sounds. While this is the least accurate of all measures of hearing sensitivity, it is often the first indication that a hearing problem may exist. Parents or caregivers are often the first to notice that the child is not responding appropriately to certain sounds.

Behavioral observation audiometry (BOA). This method of hearing assessment is used mostly with newborns and children less than one year, however, it may be sued with slightly older children. This test relies on a child's immediate response to sound of varying loudness and pitch levels. Possible responses of infants to the sounds

NIDCD Fact Sheet; March 1992.

include sudden body movements, a change in sucking behavior and eye blinks. Behavior of older children includes eye widening, searching, head turning or change in facial expression.

While BOA is an easy and inexpensive assessment technique, difficulty may be encountered in maintaining the child's interest, interpreting the child's response and determining the individual hearing sensitivity of each ear.

Visual reinforcement audiometry (VRA). VRA is used to test the hearing of children who are developmentally between five and 24 months of age. This method uses two concealed toys that can be visualized when a blinking light is activated. The toys are located within the child's line of vision but some distance from each other, requiring the child to turn his or her head to look from one toy to the other. During the training or conditioning phase the light is flashed simultaneously with the presentation of an auditory signal that comes from the direction of the toy. The toy is used as a visual reinforcement, training the child, who is sitting on the parent or caregiver's lap, to look in the direction of the sound. During the testing phase, the light is flashed immediately following the response of the child looking in the direction of the sound just heard. This test is conducted either through loudspeakers or earphones in a sound treated room. VRA can provide a general measure of hearing sensitivity as well as the ability to hear speech.

Conditioned play audiometry (CPA). This behavioral assessment technique is used to test the hearing of children who are developmentally between two and five years of age. CPA engages the child in a game during the testing procedure. For example, the child may be asked to drop a block in a bucket or put a peg in a pegboard each time a "beep" or a word is heard, or to point to the picture corresponding to a word that is heard. this test is usually performed with the child wearing earphones but can be conducted through loudspeakers if the child will not wear the earphones. Very accurate measures of hearing for each ear can be obtained with this test including the ability to hear and discriminate speech.

Physiologic Assessment Techniques

Physiologic assessments use objective measures to evaluate the ear and hearing nerve, bypassing the need for the infant or child to respond. The results of these measures often need to be used in conjunction with behavioral methods to obtain an accurate measure of hearing sensitivity.

Acoustic immittance audiometry. Acoustic immittance audiometry assesses middle ear function by measuring how well sound is transmitted by the ear drum. This test helps detect several middle ear problems including fluid in the middle ear, a torn ear drum, abnormal middle ear air pressure or reduced mobility of the ossicular chain or bones of the middle ear. While this assessment technique does not provide a measure of hearing sensitivity, detection of middle ear problems will suggest reduced hearing sensitivity. This is one of the most important hearing tests for children since middle ear infections occur frequently in children and are one of the most common causes of childhood hearing impairment. Acoustic immittance audiometry is usually completed in minutes with children of all ages, however, more research is needed to determine the suitability of this test for newborns. The test requires insertion of a small probe into the opening of the child's ear canal while the child sits on the parent or caregiver's lap. The probe contains a speaker, microphone and a device that is able to change the air pressure in the ear canal, allowing for several measures of middle ear function. The child, who must remain quiet and passive during the test, may hear a few brief tones or feel air pressure changes in the ear.

Auditory brainstem response (ABR) audiometry. This method of assessment is also referred to as brainstem evoked response (BSER) audiometry or brainstem auditory evoked response (BAER) audiometry. ABR is useful with infants and other children who are unable or unwilling to respond to behavioral testing methods. This test requires attaching electrodes to various locations on the child's head. While sleeping or resting quietly, sounds are presented to the child's ears through earphones. The electrodes record the electrical activity from the hearing nerve as well as other parts of the brain involved in hearing. The ABR can provide an accurate picture of how the human auditory system is working.

Otoacoustic emissions (OAE). Otoacoustic emissions are low-level, inaudible sounds that are produced by the inner ear. Spontaneous OAEs occur naturally in many normal-hearing persons. Evoked otoacoustic emissions (EOAEs) may be elicited from normal-hearing persons in response to sound introduced to the ear through a probe containing a tiny sound source. A microphone in the probe measures the EOAEs, which are thought to reflect inner ear function. While this method is still considered largely experimental, there is hope that measurement of EOAEs may be used as a quick, noninvasive and inexpensive measure of hearing at the level of the inner ear.

For more information write to: NIDCD Clearinghouse P.O. Box 37777, Washington, DC 20013-7777. The NIDCD is one of the institutes of the National Institutes of Health and is responsible for research and research training on normal mechanisms and disorders of hearing, balance, smell, taste, voice, speech and language.

Chapter 7

Childhood Ear Infections

What is an ear infection?

When people talk about ear infections, they usually mean middle ear infections, or *otitis media*. The infection is behind the eardrum in the middle ear space.

The infection can cause fluid to collect in the middle ear, and a hearing loss develops. In most cases, your child will run a fever, be fussy, and may pull on the ears at the beginning of an infection. Sometimes, infections are "silent"—your child may not appear to be ill at all.

Who gets ear infections?

Ear infections are the most common illness that doctors treat in children under age 5. Nearly every child has at least one ear infection; the average child has four to six ear infections by age 3. A few children are "otits prone" and have more ear infections than average, because of frequent illnesses, birth defects (such as cleft palate), or syndromes (such as Down syndrome).

Why do children get ear infections?

It can be very hard to pinpoint the exact cause of your child's ear infections. Here are a few of the many causes:

- Family history of ear infections
- Contact with children who are sick
- Birth defects such as cleft palate
- Smoking in the home
- Allergies
- Climate
- Bottle propping

Regardless of the causes for the ear infections, the normal function of the *Eustachian tube* is usually affected. The Eustachian tube is the passageway from the middle ear to the back of the throat. When the tube is blocked, air can't pass into the middle ear and fluid cannot drain out.

Why be concerned about ear infections?

Hearing loss. Any infection should be taken seriously. Frequent infections cause extra concern because they might result in a hearing loss in your child. The amount of loss varies and usually clears up once the fluid behind the eardrum is gone.

To get an idea of how speech sounds to a child with an ear infection, plug your ears with your fingers and listen to someone talk. Sounds have a remote, underwater quality. With a middle ear full of fluid, the sounds your child hears are muffled and unclear. You may find yourself talking in a loud voice so your child can hear you clearly. This is because sounds have to be louder than normal to get from the eardrum through the fluid and to the hearing nerve.

Speech and language problems. Children with ear infections are more likely to have speech and language problems. Ear infections occur most frequently between birth and age 3, which is also the critical period for children to learn speech and language. It's important to clear up an ear infection as soon as possible, because hearing loss caused by frequent ear infections can interfere with normal speech and language development.

What will the doctor do about my child's ear infections?

To get information about your child's medical history, the doctor will ask you questions such as:

- How does your child behave when there is an ear infection?
- How many ear infections has your child had?
- How have the ear infections been treated in the past?
- Do you think your child has a hearing loss?
- Do you think your child's speech and language is normal or delayed?

The doctor will examine your child to see if there is an ear infection. Using a special light—called an *otoscope*—the doctor can see your child's eardrums to diagnose whether there is an infection or fluid present in your child's middle ears.

The doctor may prescribe medication to clear an infection. But if the infections and hearing loss continue, the doctor may refer your child to specialists for other treatments. Your child may see:

- A doctor who specializes in treating the ear, nose and throat— an *ENT* or *otolaryngologist*.
- An *audiologist* who is trained to test children's hearing.
- A *speech-language pathologist*, to evaluate your child's speech and language development.

Other methods of treating ear infections include long-term use of antibiotics and the insertion of ventilation tubes through your child's eardrums.

How can I help?

Understand the nature of ear infections.

- An ear infection is just one of many things that will happen in your child's life. Most children have ear infections, and few ear infections are dangerous.
- Your child may outgrow ear infections.
- There is little you can do to prevent ear infections.
- Discuss the information in this article with the doctor.

Observe your child's behavior. Every child with an ear infection acts differently. Does your child's behavior signal an ear infection or something else?

Watch your child for signs of hearing loss.

- Does your voice calm your crying child?
- Does your child ask "what?" or "huh?" frequently?
- Do you have to raise your voice to talk to your child?

Understand your child's treatment before you leave the doctor's office. Ask the doctor to clarify anything you don't understand. Make sure you know how to give your child the medications the doctor prescribes. And be sure to give your child all of the prescribed medication.

Ask your child's doctor:

- What can I do at home to relieve my child's ear pain?
- Should my child ride on an airplane when there is an ear infection?
- What is happening with my child?
- How is it being treated?
- Why was a certain type of treatment chosen?
- When do I need to bring my child back to the doctor?
- Who else needs to be involved in my child's treatment?

Have your child's doctor send reports to any specialists your child sees. And have the specialists' reports sent to the child's primary doctor.

Encourage your child. Ear infections can be annoying and frustrating for both of you.

Play with your child and read stories to stimulate your child's speech and language development. If your child has a hearing loss, hold the child close to you or talk loudly so that your child can hear better.

For more information:

Grundfast, K, and C. Carney. *Ear infections in your child: The comprehensive parental guide to causes and treatments.* Hollywood, FL: Compact Books, 1987.

—*by Melinda M. Heald, M.S., CCC-A*

Chapter 8

Questions and Answers about Otitis Media, Hearing, and Language Development

What is otitis media?

Otitis media is an inflammation in the middle ear (the area behind the eardrum) that is usually associated with a buildup of fluid. The fluid may or may not be infected.

Symptoms, severity, frequency, and length of the condition vary. At one extreme is a single short period of thin, clear, noninfected fluid without any pain or fever but with a slight decrease in hearing ability. The other extreme is repeated bouts with infection, thick "glue-like" fluid, and possible complications such as permanent hearing loss.

Fortunately, with early identification, serious medical complications can be controlled with medicine or surgery. However, there is one problem that nearly always occurs with all types of otitis media—fluctuating hearing loss.

How common is otitis media?

Otitis media occurs most frequently in children. In fact, it ranks second to the common cold as the most common health problem in preschool children. Fifty percent of children have had at least one episode by one year of age. Between one and three years, 35% will have had repeated episodes. For school children, an estimated 5 million school days are missed every year due to otitis media.

Why is otitis media so common in children?

The Eustachian tube, a passage between the middle ear and the back of the throat, is smaller and more nearly horizontal in children than in adults. Therefore, it can be more easily blocked by conditions such as large adenoids and infections. Until the Eustachian tube changes in size and angle, children are more susceptible to otitis media.

How can otitis media cause a hearing loss?

Three tiny bones in the middle ear carry sound vibrations from the eardrum to the inner ear. When fluid is present, the vibrations are not transmitted efficiently and sound energy is lost.

The result may be a mild or even a moderate hearing loss. Therefore, some speech sounds may be muffled or inaudible.

Generally, this type of hearing loss is temporary. However, when otitis media occurs over and over again, damage to the eardrum, the bones of the ear, or even the hearing nerve can occur and cause permanent hearing loss.

Can hearing loss due to otitis media cause speech and language problems?

Children learn speech and language from listening to other people talk. The first few years of life are especially critical for this development.

If a hearing loss exists, a child does not get full benefit of language learning experiences. Consequently, critical delays in speech and language development may occur.

Otitis media without infection presents a special problem because symptoms of pain and fever are usually not present. Therefore, weeks, and even months, can go by before parents suspect a problem. During this time, the child may miss out on hearing the speech and language needed for normal development.

How can I tell if my child might have otitis media?

Even if there is no pain or fever, there are other signs you can look for that may indicate chronic or recurring fluid in the ear: inattentiveness, wanting the television or radio louder than usual, misunderstanding directions, listlessness, unexplained irritability, pulling or scratching the ears.

What should I do if I think that otitis media is causing a hearing, speech, or language problem?

A physician should handle the medical treatment. Ear infections require immediate attention, most likely from a pediatrician or otolaryngologist (ear doctor). If your child has frequently recurring infections and/or chronic fluid in the middle ear, two additional specialists should be consulted: an audiologist and a speech-language pathologist.

An audiologist's evaluation will assess the severity of any hearing impairment, even in a very young or uncooperative child, and will indicate if a middle ear disorder is present.

A speech-language pathologist measures your child's specific speech and language skills and can recommend and/or provide remedial programs when they are needed.

Will my physician refer my child for these special evaluations?

As a parent, you are the best person to look for signs that suggest poor hearing. The American Academy of Pediatrics recognizes this when it states, "Any child whose parent expresses concern about whether the child hears should be considered for referral for behavioral audiometry without delay."

Parents should not be afraid to let their instincts guide them in requesting or independently arranging for further evaluation whenever they are concerned about their children's health or development.

How can I find an audiologist or speech-language pathologist?

For a complete listing of professional services in audiology and speech-language pathology in your state, write or call:

American Speech-Language-Hearing
Association (ASHA)
10801 Rockville Pike
Rockville, Maryland 20852
800-638-8255 or 301-897-8682
(Voice or TDD).

Chapter 9

Some Facts about Otitis Media

Otitis media means fluid in the middle ear. A child with otitis media often experiences a temporary hearing loss. While such a hearing loss is usually mild and fluctuating, it may be a major cause of language delay in the preschool years when the growth of normal language development is at its peak.

The following information about otitis media may be helpful in identifying and helping young children with this middle ear problem.

- Otitis media is one of the most common diseases of early childhood.

- Otitis media usually occurs before a child is two and is common throughout the preschool years.

- When otitis media occurs frequently within a year's time, it is referred to as recurrent otitis media.

- About two-thirds of all preschool children have at least one episode of otitis media.

NICD Publication 468. Developed by and reprinted with permission of Project Preschool C.H.I.L.D. Although this project is no longer in existence, materials and services are currently available from the Toledo Public Schools Early Childhood Program.

- About 12% of all preschool children experience six or more episodes of otitis media before the age of six.

- Otitis media occurs more frequently in winter than in summer.

- Symptoms of otitis media may include the following: fever, earache, inconsistent response to sound, inconsistent behavior patterns, delayed speech and language development, and irritability.

- Prompt medical intervention is very important in the case of otitis media, not only because it often interferes with a child's hearing at a crucial period in speech and language development, but also because, if left untreated, otitis media may result in a permanent hearing impairment.

- Impedance audiometry represents the most effective means of detecting middle ear disease.

- Young children with recurrent otitis media often require educational as well as medical intervention. Such educational intervention should focus on language stimulation and the development of auditory (listening) skills.

- Otitis media can be difficult to detect because it can be present without pain, fever, or any other noticeable symptom.

- Otitis media is a major cause of hearing impairment in the preschool and school age population.

- Young children with recurrent otitis media sometimes exhibit social and emotional problems, as well as specific language and learning deficits. Such problems may result from the inconsistency they experience in their auditory environments.

Typical Characteristics of the Middle Ear—Language Impaired Child

- Difficulty remembering names and places
- Distractibility by outside noises
- Difficulty with speech and language
- Inabiliy to discriminate between words that sound alike
- Difficulty repeating sounds, letters, and numbers in proper sequence
- Frequent need for repetition of directions and important information
- Attention to only part of what is said (e.g., understanding only the first or last part of a message)
- Difficulty locating the source of sounds not in line with vision
- Inability to follow, or attend to, stories read aloud
- Use of gestures rather than verbal expression
- Inconsistent behavior on a day-to-day basis

A Glossary of Selected Terms Related to Otitis Media Language Development/Auditory Processing

Otitis media: a disorder of the middle ear usually characterized by the presence of fluid in the middle ear cavity.

Recurrent otitis media: repeated bouts of inflammation and/or the accumulation of fluid in the middle ear.

Acute otitis media: a severe, but usually brief, bout of otitis media.

Chronic otitis media: persistent and long-lasting bouts of otitis media.

Serous otitis media: the accumulation of fluid in the middle ear.

Impedance audiometry: an objective screening technique used to identify disorders of the middle ear.

Otolaryngologist: a physician who specializes in disorders of the ear, nose and throat (ENT).

Myringotomy: the surgical procedure of making an incision in the eardrum for the purpose of providing ventilation to the middle ear cavity.

Tympanostomy tubes: very small polyurethane tubes inserted in the eardrum to provide ventilation to the middle ear.

Chapter 10

Managing Severe Otitis Media

Abstract

Background: Otitis media is one of the most common pediatric diseases encountered by family physicians. While isolated, acute episodes pose little clinical difficulty, recurrent infections and persistent middle ear effusions can be perplexing problems.

Methods: This review presents a clinical approach to the management of recurrent and persistent middle ear disease.

Results and Conclusions: Recurrent infections can be treated with a trial of daily prophylactic antibiotics to decrease the rate of recurrence. Should infections continue to recur despite the daily prophylaxis, polyethylene tube placement is warranted to drain surgically the middle ear effusions that give rise to the recurrent infections. Acute episodes of otitis media are commonly followed by prolonged, asymptomatic periods of middle ear effusion. Patients with this disease have decreased hearing leading to potential deficits in their speech and academic development. If such effusions do not spontaneously resolve within 2 months, repeated courses of antibiotics with the possible addition of a course of oral steroids are warranted to speed resolution of the effusion before proceeding to placement of polyethylene tubes.

This document was originally published as "An Approach to Difficult Management Problems In Otitis Media In Children" in *The Journal of the American Board of Family Practice*, September/October 1991. Used by permission.

Introduction

Otitis media is one of the most common diseases encountered in primary care.[1] Furthermore, the frequency of medical visits and surgery for this disease continue to increase.[2] While isolated, acute episodes pose little therapeutic difficulty, recurrent or persistent infections give rise to a multitude of controversial questions. What is the proper role of the new, potent, but more expensive antibiotics? When and how should one use daily antibiotic prophylaxis? When is the placement of polyethylene tubes warranted? Because little uniformity of opinion exists on these topics, no universally accepted guidelines can be offered to the family physician. By applying what is known about the causes and natural history of middle ear disease, however, a schematic framework can be devised upon which the family physician can begin to address these issues and develop a therapeutic plan for an individual patient.

Basic Approach

The basic approach to middle ear disease begins with two important questions. First, what is in the child's middle ear cavity at the time of examination? Second, at what stage is the child's condition in the natural history of middle ear disease? By answering these two questions, an appropriate plan for managing the patient's middle ear disease can be derived.

What Is In the Middle Ear?

Three substances can exist within the middle ear cavity: air, pus, or a noninflammed effusion. The most precise way to distinguish among these three substances is to perform a tympanocentesis on all patients with suspected middle ear disease. A Gram stain and culture of any fluid obtained would then provide an accurate description of the contents of the middle ear cavity. Although this approach is precise, it is hardly practical for most patients. Thus, we are left with indirect methods based upon physical examination and patient history to diagnose middle ear disease. One such method is presented in Figure 10.1.

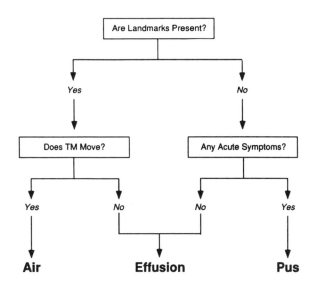

Figure 10.1. A clinical approach to middle ear diagnosis.

Physicians are accustomed to inspecting the tympanic membrane directly to diagnose middle ear diseases. Accordingly, as outlined in Figure 10.1, physical examination of the tympanic membrane forms the basis of the attempt to determine clinically what is present in the middle ear cavity. Unless scarred from prior infections, the inferior portion of the normal tympanic membrane is translucent, and the handle of the malleus is clearly identifiable as a bony ridge upon its surface (bony landmark). Unfortunately, clear effusions within the middle ear cavity can also retain the translucency of the membrane's surface, resulting in a tympanic membrane that appears to be perfectly normal. When an examination reveals the normal handle of the malleus upon the tympanic membrane, an assessment of membrane mobility is required to differentiate between those middle ear cavities that contain air and those that contain clear effusions. Normal mobility implies the presence of air in the middle ear cavity. Clear effusions in the middle ear cavity will cause the tympanic membrane to be immobile despite its apparent normalcy on inspection.

Tympanic membrane mobility is most commonly assessed using a pneumatic bulb attached to the otoscope head. The degree of tympanic membrane motion is observed directly as air is pumped back and forth in the external canal. While simple, this procedure can be awkward to perform in a restless child, and subjective interpretation is often required. More definitive quantification of tympanic membrane mobility can be obtained with a tympanometer. This instrument contains a probe that fits into the patient's external auditory canal in much the same way as does the head of an otoscope. The probe emits pressure impulses into the external canal and then measures the mobility of the tympanic membrane in response to these impulses. Earlier versions of these devices required relatively large, stationary measuring instruments attached to the probe by means of a connecting tube. Fortunately, more recent versions of this instrument combine the probe and measuring instrument into a single hand-held unit, are no more difficult to use than an otoscope, and can give simple, accurate, reliable assessments of tympanic membrane mobility. The hand-held tympanometer should take its place beside the otoscope and stethoscope as basic instruments found in all primary care offices in which pediatric middle ear disease is being managed.

Both pus and effusion within the middle ear cavity can dull the surface of the tympanic membrane and cause its normally translucent surface to become indistinguishable from the handle of the malleus loss of bony landmarks). Unless the tympanic membrane is scarred from prior infections, failure to identify the handle of the malleus upon the membrane implies that either pus or effusion is present. Differentiation between these two disease processes is based on the patient's immediate clinical history. Does the patient have acute symptoms of middle ear disease? Acute symptoms are chiefly respiratory with a history of recent onset of ear pain being especially indicative of middle ear infection. Chronic respiratory symptoms in allergic children are not of concern unless there has been a recent change in the symptom pattern. Younger children can exhibit nonspecific symptoms, such as recent fussiness, irritability, or ear pulling. Fever will not be present in all cases. Thus, a tympanic membrane on which no landmarks are seen in a child who has a history of acute symptoms suggests that pus is present in the middle ear cavity. On the other hand, a tympanic membrane with no landmarks in a child who is otherwise well and who has no acute symptoms most likely indicates the presence of a middle ear effusion.

Other common, but less useful, physical findings are also used to determine what is present in a patient's middle ear. Acute infection can impart a red color to the tympanic membrane; however, so can a crying child. Although bubbles and air fluid levels behind the tympanic membrane imply the presence of effusions, they are often difficult to identify with hand-held otoscopes. Tympanic membrane bulging or retraction can be helpful if it can be seen in the extreme; however, the assessment of intermediate degrees of these findings is somewhat subjective. The presence or absence of landmarks and the degree of tympanic membrane mobility therefore form the foundation upon which family physicians can determine what is present in the middle ear.

Much of the terminology surrounding middle ear disease is an attempt to describe what is present in the middle ear cavity. Acute otitis media implies that pus is present. Both serous otitis media and otitis media with effusion imply the presence of an effusion. Because of their common use and acceptance, this review retains the terms acute otitis media (AOM) and otitis media with effusion (OME) as described. It is important to emphasize, however, that these terms are useful only to the extent that they describe what is present in the middle ear cavity at any one time.

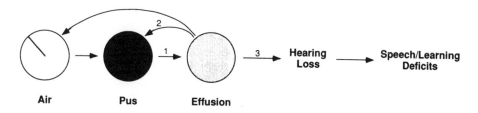

Figure 10.2. Natural history of middle ear disease.

At What Stage Is the Child's Condition in the Natural History of Middle Ear Disease

The identification of the substance present in the middle ear cavity is important because it provides a starting point from which the physician can determine the child's stage within the natural history of middle ear disease. This knowledge then forms the basis for the therapeutic plan to be used.

A schematic summary of the natural history of middle ear disease is shown in Figure 10.2. The ability of the middle ear cavity to fill with pus and become acutely infected is well known; however, the tendency of this pus to evolve into a thick, noninflamed effusion that may last for months is less well appreciated. Several investigators have studied the natural history of effusions following AOM.[3,4] Although they found that many of the post-AOM effusions resolved within 1 month, a substantial number persisted up to 3 months, and rare cases were not resolved after even longer periods of observation. Thus, episodes of pus in the middle ear cavity commonly evolve into relatively prolonged periods of noninflamed middle ear effusions (Figure 10.2, Arrow 1) before reverting back to the normal, air-filled middle ear state.

In addition to the effusion stage, two other clinically important pathways can occur. In the first, the child can experience a recurrence of AOM within weeks to months after successful treatment of the preceding acute infection. In some cases, the effusion stage of the preceding infection resolves, and an air-filled stage exists before becoming reinfected. In other cases (Figure 10.2, Arrow 2), the effusion can become reinfected, and the middle ear contents revert to the pus stage before returning to the air-filled state. In such cases, warm, moist, prolonged post-AOM middle ear effusions provide excellent culture media for bacterial growth, thus causing recurrent acute infections. Children with persistent effusions are often caught in a vicious cycle in which pus resolves to effusion after acute therapy only to be followed by later reinfection of the effusion before it has a chance to return to the normal, air-filled stage.

The second pathway (Figure 10.2, Arrow 3) is found in those rare patients who do not spontaneously resolve their effusions within 1 to 3 months after an episode of AOM. While such children have no symptoms and appear well, this condition is of concern because their tympanic membranes are immobile, leading to potential hearing impairment.[5] Although controversial, some theorize that such impaired hearing can lead to speech and learning difficulties.[6,7]

Clinical Problems

The above ideas are applied to the four clinical situations most commonly encountered in children with complicated otitis media.

Clinically Unresponsive Acute Otitis Media

Children with unresponsive AOM initially have loss of tympanic membrane landmarks in association with the recent onset of new

Figure 10.3. Approach to Nonresponsive Acute Otitis Media

Steps	Notes
1. Rule out associated severe disease	Usually can be done clinically, and rarely requires invasive workup
2. Inquire about compliance with prescribed medication	
3. Change to a broader spectrum antibiotic	
a. Amoxicillin	First-line therapy
b. Sulfa-containing antibiotics	Beware of Stevens-Johnson reaction
–Trimethoprim-sulfamethoxazole (Septra™ Bactrim™)	
–Erythromycin-sulfisoxazole (Pediazole™)	
c. Amoxicillin clavulanate (Augmentin™) Cefaclor (Ceclor™) Cefuroxime axetil (Oral Zinacef™) Cefixime (Suprax™)	All are expensive and have gastrointestinal side effects
4. Refer to otolaryngologist for surgical drainage	Therapeutic and provides definitive diagnosis of middle ear pathogen (culture and stain for fungus as well as bacteria)

77

symptoms. They are assessed as having pus within their middle ear cavity and are placed on antibiotics. They then return within 2 to 3 days with no change in their clinical status. Their continued symptoms and continued loss of landmarks indicate that pus is still present in their middle ear cavity.

While antimicrobial resistance to the prescribed antibiotic is commonly suspected in these settings, only a minority of organisms obtained by tympanocentesis from such patients have been found to be resistant to the antibiotic initially chosen.[8] Other factors, such as patient noncompliance with therapy and concurrent viral infection, probably are instrumental in the patient's failure to undergo clinical improvement.[9] Though rare, associated infections (especially meningitis) must also be excluded as diagnostic possibilities.

Based upon these considerations, a suggested approach to clinically unresponsive AOM is presented in Figure 10.3. In all cases, the possibility of a life-threatening disease must be ruled out. In a majority of these cases, this can be done clinically. Rarely, laboratory evaluations, including lumbar puncture, are required. After serious disease has been ruled out, the child's guardians should be questioned closely about their compliance with the therapy previously prescribed. In the event that compliance has been good, the antibiotic should be changed to cover possible microbial resistance to the initial antibiotic.

Figure 10.3 provides a list of antibiotics suggested for cases of acute otitis media that are clinically unresponsive to initial therapy. Currently, the incidence of ß-lactamase-producing *Haemophilis influenzae* and *Moraxella Catarrhalis* is still sufficiently low to warrant amoxicillin as first-line therapy for AOM.[10] Should microbial resistance to this antibiotic be suspected, a second-line, sulfa-containing antibiotic is recommended.[8] Should the patient continue without clinical improvement, and serious disease or noncompliance has been eliminated as a diagnostic possibility, a third-line antibiotic is warranted. Finally, should the patient demonstrate clinical resistance to even third-line medical therapy, immediate referral to an otolaryngologist is required for surgical drainage of the infected middle ear cavity both as a therapeutic maneuver and to obtain material for specific bacteriologic diagnosis.

Frequently Recurrent Otitis Media

The second clinical problem occurs in those children who have frequent recurrences of AOM. These children initially have abnormal tympanic membranes in association with acute symptoms. Pus is thought to be present in the middle ear, and antibiotic therapy is started. Unlike the children with resistant AOM, however, these children improve clinically and their symptoms resolve, implying that the acute infection has also resolved. Within weeks to months, however, the child again becomes acutely symptomatic with abnormal tympanic membranes, suggesting that the infection in the middle ear has returned to a pus-producing stage.

Although it is commonly presumed that such cases represent resistance to the initial antibiotic used, investigators have reported that the majority of cases that recurred within 1 week to 1 month after termination of the initial antibiotic were caused by organisms sensitive to the original antibiotic.[11,12] Thus, isolated, 10-day courses of the broader-spectrum antibiotics will likely add little to the management of these children. Two therapeutic maneuvers, however, are helpful in this clinical situation: daily antibiotic prophylaxis and placement of polyethylene tubes.

Daily antibiotic prophylaxis has been shown to decrease the rate of reinfection in children with recurrent AOM.[13-15] The diagnostic criteria and antibiotic regimens used in some of these studies are summarized in Figure 10.4. As no uniform opinion exists regarding the proper time to instigate prophylaxis or which antibiotic regimen to use, practitioners are free to choose among the approaches outlined.

While daily antibiotic prophylaxis is beneficial in many cases, some acute infections do recur despite this therapeutic approach. In such cases, the only currently recommended course of action is the placement of polyethylene tubes. The tubes keep the middle ear free of fluid during the time that they are in place, thereby eliminating the chronic effusion that gives rise to many of these recurrent infections.

Persistent Middle Ear Effusions

This disease process occurs in those children who do not spontaneously clear their effusions after an episode of acute purulent otitis media. Clinically, the children are well and without symptoms; however, their tympanic membranes are either dulled with loss of landmarks, or the landmarks are seen but the tympanic membrane has lost mobility. The effusion persists and hearing decreases, leading to possible speech and learning defects—all in children who appear outwardly well and who may even have normal tympanic membranes on

Figure 10.4. Approach to Frequently Recurrent Acute Otitis Media (AOM).

Study	When Started	Regimen Used
1. Begin daily antibiotic prophylaxis		
Liston, et al.[13]	At least 3 AOM episodes occuring at a frequency of at least once every 2 months (6 months–5 years)	Sulfisoxazole, 75 mg/kd/d bid for 3 months
Perrin, et al.[14]	3 or more AOM episodes within the last 18 months or a total of 5 in whole life (11 months–8 years)	Sulfisoxazole, 1000 mg/d bid for 3 months
Lampe and Weir[15]	4 or more AOM episodes within the last 12 months or 3 episodes within the last 6 months (birth–6 years)	Erythromycin, 20 mg/kd/d bid for 2–3 months (found to be more effective than sulfisoxazole, 1000 mg/d bid for 2–3 months)
Marchant[16]	3 or more AOM episodes within the last 18 months	Amoxicillin, 20 mg/kg/d bid or sulfisoxazole, 80 mg/kd/ d bid during the winter and spring months
Bluestone[10]	3 or more AOM episodes in 6 months or 4–5 episodes in 12 months	Amoxicillin, 20 mg/kg/d qd or sulfisoxazole, 50 mg/kg/ d qd during the "respiratory season"
2. Refer to otolaryngologist for possible polyethylene tube placement if acute infections recur while on daily antibiotic therapy.		

gross inspection. Thus, persistent middle ear effusions are worrisome because they are unheralded by clinical symptoms that bring these children to medical attention.

Whereas the majority of middle ear effusions resolve spontaneously within 3 months, several forms of therapy have been studied to hasten the resolution of these effusions and decrease their potential impact upon the child's hearing and learning. Although popular in the past, decongestants and antihistamines have now been shown to be of no benefit in aiding the resolution of persistent effusions.[17] On the other hand, antibiotics have been found to have at least a temporary beneficial effect,[18, 19] and broader spectrum antibiotics may be even more useful.[20] Recently, the addition of a short-term course of oral steroids to antibiotic therapy was beneficial in hastening the resolution of persistent effusions and is discussed below.

Figure 10.5 offers a clinical approach to persistent OME. After an episode of AOM, the child is seen monthly until resolution of the resultant effusion is documented by the return of tympanic membrane mobility. Should this resolution not occur by the second monthly visit, a 10- to 14-day trial of amoxicillin can be prescribed. If the effusion persists despite the amoxicillin therapy, a 10- to 30-day trial of a broader spectrum antibiotic can then be undertaken as final medical therapy prior to consideration of polyethylene tube placement. Use of polyethylene tubes is most imperative if the child has deficits in hearing or speech development that are associated with the persistent effusion. On the other hand, if the child's hearing and speech development are normal, some authors would recommend only continued observation for spontaneous resolution of the effusion.[21]

Incidentally Noted Effusions

While this review has focused on middle ear disease caused by AOM, middle ear effusions can occur in children at other times as well. Any process that affects the eustachian tube, such as upper respiratory tract infections and respiratory tract allergy, can result in a buildup of effusion within the middle ear. Such effusions commonly are found in children during routine well-child visits.[4] Casselbrant and coworkers[22] looked at the natural history of these effusions in children and found that approximately one-half of all children observed for 1 year experienced an episode of effusion. Similar to effusions following episodes of AOM, these effusions were largely self-limited, resolving

Figure 10.5. *Approach to Persistent Middle Ear Effusions in an Asymptomatic Child.*

Time Interval After Episode of Acute Otitis Media	Approach
Effusion persistent at 1-month follow-up	Observe
	Recheck in 1 month
Effusion persistent at 2-month follow-up	10- to 14-day trial of amoxicillin (or sulfa-containing antibiotic if allergic to penicillin compounds)
Effusion persistent after first antibiotic trial	14- to 30-day trial of step 3c antibiotic (as defined in Table 1)
	Consider concurrent 7-day course of oral prednisone
Effusion persistent after second antibiotic trial	Consider otolaryngology referal for possible polyethylene tube placement
	Tube placement most imperative with associated hearing or speech delay
	May consider continued observation if hearing and speech are normal

within 3 months, with rare examples lasting up to 6 months. These effusions, when found, warrant the close monthly management outlined in Figure 10.5.

Surgical Issues

Although current approaches to the therapy of middle ear disease in children emphasize the role of polyethylene tubes in those cases that do not respond to medical management, family physicians should be aware that controversy exists about the use of these tubes.[23] Much of the controversy has centered on the fear that placement of polyethylene tubes will lead to tympanic membrane damage and associated iatrogenic hearing loss. Indeed, infrequent instances of severe sequelae, such as persistent tympanic membrane perforations and cholesteatomas, have been documented.[24] Postoperative hearing loss has also been reported in a certain percentage of those children for whom multiple polyethylene tube placements were required.[25] On the other hand, the most common surgical sequela, tympanosclerosis, has only rarely been associated with significant hearing loss following single polyethylene tube insertions.[26]

In addition to the fears about possible surgical side effects, some physicians doubt the benefits to be gained by polyethylene tube use. Although polyethylene tube placement does result in normalization of hearing,[27] this effect appears to be transient, and little difference in hearing has been found between children with surgically treated and untreated ears after as little as 3 to 6 months of follow-up.[28-30] From a strict audiologic standpoint, therefore, polyethylene tube placement appears to gain 3 to 6 months of improved hearing before the child's hearing improves on its own. Whether this transient period of improved hearing necessarily results in enhanced long-term speech and intellectual development remains to be determined.

Clearly, the role of polyethylene tubes in the treatment of middle ear disease has yet to be elucidated fully. Single tube insertions appear to be safe in most cases and result in immediate benefits, but long-term benefits are uncertain. It would seem judicious to consider surgical therapy only after time and maximal medical therapy have failed to ameliorate the patient's middle ear disease. In particular, those children who have speech and learning deficits associated with their middle ear disease would be candidates for surgical therapy after all other attempts fail. Further study is needed to define better the role of polyethylene tube placement in children with middle ear disease.

Future Trends

The preceding approaches to the management of complicated otitis media are based upon current knowledge of the causes and natural history of middle ear disease. Conflicting ideas in the contemporary otitis literature can lead to future alterations in these present recommendations.

The usual treatment of isolated, acute cases of otitis media in the United States consists of a 7- to 10-day course of oral antibiotics. This therapy is based upon bacteriologic studies of the middle ear fluid obtained from children with AOM in which a bacterial pathogen was found in up to 89 percent of cases.[10] On the other hand, European researchers have reported that these infections have a high rate of spontaneous resolution and have recommended antibiotic therapy only in those cases that do not clinically resolve within 3 to 4 days of onset.[31, 32] Using this protocol, more than 90 percent of the children studied were managed successfully without antibiotics. No increase in the rate of suppurative complications, such as meningitis or mastoiditis, was noted. Nevertheless, until further data are available, antibiotic therapy should remain the standard for AOM in the United States. If these experimental findings are replicated in the US population, however, we may need to rethink the entire role of antibiotics in the management of middle ear disease.

It is the recommendation of this review to wait 2 months for persistent effusions to clear before introducing antibiotic trials in the presurgical management of OME. Another medical treatment that has been studied before pursuing surgical intervention is the short-term administration of oral steroids. Prospective studies of the use of steroids alone to treat persistent OME have not found such therapy to be beneficial.[33-35] When used in combination with antibiotic therapy, however, oral steroids taken for 7 to 14 days led to increases in the rate of OME resolution that were greater than the increases achieved with antibiotic use alone.[36-38] The steroid-antibiotic combination had no increase in side effects and resulted in low OME recurrence rates. Adding steroids to antibiotic management can be considered, therefore, for any child in whom one wishes to try all possible medical therapies before proceeding to surgery, especially if an allergic diathesis is thought to underlie the persistent OME. Should future research continue to substantiate the value of the steroid-antibiotic combination in the medical treatment of persistent OME, short-term oral steroid therapy may become a routine part of the management of all patients with OME.

At present, most children undergoing surgery for persistent OME receive placement of polyethylene tubes. Since the introduction of these tubes in the 1950s, however, numerous other surgical approaches to the treatment of persistent effusions have been studied, including varying combinations of myringotomy without polyethylene tube placement, tonsillectomy with adenoidectomy, and adenoidectomy alone.[39-42] From this body of data, it should be noted that polyethylene tube placement has never been shown to be consistently superior to the other surgical procedures studies. In fact, the most recent study in this series found myringotomy plus adenoidectomy to be superior to polyethylene tube placement in terms of increased postoperative auditory acuity and reduced need for repeat surgery.[42] As in all surgical fields, the best approach is probably the one with which the particular surgical consultant is most familiar and comfortable. It is important to know, however, that surgical techniques other than insertion of polyethylene tubes are acceptable therapy at this time and may replace polyethylene tube placement as more experience is acquired. Much of the discussion in this review has been based upon the assumption that the hearing loss associated with persistent middle ear effusions is detrimental to the patient and can lead to subsequent speech and learning difficulties. The extent to which these sequelae actually occur is a subject of controversy, and ample data are available to support both sides of the issue.[6,7] Should future research not substantiate an association between persistent OME and speech and learning difficulties, persistent OME may then be viewed as a benign, self-limiting condition that does not warrant the medical therapies and surgical procedures currently applied in its management. Until further research resolves this issue, however, family physicians must expect that some children with middle ear effusions can suffer significant speech and learning deficits from the hearing loss associated with those effusions. Thus, close monthly monitoring is warranted.

Summary

Importance of Patient's History

Whereas physical examination of the tympanic membrane is important to determine a course of action for patients with middle ear disease, inspection alone is insufficient evidence on which to base therapy. Knowledge of the patient's history of middle ear pathology is equally important. A patient with loss of landmarks but no symptoms 1 month after an episode of AOM has an effusion and requires nothing more than observation. On the other hand, a patient whose tympanic membrane is normal with good mobility may warrant the instigation of antibiotic prophylaxis if there have been recurrent infections in the past year.

Natural History of Otitis Media with Effusion

OME commonly follows AOM and other processes that interfere with the function of the eustachian tube. Middle ear effusions are frequently found during childhood. Fortunately, the majority of these effusions will resolve spontaneously. Close observation is warranted, however, to diagnose those cases that persist, leading to potential hearing, speech, and learning deficits.

Use of Broader Spectrum Antibiotics

Only a minority of cases of middle ear disease are due to microbes bacteriologically resistant to first-line antibiotics. The broader spectrum antibiotics are warranted only in those cases of AOM that do not respond clinically to first-line antibiotics. They can also be used in a last-ditch effort to resolve persistent middle ear effusions medically before recommending polyethylene tube placement.

Indications for Polyethylene Tube Placement

Currently, there are two indications for polyethylene tube placement: (1) frequently recurrent AOM that is not responsive to prophylactic antibiotics, and (2) OME that does not resolve within 3 months of observation despite repeated antibiotic treatments. Because the long-term benefits of polyethylene tubes are uncertain, these clinical indications for polyethylene tube placement may change as we gain greater understanding of middle ear disease.

References

1. Kirkwood C. R., H. R. Clure, R. Brodsky, G. H. Gould, R. Knaak, M. Metcalf, et al. "The Diagnostic Content of Family Practice: 50 Most Common Diagnoses Recorded in the WAE Community Practices." *J Fam Pract*. Vol. 15 (1982):485-92.

2. Croteau, N., V. Hai, I. B. Pless, C. Infante-Rivard. "Trends in Medical Visits and Surgery for Otitis Media Among Children." *Am J Dis Child*. Vol. 144 (1990): 535-8.

3. Shurin, P. A., S. I. Pelton, A. Donner, J. O. Klein. "Persistence of Middle-Ear Effusion after Acute Otitis Media in Children." *N EnglJ Med*. Vol. 300 (1979): 1121-3.

4. Marchant, C. D., P. A. Shurin, W. A. Turczyk, D. E. Wasikowski, M. A. Tutihasi, S. E. Kinney. "Course and Outcome of Otitis Media in Early Infancy: A Prospective Study." *J Pediatr*. Vol. 104 (1984): 826-31.

5. Bluestone, C.D., Q. C. Beery, J. L. Paradise. "Audiometry and Tympanometry in Relation to Middle Ear Effusions in Children." *Laryngoscope*. Vol. 83 (1973): 594-604.

6. Teele, D. W., J. O. Klein, B. A. Rosner. "Otitis Media with Effusion during the First Three Years of Life and Development of Speech and Language." *Pediatrics*. Vol 74 (1984): 282-7.

7. Wright P. F., S. H. Sell, K. B. McConnell, A. B. Sitton, J. Thompson, W. K. Vaughn, et al. "Impact of Recurrent Otitis Media on Middle Ear Function, Hearing, and Language." *J Pediatr*. Vol. 113 (1988): 581-7.

8. Teele, D. W., S. I. Peltono, J. O. Klein. "Bacteriology of Acute Otitis Media Unresponsive to Initial Antimicrobial Therapy." *J Pediatr*. Vol 98 (1981): 537-9.

9.   Arola, M., T. Ziegler, O. Ruuskanen. "Respiratory Virus Infection as a Cause of Prolonged Symptoms in Acute Otitis Media." *J Pediatr*. Vol 116 (1990): 697-701.

10. Bluestone, C. D. "Modern Management of Otitis Media." *Pediatr Clin North Am*. Vol. 36 (1989): 1371-87.

11. Harrison, C. J., M. I. Marks, D. F. Welch. "Microbiology of Recently Treated Acute Otitis Media Compared with Previously Untreated Acute Otitis Media." *Pediatr Infect Dis J*. Vol. 4 (1985): 641-6.

12. Carlin, S. A., C. D. Marchant, P. A. Shurin, C. E. Johnson, D. Murdell-Panek, S. J. Barenkamp. "Early Recurrences of Otitis Media: Reinfection or Relapse?" *J Pediatr*. Vol. 110 (1987): 20-5.

13. Liston, T. E., W. S. Foshee, W. D. Pierson. "Sulfisoxazole Chemoprophylaxis for Frequent Otitis Media." *Pediatrics*. Vol 71 (1983): 524-30.

14. Perrin, J. M., E. Charney, J. B. Mac Whinney, Jr., T. K. McInerny, R. L. Millr, L. F. Nazarian. "Sulfisoxazole as Chemoprophylaxis for Recurrent Otitis Media. A Double-blind Crossover Study in Pediatric Practice." *N EnglJ Med*. Vol 291 (1974): 66-7.

15. Lampe, R. M., M. R. Weir. "Erythromycin Prophylaxis for Recurrent Otitis Media." *Clin Pediatr*. Vol 25 (1986): 510-5.

16. Marchant, C. D. "Otitis Media Today." *Pediatr Consultant*. Vol 8 (1990): 1-8.

17. Cantekin, E. I., E. M. Mandel, C. D. Bluestone, H. E. Rockette, J. L. Paradise, S. E. Stool, et al. "Lack of Efficacy of a Decongestant-Antihistamine Combination for Otitis Media with Effusion ("Secretory" Otitis Media) in Children. Results of a Double-blind, Randomized Trial." *N EnglJ Med*. Vol 308 (1983): 297-301.

18. Mandel E. M., H. E. Rockette, C. D. Bluestone, J. L. Paradise, R. J. Nozza. "Efficacy of Amoxicillin with and without Decongestant-Antihistamine for Otitis Media with Effusion in Children. Results of a Double-blind, Randomized Trial." *N Engl J Med.* Vol. 316 (1987): 432-7.

19. Thomsen, J., J. Sederbert-Olsen, V. Balle, R. Vejlsgaard, S. E. Stangerup, G. Bondesson. "Antibiotic Treatment of Children with Secretory Otitis Media. A Randomized, Double-blind, Placebo-controlled Study." *Arch Otolaryngol Head Neck Surg.* Vol. 115 (1989): 447-51.

20. Chan, K. H., E. M. Manden, H. E. Rockette, C. D. Bluestone, L. W. Bass, M. M. Blatter, et al. "A Comparative Study of Amoxicillin-Clavulanate and Amoxicillin. Treatment of Otitis Media with Effusion." *Arch Otolaryngol Head Neck Surg.* Vol. 114 (1988): 142-6.

21. Callahan, C. W., Jr., S. Lazoritz. "Otitis Media and Language Development." *Am Fam Physician.* Vol. 37 (1988): 186-90.

22. Casselbrant, M. L., L. M. Brostoff, E. I. Cantekin, M. R. Flaherty, W. J. Doyle, C. D. Bluestone, et al. "Otitis Media with Effusion in Preschool Children." *Laryngoscope.* Vol. 95 (1985): 428-36.

23. Paradise, J. L., K. D. Rogers. "On Otitis Media, Child Development, and Tympanostomy Tubes: New Answers or Old Questions?" *Pediatrics.* Vol. 77 (1986): 88-92.

24. Bluestone C. "Surgical Management of Otitis Media with Effusion: State of the Art." In *Recent Advances in Otitis Media with Effusion.* Edited by D. Lim. Philadelphia: BC Decker, 1984.

25. Pichichero, M. E., L. R. Berghash, A. S. Hengerer. "Anatomic and Audiologic Sequelae after Tympanostomy Tube Insertion or Prolonged Antibiotic Therapy for Otitis Media." *Pediatr Infect Dis J.* Vol. 8 (1989): 780-7.

26. Tos, M., S. E. Stangerup. "Hearing Loss in Tympanosclerosis Caused by Grommets." *Arch Otolaryngol Head Neck Surg.* Vol. 115 (1989): 931-5.

27. Richards, S. H., J. D. Shaw, D. Kilby, H. Campbel. "Grommets and Glue Ears: A Clinical Trial." *J Laryngol Otol.* Vol. 85 (1971): 17-22.

28. Kilby D., S. H. Richards, G. Hart. "Grommets and Glue Ears: Two-Year Results." *J Laryngol Otology.* Vol. 86 (1972): 881-8.

29. Brown M., S. Richards, A. Ambegaokar. "Grommets and Glue Ear a Five-Year Follow Up of a Controlled Trial." *J Royal Soc Med.* Vol. 71 (1978): 353-6.

30. Lildholdt, T. "Unilateral Grommet Insertion and Adenoidectomy in Bilateral Secretory Otitis Media: Preliminary Report on the Results in 91 Children." *Clin Otolaryngol.* Vol. 4 (1979): 87-93.

31. VanBuchem, F.V., M. F. Peeters, Van't Hof MA. "Acute Otitis Media: A New Treatment Strategy." *Br Med J.* Vol. 290 (1985): 1033-7.

32. Bollag, U., E. Bollag-Albrecht. "Otitis Media in Practice. A Different Approach to Management." *Clm Pediatr.* Vol. 29 (1990): 24-5.

33. Macknin, M. L., P. K. Jones. "Oral Dexamethasone for Treatment of Persistent Middle Ear Effusion." *Pediatrics.* Vol. 75 (1985): 329-35.

34. Mederman, L., V. Walter-Buckholtz, T. Jabalay. "A Comparative Trial of Steroids vs. Placebo for Treatment of Chronic Otitis Media with Effusion." In *Recent Advances in Otitis Media with Effusion.* Edited by D. Lim. Philadelphia: BC Decker, 1984.

35. Giebink, G. S., P. B. Batalden, C. T. Le, F. M. Lassman, D. J. Buran, A. E. Seltz. "A Controlled Trial Comparing Three Treatments for Chronic Otitis Media with Effusion." *Pediatr Infect Dis J.* Vol. 9 (1990): 33-40.

36. Persico, M., L. Podoshin, M. Fradis. "Otitis Media with Effusion: A Steroid and Antibiotic Therapeutic Trial Before Surgery." *Ann Otol Rhinol Laryngol.* Vol. 87 (1978): 191-6.

37. Berman, S., J. Grose, G. O. Zerbe. "Medical Management of Chronic Middle-Ear Effusion. Results of a Clinical Trial of Prednisone Combined with Sulfamethoxazole and Trimethoprim." *Am J Dis Child.* Vol. 141 (1987): 690-4.

38. Berman, S., K. Grose, R. Nuss, C. Huber-Navin, R. Roark, S. A. Gabbard, et al. "Management of Chronic Middle Ear Effusion with Prednisone Combined with Trimethoprim-Sulfamethoxazole." *Pediatr Infect Dis J.* Vol. 9 (1990): 533-8.

39. Leek, J. "Middle Ear Ventilation in Conjunction with Adenotonsillectomy." *Laryngoscope.* Vol. 89 (1979): 1760-3.

40. Roydhouse, N. "Adenoidectomy for Otitis with Mucoid Effusion." *Ann Otol Rhinol Laryngol Suppl.* Vol. 89 (1980): 312-5.

41. Maw, A. R., F. Herod. "Otoscopic, Impedance, and Audiometric Finding in Glue Ear Treated by Adenoidectomy and Tonsillectomy." *Lancet.* Vol 1 (1986): 1399-402.

42. Gates, G. A., C. A. Avery, T. J. Prihoda, J. C. Cooper, Jr. "Effectiveness of Adenoidectomy and Tympanostomy Tubes in the Treatment of Chronic Otitis Media with Effusion." *N Engl J Med.* Vol. 317 (1987): 1444-51.

My thanks to Dr. Michael Foulds and Dr. Anita Bowes for their critical review of this manuscripts.

—*by James D. Legler, M.D.*

Chapter 11

Genetics and Deafness

Note to the Reader:

There are many terms used to describe people who have some degree of hearing loss: **"deaf"** and **"hard of hearing"** are two of them. For the sake of simplicity, this booklet uses the word **"deaf"** to cover all degrees of hearing loss ranging from profound to mild. This booklet is written for parents of deaf children, deaf people and their families, and professionals who wish to learn more about the relationship between heredity and deafness.

Why can two hearing parents have a deaf child?
Why can two deaf parents have a hearing child?
What caused your child's deafness?
What caused your deafness?

Finding answers to these questions is not easy. No two people are alike. Yet there are answers. One of the best ways to find the answers is through genetic counseling.

This fact sheet was prepared by the Gallaudet University Genetic Services Center and the National Information Center on Deafness. (No. 91-12-139; [293] 11/90-5M 050).

What Causes Deafness?

The causes of deafness can be grouped into two categories: environmental causes and genetic causes. It is estimated that approximately 50 percent of deafness occurs from environmental causes and 50 percent from genetic causes. Environmental causes of deafness include:

- some illnesses that the mother may have had while she was pregnant, such as rubella (German measles);
- premature birth of the baby;
- illnesses that the child can get after birth, such as meningitis or some viruses; and
- some medicines

Environmental types of deafness cannot be inherited.

Genetic deafness is inherited, it is passed from parents to their children. This also is called hereditary deafness. There are about 200 different types of genetic deafness. Often, a person with a genetic type of deafness inherited it from parents who had normal hearing. It is possible for hearing parents to have a deaf child from genetic causes even when no other family member is deaf.

What Is Genetics?

Genetics is the study of inheritance—how characteristics (traits) such as eye color, hair color, blood type, and deafness are passed from parents to their children.

To understand better about the ways deafness can be passed from parents to children, it is important to understand more about genetics. Genetics is a very complex subject. New discoveries are being made rapidly. The following pages provide basic information about genetics.

Our bodies are made of millions of cells. Each cell contains a total of 46 thread-like structures called chromosomes. Each chromosome has thousands of genes on it. The genes are the part of the cell that contains hereditary information. These tiny genes provide all the information about inherited traits such as the color of hair, eyes, and skin; the shape and size of the nose, feet, and hands; height; and so on.

We all started as a single cell formed from the union of an egg from our mother and a sperm from our father. Both the egg cell and the sperm cell are special cells. Instead of having 46 chromosomes, like all the other cells in the body, the egg and sperm cells each have only 23 chromosomes. The genes on the 23 chromosomes from the mother's egg cell carry genetic information from the mother to the child. The genes on the 23 chromosomes from the father's sperm cell carry genetic information from the father to the child. The 23 chromosomes from the mother and the 23 chromosomes from the father form the 46 chromosomes in the cell that will eventually become the baby. So each parent contributes one-half of the 46 chromosomes and therefore, one-half of the genes inherited by the child.

What Do Genes Do?

The thousands of genes on the chromosomes are so small that we cannot see them even with the most powerful microscope, but despite their size, scientists have learned what genes do. As mentioned before, they provide instructions for specific traits or characteristics such as blood type, eye color, hair color, and in some instances, a type of deafness. Hundreds of genes determine how the ear is made and how it functions. One change in a single gene controlling the development or functioning of the ear can result in deafness.

Genes work in pairs. Each of the 200 or so different types of genetic deafness is caused by its own pair of genes. Two factors influence how a person can inherit genetic deafness: the combination of genes the person has and how the specific kind of deafness is inherited. This is what geneticists call the "pattern of inheritance." In some families with genetic deafness, there are several generations of deaf members. In other families with genetic deafness, there may be only one deaf person. It all depends on the combination of gene pairs and the pattern of inheritance of the specific type of deafness.

What Are the Patterns of Inheritance?

Deafness can be inherited in one of three patterns: dominant, recessive, or, in rare cases, X-linked. To make this information easier to understand, we will refer to these patterns as "dominant genes" and "recessive genes." Each type of genetic deafness is controlled by its own pair of genes. The inheritance of dominant, recessive and X-linked genes for deafness is explained later in this publication.

What Is Genetic Counseling?

Genetic counseling is the process of obtaining information about traits that run in families. Much can be learned about the cause of deafness through genetic counseling. Genetic counseling is provided by a team of professionals who have special training in genetics. These professionals include genetics doctors, counselors, nurses, and social workers.

What Happens During Genetic Counseling?

Here are a few things you might expect to happen in a genetic counseling session, which lasts approximately one to two hours.

One of the first things a genetic counselor needs to know is your family history. The genetics team—the genetics doctor and the genetic counselor—will ask questions about both your mother's and father's sides of the family. The genetics team also will ask specific questions about the health of your family members and about traits that occur in your family. They also will want to know if anyone else in the family is deaf.

The genetics doctor will give you, and perhaps your child, a physical examination. Sometimes, several family members will be given a brief physical examination. During the examination the genetics doctor will take several measurements such as head size and the distance between the eyes. These measurements and other physical characteristics sometimes offer the geneticist clues about the type of deafness present. Usually a blood test will not be done because there is no simple blood test to discover genes for deafness. However, sometimes the genetics doctor will recommend some medical tests or refer you to other medical specialists to help determine the cause of deafness. A hearing test (audiogram) cannot by itself be used to determine the cause of deafness. However, the hearing test—along with medical records and the physical examination—can offer additional clues about the cause of deafness.

Two-thirds of all genetic types of deafness result in only deafness. In such cases there are no other specific physical or medical conditions. One-third of all genetic types of deafness include other specific physical characteristics or medical conditions such as vision changes heart trouble. These combined conditions are called syndromes. It is important to know if your deafness is part of a syndrome so proper information and necessary medical treatment can be obtained.

During a genetic counseling session, the geneticist also will review your medical history, asking for information about illnesses you had as a child or problems that may have existed at the time of birth. Sometimes the geneticist will need to review other records. such as X-rays, audiograms, and medical tests.

After genetics team members have completed this complex investigation, they will meet with you and your family. In this meeting, they will explain what they have found and answer your questions. Sometimes the genetics team can determine whether the deafness is genetic or environmental and exactly what caused it. If the cause is environmental, the deafness is not inherited. If the deafness is genetic, the genetics team will explain the pattern of inheritance and what chance future children have to inherit the genes for deafness. In some cases, geneticists may not be able to determine if the deafness is due to environmental or genetic factors; the cause of deafness remains an "unknown" factor. However, when the genetics team cannot determine exactly what caused the deafness, they can still exclude many possible causes and associated medical conditions.

What Is Dominant Inheritance?

Genes come in pairs, one from each of the parents. In dominant inheritance, a person will be deaf when only one gene of a pair codes for deafness. About 20 percent of genetic types of deafness are dominant. As shown, the most common pattern in dominant types of deafness is for the person to have one dominant gene for deafness (D) and the other gene of the pair for normal hearing (d). However, because the dominant gene (D) is a strong gene, the person will be deaf. Both males and females can have dominant types of deafness.

When a person with a dominant gene for deafness has a child, the child will inherit either the dominant gene for deafness (D) or the gene for hearing (d). In other words, there is a 50 percent chance that the child will inherit the dominant gene for deafness and be deaf. There is no way to control which of the two genes in the pair the child will inherit. It is a matter of chance, just like flipping a coin. A child with a dominant type of deafness almost always has a deaf parent, and there are usually several generations of relatives who are deaf.

What Is Recessive Inheritance?

Nearly 80 percent of genetic types of deafness are recessive. A person who has a recessive type of deafness has a matched pair of recessive genes for deafness (rr). If a person has two genes for hearing (RR), the person will have normal hearing. In recessive inheritance, a person who has one gene that codes for hearing and one gene that codes for deafness (Rr) is called a carrier. A carrier will have normal hearing, but will pass on to each of his or her children either the recessive gene for deafness or the gene for hearing. As shown, when both parents are carriers of the same gene for recessive deafness, each of their children has a 25 percent chance of inheriting a matched pair of genes for deafness (rr) and therefore, will be deaf. On the other hand, each of their children has a 75 percent chance of inheriting at least one of the genes for hearing and therefore, will be hearing.

Most people with a recessive type of deafness have hearing parents and may have both hearing and deaf brothers and sisters. Recessive deafness may not show up for many generations in a family, and the family members who carry the gene for recessive deafness often do not know they are carriers. Only when both parents pass on to their child genes for the same recessive type of deafness can a child inherit a "double dose" of the gene and be deaf.

What Is X-Linked Inheritance?

About one to two percent of genetic deafness is X-linked. In females, one pair of chromosomes is a pair of sex chromosomes} both called X. In males, the sex chromosomes are X and Y. In X-linked recessive, the gene for deafness is on the mother's X chromosome. She is a carrier and is hearing. Only male children can inherit the deafness from the mother, but female children can become carriers of the gene for deafness and pass it on to their children. X-linked inheritance of deafness is very rare.

In Summary:

By reading this booklet, you may have learned a lot of new and complex information about genetics and deafness. Deafness can result from environmental causes or genetic causes. Genetic types of deafness are inherited; that is, they are passed from parents to their children. Genetic (hereditary) deafness can be inherited in one of three patterns: "dominant," "recessive," or "X-linked." The most common type of genetic inheritance (approximately 80 percent) is recessive. A genetic counseling session includes a review of family and medical histories and a physical examination. Geneticists use all of this information to help determine the cause of deafness.

For More Information On Genetic Counseling Contact:

Genetic Services Center
Gallaudet University
College Hall
800 Florida Ave. NE
Washington, DC 20002-3695
(202) 651-5258 (V/TDD)
1-800-451-8834, ext. 5258 (V/TDD)

The Genetic Services Center (GSC) is located on the main campus of Gallaudet University. The GSC provides genetic evaluations and counseling. This service is available to deaf individuals and families who live in or are visiting the Washington, D.C., area. The GSC staff uses sign language. The GSC can also provide information about genetic services in other parts of the country.

To locate local genetic services in other areas, contact any of the following organizations:

American Society of Human Genetics
American Board of Medical Genetics
9650 Rockville Pike
Bethesda, MD 20814
(301) 571-1825 (V)

National Society of Genetic Counselors
233 Canterbury Drive
Wallingford, PA 19086
(215) 872-7608 (V)

March of Dimes Birth Defects Foundation
Professional Education
1275 Mamaroneck Avenue
White Plains, NY 10605
(914) 428-7100 (V)

In addition, many large universities and hospitals have clinical genetic services. Ask your doctor or your local health department for a list of genetic service providers. The cost of genetic services and insurance coverage will vary.

For More Information on Deafness and Hearing Loss Contact:

Alexander Graham Bell Association for the Deaf, Inc.
3417 Volta Place, NW
Washington, DC 20007
(202) 337-5220 (V/TDD)

American Society for Deaf Children
814 Thayer Ave.
Silver Spring, MD 20910
(301) 585-5400 (V/TDD)

American Speech-Language-Hearing Association
10801 Rockville Pike
Rockville, MD 20852
(301) 897-5700 (V/TDD)
(800) 638-8255 (V/TDD)

Association of Late-Deafened Adults
1027 Oakton
Evanston, IL 60202
(312) 604-4192 (TDD)

National Association of the Deaf
814 Thayer Ave.
Silver Spring, MD 20910
(301) 587-1788 (V/TDD)

National Information Center on Deafness
Gallaudet University
800 Florida Ave. NE
Washington, DC 20002-3695
(202) 651-5051 (V) or (202) 651-5052 (TDD)

Registry of Interpreters for the Deaf, Inc.
8719 Colesville Road, Suite 310
Silver Spring, MD 20910
(301) 608-0050 (V/TDD)

Self Help for Hard of Hearing People, Inc.
7800 Wisconsin Ave.
Bethesda, MD 20814
(301) 657-2248 (V) or (301) 657-2249 (TDD)

—by Dorothy Smith

Chapter 12

Facts on Hereditary Deafness

What Is Hereditary Deafness?

Hereditary deafness is hearing loss that is inherited or passed down from parents to their children. This type of hearing loss may be inherited from one or both parents who may or may not have a loss of hearing themselves.

Hereditary material or genes are located on chromosomes which are found in each cell of the body. Genes provide instructions for specific traits or characteristics such as hair color or blood type. Defective genes can also pass along traits such as hearing loss or speech and language disorders.

The hereditary hearing loss that results from defective genes may be syndromic or nonsyndromic, dominant or recessive. Syndromic hearing loss is associated with specific traits additional to hearing impairment. For example, hearing, balance and visual problems occur in Usher syndrome. Nonsyndromic hearing impairment has hearing loss as its only characteristic. Dominant transmission of deafness requires only one faulty gene, from either the mother or father to cause the hearing loss, whereas recessive transmission of deafness requires a faulty gene from both the mother and father.

Of the more than 4,000 infants born deaf each year, more than half have a hereditary disorder. However, not all hereditary hearing

Published by the National Institute on Deafness and Other Communication Disorders.

loss is present at birth. Some infants may inherit the tendency to acquire hearing loss later in life.

Scientists supported by the National Institute on Deafness and Other Communication Disorders (NIDCD) are on the forefront of research on the molecular bases of hearing and deafness, continuing to explore the genetics of hearing loss in a variety of disorders, including Waardenburg syndrome, Usher syndrome, nonsyndromic hereditary deafness, otosclerosis, adult-onset hearing loss and presbycusis, and the hereditary predisposition to noise-induced hearing loss and otitis media. This research should lead to a better understanding of how hearing impairment or deafness is transmitted from parent to child, making it possible to identify and characterize the genes in which changes or mutations cause hearing impairment. Through these efforts it may be possible to discover how genes work, what proteins they manufacture and the role they play in the development and maintenance of normal hearing. These discoveries should lead to early diagnosis, prevention and treatment, such as gene transfer therapy.

Research on Hereditary Deafness Syndromic Hearing Impairment

There are more than 200 forms of syndromic hereditary hearing impairment. NIDCD-supported scientists have been able to map or locate the abnormal genes on their chromosomes for three of these hereditary syndromic forms of hearing loss: Waardenburg syndrome (WS) type 1 and Usher syndrome types 1 and 2. WS type 1, which accounts for two to three percent of all cases of congenital deafness, has been mapped to a narrow band on the long arm of chromosome 2. Usher syndrome type 2 has been mapped to chromosome 1 and type 1 has been mapped to chromosome 11. These two types account for approximately ten percent of all cases of congenital deafness.

Both Usher syndrome types 1 and 2 are recessive disorders which cause congenital hearing loss and late-onset blindness due to retinitis pigmentosa. Usher syndrome type 1 is characterized by severe hearing loss, complete loss of balance and blindness. Usher syndrome type 2 is characterized by moderate hearing loss, normal balance function and blindness. More than half of the approximately 16,000 deaf and blind people in the United States are believed to have Usher syndrome.

WS types 1 and 2 are dominant disorders which are often characterized by hearing impairment and changes in skin and hair pigmentation. Hearing impairment is present in approximately 20 percent of those with WS type 1. In addition, individuals with WS type 1 have an unusually wide space between the inner corners of their eyes. In contrast, approximately 50 percent of individuals with WS type 2 have hearing impairment but they do not have the wide spacing between the inner corners of their eyes.

To accelerate research on WS, an international consortium was formed by the NIDCD in September 1990. The consortium consists of the following six research teams: Boston University Medical School Center for Human Genetics, Boston Massachusetts; Michigan State University Department of Zoology, East Lansing, Michigan; Laboratory of Molecular Biology, NIH-NIDCD, Bethesda, Maryland; Department of Medical Genetics, University of Manchester, United Kingdom; Molecular Genetics Laboratory, Virginia Commonwealth University, Richmond, Virginia; and Department of Human Genetics, University of Cape Town Medical School, Cape Town, South Africa.

One team from the consortium recently studied 60 members from six generations of a Brazilian family, 26 of whom were diagnosed with WS type 1. This team discovered that each affected family member had a defect in the gene called PAX 3 on chromosome 2. This defect was due to one amino acid substitution in the gene that was not found in 17 other WS type 1 families unrelated to the Brazilian family, indicating that other mutations may cause the syndrome in other families. Seventy-eight percent of the members of this Brazilian family had noticeable hearing loss which is well above the 20 percent found in most WS type 1 cases, placing additional importance on the significance of this gene in the development of hearing loss in WS.

A group of scientists has discovered a defective gene in disordered mice referred to as Pax-3 (lower case to distinguish it from the human symbol PAX 3). These mice have hearing loss, pigmentary disturbances and facial changes. The Pax-3 gene, which regulates early development of the mice in the womb, is comparable to the PAX 3 gene found on chromosome 2 in humans. Another team from the consortium has found another mutation in the PAX 3 gene in several families with WS type 1.

Nonsyndromic Recessive Hearing Impairment

Approximately 80 percent of the nonsyndromic hereditary hearing disorders are recessive. Another international collaboration will provide NIDCD scientists with a rare opportunity to study nonsyndromic recessive hearing impairment in a large segment of the population in southern India where scientists report that 40 to 50 percent of the children in schools for the deaf have this type of hearing impairment. This type of hearing loss has been difficult to study in the United States because of the difficulty in making a definitive diagnosis.

Nonsyndromic Dominant Hearing Impairment

A team of NIDCD-supported scientists has located the gene responsible for a nonsyndromic dominant form of hearing impairment in a large family from Costa Rica who develop hearing impairment in late childhood. Hearing loss for the affected members of this family becomes severe between 30 and 40 years of age. These scientists were able to analyze the genetic material of 86 descendants of Felix Monge, an 18th century ancestor who had a hearing loss similar to his 20th century descendants. The gene is located on a specific portion of chromosome 5. Since hearing loss in this family begins later in childhood, rather than at birth, it is possible that this gene is responsible for the maintenance of auditory hair cells during early life.

About the NIDCD

The NIDCD is one of the institutes of the National Institutes of Health (NIH). The NIDCD conducts and supports biomedical and behavioral research and research training on normal and disordered mechanisms of hearing, balance, smell, taste, voice, speech and language.

About the Recent Research Series

This series is intended to inform health professionals, patients, and the public about progress in understanding the normal and disordered processes of human communication through recent advances made by NIDCD-supported scientists in each of the Institute's seven program areas of hearing, balance, smell, taste, voice, speech, and language.

For additional information on hereditary deafness, write to:

National Institute on Deafness and Other Communication Disorders
NIDCD Clearinghouse
P.O. Box 37777
Washington, DC 20013-7777

Chapter 13

NIH Consensus Statement on Noise and Hearing Loss

Introduction

Hearing loss afflicts approximately 28 million people in the United States. Approximately 10 million of these impairments are at least partially attributable to damage from exposure to loud sounds. Sounds that are sufficiently loud to damage sensitive inner ear structures can produce hearing loss that is not reversible by any presently available medical or surgical treatment. Hearing impairment associated with noise exposure can occur at any age, including early infancy, and is often characterized by difficulty in understanding speech and the potentially troublesome symptom, tinnitus (i.e., ringing in the ears). Very loud sounds of short duration, such as an explosion or gunfire, can produce immediate, severe, and permanent loss of hearing. Longer exposure to less intense but still hazardous sounds, commonly encountered in the workplace or in certain leisure time activities, exacts a gradual toll on hearing sensitivity, initially without the victim's awareness. More than 20 million Americans are exposed on a regular basis to hazardous noise levels that could result in hearing loss. Occupational noise exposure, the most common cause of noise-induced hearing loss (NIHL), threatens the hearing of firefighters, police officers, military personnel, construction and factory workers, musicians, farmers, and truck drivers, to name a few. Live or recorded

NIH Consensus Statement; NIH Consensus Development Conference, January 22-24, 1990; Volume 8, Number 1.

high-volume music, recreational vehicles, airplanes, lawn-care equipment, woodworking tools, some household appliances, and chain saws are examples of nonoccupational sources of potentially hazardous noise. One important feature of NIHL is that it is preventable in all but certain cases of accidental exposure. Legislation and regulations have been enacted that spell out guidelines for protecting workers from hazardous noise levels in the workplace and consumers from hazardous noise during leisure time pursuits. Inconsistent compliance and spotty enforcement of existing governmental regulations have been underlying causes for their relative ineffectiveness in achieving prevention of NIHL. A particularly unfortunate occurrence was the elimination of the Office of Noise Abatement and Control within the Environmental Protection Agency in 1982.

On January 22-24, 1990, the National Institute on Deafness and Other Communication Disorders, together with the Office of Medical Applications of Research of the National Institutes of Health convened a Consensus Development Conference on Noise and Hearing Loss. Co-sponsors of the conference were the National Institute of Child Health and Human Development, the National Institute on Aging, and the National Institute for Occupational Safety and Health of the Centers for Disease Control. The effects of environmental sounds on human listeners may include:

- Interference with speech communication and other auditory signals.
- Annoyance and aversion.
- Noise-induced hearing loss.
- Changes in various body systems.
- Interference with sleep.

This conference was entirely centered on NIHL. The panel focused on five questions related to noise and hearing loss:

- What is noise-induced hearing loss?
- What sounds can damage hearing?
- What factors, including age, determine an individual's susceptibility to noise-induced hearing loss?
- What can be done to prevent noise-induced hearing loss?
- What are the directions for future research?

110

Following a day and a half of presentations by experts in the relevant fields and discussion from the audience, a consensus panel comprising specialists and generalists from the medical and other related scientific disciplines, together with public representatives, considered the evidence and formulated a consensus statement in response to the five previously stated questions.

What Is Noise-Induced Hearing Loss?

Sounds of sufficient intensity and duration will damage the ear and result in temporary or permanent hearing loss. The hearing loss may range from mild to profound and may also result in tinnitus. The effect of repeated sound overstimulation is cumulative over a lifetime and is not currently treatable. Hearing impairment has a major impact on one's communication ability and even mild impairment may adversely affect the quality of life. Unfortunately, although NIHL is preventable, our increasingly noisy environment places more and more people at risk.

Studies of NIHL

Most studies of the association between sound exposure and hearing loss in humans are retrospective measurements of the hearing sensitivities of numerous individuals correlated with their noise exposures. The variability within these studies is usually large; thus, it is difficult to predict the precise magnitude of hearing loss that will result from a specific sound exposure. Prospective studies of selected workers' hearing levels over a long time while their sound exposures are carefully monitored are costly and time-consuming and, due to attrition, require a large number of subjects. When significant hearing loss is found, for ethical reasons, exposures must be reduced, interfering with the relationships under study. Although studies of NIHL in humans are difficult, they provide valuable information not available from animal studies and should be continued.

In prospective animal studies, sound exposures can be carefully controlled, and the anatomic and physiologic correlates of NIHL can be precisely defined. Although there may be interspecies differences with respect to the absolute sound exposure that will injure the ear, the basic mechanisms that lead to damage appear to be similar in all mammalian ears.

111

Anatomic and Physiologic Correlates of NIHL

Two types of injury are recognized: acoustic trauma and NIHL. Short-duration sound of sufficient intensity (e.g., a gunshot or explosion) may result in an immediate, severe, and permanent hearing loss, which is termed acoustic trauma. Virtually all of the structures of the ear can be damaged, in particular the organ of Corti, the delicate sensory structure of the auditory portion of the inner ear (cochlea), which may be torn apart. Moderate exposure may initially cause temporary hearing loss, termed temporary threshold shift (TTS). Structural changes associated with TTS have not been fully established but may include subtle intracellular changes in the sensory cells (hair cells) and swelling of the auditory nerve endings. Other potentially reversible effects include vascular changes, metabolic exhaustion, and chemical changes within the hair cells. There is also evidence of a regional decrease in the stiffness of the stereocilia (the hair bundles at the top of the hair cells), which may recover. This decrease in stereocilia stiffness may lead to a decrease in the coupling of sound energy to the hair cells, which thereby alters hearing sensitivity.

Repeated exposure to sounds that cause TTS may gradually cause permanent NIHL in experimental animals. In this type of injury, cochlear blood flow may be impaired, and a few scattered hair cells are damaged with each exposure. With continued exposure, the number of damaged hair cells increases. Although most structures in the inner ear can be harmed by excessive sound exposure, the sensory cells are the most vulnerable. Damage to the stereocilia is often the first change, specifically, alteration of the rootlet structures that normally anchor the stereocilia into the top of the hair cell. Once destroyed, the sensory cells are not replaced. During the recovery period between some sound exposures, damaged regions of the organ of Corti heal by scar formation. This process is very important because it reestablishes the barrier between the two fluids of the inner ear (perilymph and endolymph). If this barrier is not reestablished, degeneration of hair cells may continue. Further, once a sufficient number of hair cells are lost, the nerve fibers to that region also degenerate. With degeneration of the cochlear nerve fibers, there is corresponding degeneration within the central nervous system. The extent to which these neural changes contribute to NIHL is not clear.

With moderate periods of exposure to potentially hazardous high frequency sound, the damage is usually confined to a restricted area in the high-frequency region of the cochlea. With a comparable exposure to low-frequency noise, hair cell damage is not confined to the low-frequency region but may also affect the high-frequency regions. The predominance of damage in different cochlear regions with different frequency exposures reflects factors such as the resonance of the ear canal, the middle ear transfer characteristics, and the mechanical characteristics of the organ of Corti and basilar membrane.

Assessment of NIHL

Hearing loss is measured by determining auditory thresholds (sensitivity) at various frequencies (pure-tone audiometry). Complete assessment should also include measures of speech understanding and middle-ear status (immittance audiometry). Pure-tone audiometry is also used in industrial hearing conservation programs to determine whether adequate protection against hazardous sound levels is provided.

The first audiometric sign of NIHL resulting from broadband noise is usually a loss of sensitivity in the higher frequencies from 3,000 through 6,000 Hertz (Hz) (i.e., cycles per second), resulting in a characteristic audiometric "notch." With additional hearing loss from noise or aging, the threshold at 8,000 Hz may worsen and eliminate this characteristic audiometric pattern. Thus, the presence or absence of NIHL cannot be established on the basis of audiometric shape, per se. The hearing loss is usually bilateral, but some degree of asymmetry is not unusual, especially with lateralized noise sources such as rifles. After moderate sound exposure, TTS may occur, and, during a period of relative quiet, thresholds will return to normal levels. If the exposure continues on a regular basis, permanent threshold shifts (PTS) will result, increasing in magnitude and extending to lower and higher frequencies. If the exposures continue, NIHL increases, more rapidly in the early years. After many years of exposure, NIHL levels off in the high frequencies, but continues to worsen in the low frequencies. Although TTS and PTS are correlated, the relation is not strong enough to use TTS to predict the magnitude of permanent hearing loss.

An important consequence of the sensitivity loss associated with NIHL is difficulty in understanding speech. Whereas a large proportion of the energy in speech is contained within the low frequency range, much of the information required to differentiate one speech sound from another is contained within the higher frequencies. With significant hearing loss in the high frequencies, important speech information is often inaudible or unusable. Other interfering sounds such as background noise, competing voices, or room reverberation may reduce even further the hearing-impaired listener's receptive communication ability. The presence of tinnitus may be an additional debilitating condition.

NIHL may interfere with daily life, especially those social activities that occur in noisy settings. Increased effort is required for understanding speech in these situations, which leads to fatigue, anxiety, and stress. Decreased participation in these activities often results, affecting not only hearing-impaired individuals but also friends and family members. Hearing loss is associated with depression in the elderly and may be related to dementia and cognitive dysfunction. Systematic study of the effects of hearing loss on the quality of life have only lately focused specifically on individuals with NIHL; therefore, continued studies of this kind are desirable.

The impairment in hearing ability resulting from NIHL may vary from mild to severe. An individual's ability to communicate and function in daily life varies with the degree of loss and the individual's communication needs although these relationships are complex. The magnitude of the effect on communication ability may be estimated by a variety of scales, which are often used in disability determinations. These scales, which vary substantially in the frequencies used, the upper and lower limits of impairment, age correction, and adjustment for asymmetric hearing loss, attempt to predict the degree of communication impairment (understanding of speech) on the basis of pure-tone thresholds. There is no consensus about the validity or utility of the scales, which scale should be used, whether measures of speech understanding should be included, or whether self-assessment ratings should be incorporated into either impairment rating scales or disability determinations.

What Sounds Can Damage Hearing?

Some sounds are so weak physically that they are not heard. Some sounds are audible but do not have any temporary or permanent after-effects. Some sounds are strong enough to produce a temporary hearing loss from which there may appear to be complete recovery.

Damaging sounds are those that are sufficiently strong, sufficiently long-lasting, and involve appropriate frequencies so that permanent hearing loss will ensue.

Most of the sounds in the environment that produce such permanent effects occur over a very long time (for example, about 8 hours per workday over a period of 10 or more years). On the other hand, there are some particularly abrupt or explosive sounds that can cause damage even with a single exposure.

The line between these categories of sounds cannot be stated simply because not all persons respond to sound in the same manner. Thus, if a sound of given frequency bandwidth, level, and duration is considered hazardous, one must specify for what proportion of the population it will be hazardous and, within that proportion, by what criterion of damage (whether anatomical, audiometric, speech understanding) it is hazardous.

The most widely used measure of a sound's strength or amplitude is called "sound level," measured by a sound-level meter in units called "decibels" (dB). For example, the sound level of speech at typical conversational distances is between 65 and 70 dB. There are weaker sounds, still audible, and of course much stronger sounds. Those above 85 dB are potentially hazardous.

Sounds must also be specified in terms of frequency or bandwidth, roughly like the span of keys on a piano. The range of audible frequencies extends from about 20 Hz, below the lowest notes on a piano, to at least 16,000 or 20,000 Hz, well above the highest notes on a piccolo. Most environmental noises include a wide band of frequencies and, by convention, are measured through the "A" filter in the sound-level meter and thus are designated in dB(A) units. It is not clear what effect, if any, sound outside the frequency range covered in dB(A) measurements may have on hearing. At this time, it is not known whether ultrasonic vibration will damage hearing. To define what sounds can damage hearing, sound level, whether across all frequency bands or taken band by band, is not enough. The duration of exposure—typical for a day and accumulated over many years—is critical. Sound levels associated with particular sources such as snowmobiles, rock music, and chain saws, are often cited, but predicting the likelihood of NIHL from such sources also requires knowledge of typical durations and the number of exposures.

There appears to be reasonable agreement that sound levels below 75 dB(A) will not engender a permanent hearing loss, even at

4000 Hz. At higher levels, the amount of hearing loss is directly related to sound level for comparable durations.

According to some existing rules and regulations, a noise level of 85 dB(A) for an 8-hour daily exposure is potentially damaging. If total sound energy were the important predictor, an equivalent exposure could be as high as 88 dB(A) if restricted to 4 hours. (A 3-dB increase is equivalent to doubling the sound intensity.) This relation, enshrined in some standards and regulations, is a theory based on a dose or exposure defined by total energy.

In spite of the physical simplicity of a total-energy concept other principles have been invoked to define equivalent exposures of different sound levels and durations. Early research suggested that NIHL after 10 years could be predicted from temporary threshold shifts (TTS) measured 2 minutes after a comparable single-day exposure. Those results, however, were taken to indicate that a halving of duration could be offset by a 5-dB change in sound level rather than a 3-dB change. This 5-dB rule is implemented in the Walsh-Healey Act of 1969 and subsequent Occupational Safety and Health Administration regulations for the purpose of requiring preventive efforts for noise-exposed workers. The 3-dB trading rule is agreed to in International Standards Organization (ISO) Standard 1999.2 (1989) for the purpose of predicting the amount of noise-induced hearing loss resulting from different exposures. There is no consensus concerning a single rule to be used for all purposes in the United States.

Generally, for sound levels below about 140 dB, different temporal forms of sound, whether impulse (gunshot), impact (drop forge) or steady state (turbine), when specified with respect to their level and duration, produce the same hearing loss. This does not appear to follow at levels above 140 dB, where impulse noise creates more damage than would be predicted. This may imply that impulse noise above a certain critical level results in acoustic trauma from which the ear cannot recover.

Although sound exposures that are potentially hazardous to hearing are usually defined in terms of sound level, frequency bandwidths, and duration, there are several simple approximations that indicate that a sound exposure may be suspected as hazardous. These include the following: If the sound is appreciably louder than conversational level, it is potentially harmful, provided that the sound is present for a sufficient period of time. Hazardous noise may also be suspected if the listener experiences: (a) difficulty in communication while in the sound, (b) ringing in the ear (tinnitus) after exposure to the sound, and/or (c) the experience that sounds seem muffled after leaving the sound-exposure area.

In the consideration of sounds that can damage hearing, one point is clear: it is the acoustic energy of the sound reaching the ear, not its source, which is important. That is, it does not matter if the hazardous sound is generated by a machine in the workplace, by an amplifier/loudspeaker at a rock concert, or by a snowmobile ridden by the listener. Significant amounts of acoustic energy reaching the ear will create damage—at work, at school, at home, or during leisure activities. Although there has been a tendency to concentrate on the more significant occupational and transportation noise, the same rules apply to all potential noise hazards.

What Factors, Including Age, Determine an Individual's Susceptibility to Noise Induced Hearing Loss?

One thoroughly established characteristic of NIHL is that, on the average, more intense and longer-duration noise exposures cause more severe hearing loss. A second is that there is a remarkably broad range of individual differences in sensitivity to any given noise exposure. Several factors have been proposed to explain differences in NIHL among individuals; others may be associated with differences over time within the same individual. It is important to distinguish those factors whose roles in determining susceptibility are supported by a consistent body of theory and empirical evidence from other factors whose roles have been proposed but for which theory, data, or both are less conclusive.

Differences Among Individuals

Both temporary threshold shift (TTS) and permanent threshold shift (PTS) in response to a given intense noise may differ as much as 30 to 50 dB among individuals. Both animal research and retrospective studies of humans exposed to industrial noise have demonstrated this remarkable variation in susceptibility. The biological bases for these differences are unknown. A number of extrinsic factors (e.g., characteristics of the ear canal and middle ear, drugs, and prior exposure to noise) may influence an individual's susceptibility to NIHL. However, animal studies that have controlled these variables suggest that individual differences in inner ear anatomy and physiology also may be significant. Additional research is necessary to determine whether vascular, neural feedback (efferent system), or other mechanisms can account for and predict such individual variation.

One factor that may be associated with decreased susceptibility to NIHL is conductive hearing loss; the cochlear structures may be protected by any form of acoustic attenuation. For similar reasons, middle ear muscles, which normally serve a protective function by contracting in response to intense sound, when inoperative, can result in increased susceptibility. Among the other factors that are theoretically associated with differences in susceptibility are (a) unusually efficient acoustic transfer through the external and middle ear, as a determinant of the amount of energy coupled to the inner ear structures. and (b) preexisting hearing loss, which could imply that less additional loss would occur if the sensitive structures have already been damaged. Support for these hypotheses has been modest, in the case of the transfer function, because little empirical work has been done to test that hypothesis, and, in the case of reduced sensitivity, because several studies disagree. In general, when there is a difference in average loss to a given noise exposure, those ears with previous PTS or TTS have shown somewhat less additional loss than those not previously exposed.

Findings have sometimes implicated degree of pigmentation, both of the receptor structures (melanization) and of the eye and skin, as related to susceptibility. However, these results, too, are equivocal.

Gender. There is little difference in hearing thresholds between young male and female children. Between ages 10 and 20, males begin to show reduced high-frequency auditory sensitivity relative to females. Women continue to demonstrate better hearing than men into advanced age. These gender differences are probably due to greater exposure of males to noise rather than to their inherent susceptibility to its effects.

Differences Within Individuals

Ototoxic drugs. Among the causes of differences of susceptibility to noise exposure within individuals are ototoxic drugs and other chemicals. In animal research, certain antibiotics (aminoglycocides) appear to exacerbate the damaging effects of noise exposure. Clinical evidence of corresponding effects in human patients has not been established, but precautions should be taken with regard to noise exposures of individual patients treated with these medications. Although high doses of aspirin are widely known to cause TTS and tinnitus, aspirin has not been shown to increase susceptibility to NIHL.

Age. In certain animal models there is evidence of heightened susceptibility to noise exposure shortly after birth—a "critical period" (possibly following the time when fluids fill the middle ear but before complete development of the cochlear structures). However, it is not clear that data from such animal models can be generalized to full-term normal human infants. Premature infants in noisy environments (e.g. neonatal intensive care units), however, may be at risk. At the other extreme, increasing age has been hypothesized to be associated with decreasing susceptibility. This contention is based on the existence of presbycusis, hearing loss that increases with age and that is not known to be attributable to excessive noise exposure or other known etiology. The typical levels of presbycusis at various ages have recently been incorporated as Annex A in International Standards Organization Standard 1999.2 (1989). That standard may be used to estimate the portion of overall hearing loss that is attributable to exposure to excessive noise.

In summary, scientific knowledge is currently inadequate to predict that any individual will be safe in noise that exceeds established damage-risk criteria, nor that specific individuals will show greater-than-average loss following a given exposure. Among the many proposed explanations, the hypothesis that the resonant and transmission properties of the external and middle ear affect individual susceptibility deserves further attention. Empirical support for this hypothesis should not be difficult to obtain, but very few data have been collected on this question, both for TTS (experimentally) and PTS (retrospectively). Differences in susceptibility of the cochlear structures to NIHL may exist, but no practical approach to predicting them is yet available. Identification of susceptible humans will almost certainly be delayed until a successful animal model is available.

What Can Be Done to Prevent Noise-Induced Hearing Loss?

Noise-induced hearing loss occurs every day—in both occupational and nonoccupational settings. The crucial questions for prevention are as follows: (1) What can individuals do to protect themselves from NIHL? (2) What role should others, such as educators, employers, or the Government, play in preventing NIHL? (3) What general strategies should be employed to prevent NIHL? Answers to these questions have long been known, but solutions have not been effectively implemented in many cases. As a result, many people have needlessly suffered hearing loss.

Individual Protection Strategies

Hearing conservation must begin by providing each individual with basic information. NIHL is insidious, permanent, and irreparable, causing communication interference that can substantially affect the quality of life. Ringing in the ears and muffling of sounds after sound exposure are indicators of potential hazard. Dangerous sound exposures can cause significant damage without pain, and hearing aids do not restore normal hearing. Individuals should become aware of loud noise situations and avoid them if possible or properly use hearing protection. It is important to recognize that both the level of the noise and its duration (i.e., exposure) contribute to the overall risk. Certain noises, such as explosions, may cause immediate permanent damage.

Many sources, such as guns, power tools, chain saws, small airplanes, farm vehicles, firecrackers, some types of toys, and some medical and dental instruments may produce dangerous exposures. Music concerts, car and motorcycle races, and other spectator events often produce sound levels that warrant hearing protection. Similarly, some stereo headphones and loudspeakers are capable of producing hazardous exposures. Parents should exercise special care in supervising the use of personal headset listening devices, and adults and children alike should learn to operate them at safe volume settings

Nonoccupational Strategies

Hearing loss from nonoccupational noise is common, but public awareness of the hazard is low. Educational programs should be targeted toward children, parents, hobby groups, public role models, and professionals in influential positions such as teachers, physicians, audiologists and other health care professionals, engineers, architects, and legislators. In particular, primary health care physicians and educators who deal with young people should be targeted through their professional organizations. Consumers need guidance and product noise labeling to assist them in purchasing quieter devices and in implementing exposure reduction strategies. The public should be made aware of the availability of affordable, effective hearing protectors (ear plugs, ear muffs, and canal caps). Hearing protection manufacturers should supply comprehensive instructions concerning proper protector use and also be encouraged to increase device availability to the public sector. Newborn nurseries, including neonatal intensive care units, should be made quieter. Medical and dental personnel should be trained to educate their patients about NIHL.

Individuals with significant noise exposure need counseling. Basic audiometric evaluations should be widely available. The goal is to detect early noise-induced damage and interrupt its progression before hearing thresholds exceed the normal range.

Occupational Strategies

Hearing conservation programs for occupational settings must include the following interactive components: sound surveys to assess the degree of hazardous noise exposure, engineering and administrative noise controls to reduce exposures, education to inform at-risk individuals why and how to prevent hearing loss, hearing protection devices (earplugs, earmuffs, and canal caps) to reduce the sound reaching the ear, and audiometric evaluations to detect hearing changes. Governmental regulations that currently apply to most noisy industries should be revised to encompass all industries and all employees, strengthened in certain requirements, and strictly enforced with more inspections and more severe penalties for violations.

Many existing hearing conservation programs remain ineffective due to poor organization and inadequately trained program staff. Senior management must use available noise controls, purchase quieter equipment, and incorporate noise reduction in planning new facilities. Noise exposures must be measured accurately and the degree of hazard communicated to employees. Hearing protection devices must be available that are comfortable, practical for the demands of work tasks, and provide adequate attenuation. Labeled ratings of hearing protector attenuation must be more realistic so that the degree of protection achieved in the workplace can be properly estimated. Each employee must be individually fitted with protectors and trained in their correct use and care. Employees need feedback about their audiometric monitoring results annually.

Employers need to monitor program effectiveness by using appropriate techniques for analysis of group audiometric data. By detecting problem areas, managers can prioritize resource allocations and modify company policies to achieve effectiveness. Potential benefits include reduced costs for worker's compensation, enhanced worker morale, reduced absenteeism, fewer accidents, and greater productivity. Enactment of uniform regulations for awarding worker's compensation for occupational hearing loss would stimulate employers' interest in achieving effective hearing conservation programs. Equitable criteria for compensability should be developed based on scientific investigations of the difficulties in communication and other aspects of auditory function encountered in everyday life by persons with differing degrees of NIHL.

General Strategies

Both nonoccupational and occupational NIHL could be reduced by implementing broader preventive efforts. Labeling of consumer product noise emission levels should be enforced according to existing regulations. Incentives for manufacturers to design quieter industrial equipment and consumer goods are needed along with regulations governing the maximum emission levels of certain consumer products, such as power tools. Reestablishment of a Federal agency coordinating committee with central responsibility for practical solutions to noise issues is essential. Model community ordinances could promote local planning to control environmental noise and, where feasible, noise levels at certain spectator events. High-visibility media campaigns are needed to develop public awareness of the effects of noise on hearing and the means for self-protection. Prevention of NIHL should be part of the health curricula in elementary through high schools. Self-education materials for adults should be readily available.

What Are the Directions for Future Research?

The panel recommends that research be undertaken in two broad categories: (1) Studies that use existing knowledge to prevent NIHL in the immediate future, and; (2) research on basic mechanisms to prevent NIHL in the long-term future.

- Development of rationale and collection of empirical data to evaluate systems for combining sound level and duration to predict NIHL.

- Longitudinal studies to further delineate responses of the ear to noise over time in different groups of people with varying levels of exposure.

- Continued investigation of engineering noise measurement and control techniques, such as acoustic intensity measurement, active noise-cancellation systems, and cost-benefit analyses of noise reduction.

- Development and investigation of hearing protector designs that provide improved wearer comfort, usability, and more natural audition.

- Development of repeatable laboratory procedures that incorporate behavioral tests to yield realistic estimates of hearing protector attenuation performance that are accepted for device labeling purposes.

- Empirical evaluation of the efficacy of hearing conservation programs and the field performance of hearing protection devices in industry.

- Development and validation of evaluation techniques for detection of the following: (a) subtle changes in hearing resulting from noise exposure and (b) early indicators of NIHL.

- Determination of the pathophysiological correlates of TTS and PTS.

- Investigation of the anatomic and physiologic bases of presbycusis and interactive effects with NIHL.

- Investigation of genetic bases for susceptibility to NIHL, using contemporary techniques, including molecular biology.

- Further studies of drugs (e.g., vasodilating agents) and other pre-exposure conditions (e.g., activation of efferent systems or exposure to "conditioning" noise) that have been suggested in preliminary reports to protect the inner ear from NIHL and elucidation of the underlying mechanisms.

- Investigation into the physiologic mechanisms underlying the synergistic effects of certain drugs and noise exposure in animal models.

Conclusions and Recommendations

- Sounds of sufficient intensity and duration will damage the ear and result in temporary or permanent hearing loss at any age.

- NIHL is characterized by specific anatomic and physiologic changes in the inner ear.

- Sounds with levels less than 75 dB(A), even after long exposures, are unlikely to cause permanent hearing loss.

- Sounds with levels above 85 dB(A) with exposures of 8 hours per day will produce permanent hearing loss after many years.

- There is a broad range of individual differences among people in the amount of hearing loss each suffers as a result of identical exposures.

- Current scientific knowledge is inadequate to predict that any particular individual will be safe when exposed to a hazardous noise.

- Because sources of potentially hazardous sound are present in both occupational and nonoccupational settings, personal hearing protection should be used when hazardous exposures are unavoidable.

- Vigorous enforcement of existing regulations, particularly for the workplace and consumer product labeling, would significantly reduce the risk of workplace NIHL. Regulations should be broadened to encompass all employees with hazardous noise exposures.

- Application of existing technologies for source noise control, especially in the manufacture of new equipment and construction of new facilities, would significantly reduce sound levels at the ear.

- In addition to existing hearing conservation programs, a comprehensive program of education regarding the causes and prevention of NIHL should be developed and disseminated, with specific attention directed toward educating school-age children.

Chapter 14

Questions and Answers about Noise and Hearing Loss

Does noise cause hearing loss?

Yes. If you experience any or all of the following:

- a one-time exposure to extremely loud noise,
- repeated or long exposure to loud noise,
- extended exposure to moderate noise,

you have been subjected to noise that can damage your hearing. Noise-induced hearing loss is usually gradual and painless, but, unfortunately, permanent.

How does noise cause hearing loss?

Your ear receives sound waves and sends them through a delicately balanced system to the brain. Part of this remarkable system is a chamber in the inner ear filled with fluid and lined with thousands of tiny hair cells. The hair cells signal the auditory nerve to send electrical impulses to the brain. The brain interprets these impulses as sound.

When you are exposed to loud or prolonged noise, the hair cells are damaged and the transmission of sound is permanently altered.

Am I exposed to damaging noise?

Today, over 20 million people in the United States are exposed to environmental noise that can damage hearing. If you use stereo headsets, operate power tools for yard work, have a long daily commute in heavy traffic, or use a number of household appliances, you, too, may be exposed to potentially damaging noise.

Many people are exposed to hazardous noise levels at work, including: fire fighters, military personnel, disc jockeys, construction workers, farmers, industrial arts teachers, computer operators, factory workers, as well as cab, truck, and bus drivers, to name a few.

Exposure to damaging noise does not come only from the workplace. Recreational activities such as hunting, motorboating, waterskiing, snowmobiling, motorcycling, and exposure to rock music or the use of stereo headsets, also expose you to hazardous noise.

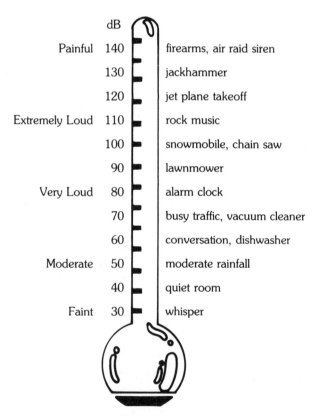

	dB	
Painful	140	firearms, air raid siren
	130	jackhammer
	120	jet plane takeoff
Extremely Loud	110	rock music
	100	snowmobile, chain saw
	90	lawnmower
Very Loud	80	alarm clock
	70	busy traffic, vacuum cleaner
	60	conversation, dishwasher
Moderate	50	moderate rainfall
	40	quiet room
Faint	30	whisper

Figure 14.1. Noise thermometer.

What is a dangerous noise level?

Both the amount of noise and the length of time, you are exposed to the noise determine its ability to damage your hearing.

Noise levels are measured in decibels (dB). The higher the decibel level, the louder the noise. Sounds louder than 80 decibels are considered potentially hazardous. The noise "thermometer" (Figure 14.1) gives an idea of average decibel levels for everyday sounds around you.

What are warning signs that noises around me are too loud?

If you experience any of the following signs, the noises around you are too loud:

- You have to raise your voice to be heard.
- You can't hear someone less than two feet away from you.
- Speech around you sounds muffled or dull after leaving a noisy area.
- You have pain or ringing in your ears after exposure to noise.

What can I do to protect myself?

First, avoid loud noise whenever possible. If you cannot avoid exposure to noise:

- Wear hearing protectors: ear plugs or earmuffs (you can probably get them from your drug store, hardware, or sporting goods store). Using cotton in your ears does not work. When using hearing protectors, you can still hear and understand voices and other sounds with ease.

- Have your hearing tested by an audiologist.

- Limit periods of exposure to noise; for example, if you are at a rock concert, walk out for a while—give your ears a break.

- Be aware of the noise in your environment and take control of it when you can. Your county may have a local noise ordinance. Find out what you can do in your community to advocate for quiet. For example, some high schools have set a decibel limit for the music played at school dances to protect the student's hearing. An audiologist can measure sound levels at a specific location and make recommendations for keeping sound levels safe.

What resources are available to me if I think I have a hearing problem?

For an evaluation of hearing abilities, an audiologist should be contacted. When hearing loss is the result of current disease, or if a medical problem is suspected, a physician should be seen. The audiologist you select should hold a Certificate of Clinical Competence (CCC) from the American Speech-Language-Hearing Association (ASHA). In many states a license is also required. For a list of audiologists in your area, contact ASHA, 10801 Rockville Pike, Rockville, MD 20852, 800-638-8255 or 301-897-8682 (Voice or TDD).

Chapter 15

Enjoy, Protect the Best Ears of Your Life

Rock musician Kathy Peck had been playing bass guitar for several years. But when her three-piece band, The Contractions, opened for Duran Duran at the Oakland Coliseum in California in 1984, Peck, then in her mid-20s, heard more than the echo of applause.

"My ears were ringing for days afterward," she remembers. Eventually Peck found she had destroyed 40 percent of her hearing from years of playing loud music.

"I was basically deaf for three years. It was very frustrating, very isolating," Peck says. It took her several years to learn to manage her handicap with hearing aids and lip reading.

"People in the music industry told me not to let anyone know about my condition because they wouldn't listen to my records or anything," she says. "People were afraid, like I had leprosy."

Hearing Loss Is Increasing Among Young People

Peck is just one of 23.3 million Americans who have hearing loss, according to a 1990 survey by the National Center for Heath Statistics. About 1.3 million of them are 18 or younger. Although statistics are lacking, anecdotal evidence suggests more young people are losing their hearing today than ever before.

DHHS Publication Number (FDA)92-1195. Some subheads that did not originally appear in this document have been added to assist the reader.

According to the National Institutes of Health, one-third of all hearing loss cases stem at least in part from the loud noises of modern life: power lawn mowers, jet engines, city traffic, loud appliances, rock music, stereo headsets.

Some 59 million Americans are exposed to urban traffic noise, 16 million to aircraft noise, and 3.1 million to highway noise, according to the U.S. Environmental Protection Agency.

Loud noises destroy the tiny hair cells in the inner ear (see Figure 15.1) that signal the auditory nerve to send sound messages to the brain. Once those cells die, they never grow back.

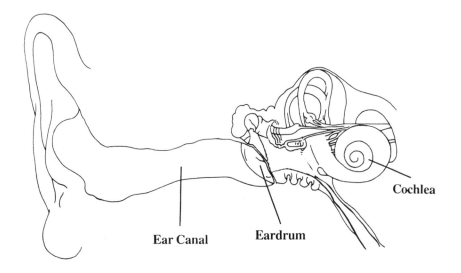

Figure 15.1. *Inside the Ear: Loud noise can damage almost any internal structure of the ear, shown above. Most noise-induced hearing loss occurs in the hair cells inside the cochlea, which signal sound impulses to the brain. Earplugs or muffs that block the ear canal can muffle loud noises and help preserve hearing.*

The result is a kind of deafness called "sensorineural hearing loss." This affects both volume and clarity, first at high pitches, then later at lower pitches where speech is heard.

Noise may also cause "tinnitus," a ringing in the ears. Besides being a constant annoyance, tinnitus often signals impending hearing loss. Although both conditions are permanent and incurable, they can be improved with hearing aids.

FDA regulates those devices, as well as equipment to diagnose hearing loss. But the agency hopes you choose an easier path to better hearing—protecting your ears while they're young.

"One of the things that bothers me is that [young people] are aging their ears before their chronological time," says audiologist David Lipscomb, who has researched hearing loss in students at the University of Tennessee.

In the fall of 1969, he tested the hearing of entering freshmen and found about 60 percent of them had hearing loss. Fourteen percent of the young men tested had hearing similar to the average 65-year-old. By comparison, only 3.8 percent of sixth-graders had hearing loss, suggesting that something—probably noise—was damaging hearing during the teen years.

"We know that the average 70-year-old will have some impairment from aging," says Lipscomb. "But for young people [exposed to loud noises], the aging process is speeded up. They're blowing their spare tires."

Modern Life: A Pain in the Ear

In the absence of loud noises, hearing doesn't appear to deteriorate much with age.

For example, deep in the Sudan bush, a primitive tribe lives in a quiet environment, surrounded by swamps and the White Nile River. A study done in the early 1960s found that people of any age in the tribe had hearing superior to that of a comparison group of American farmers. Furthermore, the old people heard as well as the young.

Modern life is much harder on hearing. According to the American Speech-Language-Hearing Association (ASHA), an estimated 20 million Americans are regularly exposed to noise at dangerous levels.

Noise is measured in decibels. Anything 80 decibels or louder, such as a loud buzzer alarm clock, is potentially dangerous, according to ASHA. The higher the decibel, the louder the noise. The accompanying noise scale shows the loudness of common sounds.

The louder the noise, the shorter the time it takes to hurt your hearing. Your ears can endure 90 decibels of noise, such as a lawn mower, for about eight hours before damage occurs. For every 5 decibels above that, it takes only half as much time for damage to begin.

A noise at 95 decibels will hurt your ears in four hours. An arcade full of video games could cause damage in two hours. The average rock concert or stereo headset set at full blast (about 110 decibels) could damage your ears in a half hour. Like Peck, most people don't notice they've lost any hearing until they develop tinnitus or they can't understand speech.

But the damage begins long before that. An individual concert, hunting trip, lawn mower, or power tool may not hurt your ears at the time, but added together over the years, they can be disastrous.

Have you ever walked away from a construction site or loud concert and everything sounds as if you're under water? Or you feel a fullness or buzzing in your ears?

That's called a "temporary threshold shift." Although it goes away, it's a signal that you've damaged some hair cells in your inner ear. The cells will probably heal, but additional damage may permanently destroy them.

Want Better Hearing? Shhhh!

The best way to safeguard your hearing is to avoid loud noises as much as possible.

How do you know if you're in danger? Lipscomb gives four clues:

- if your ears are ringing
- if things sound muffled, as if you're in a barrel
- if sounds are distorted, as if they're coming through a poor-quality speaker
- if you find yourself shouting to communicate.

The rule of thumb for listening to music is to keep it low enough so that you can hear other sounds above the tunes. If you're listening to a Walkman portable radio or similar headset, no one else should be able to hear your music.

When loud noise can't be avoided—such as when you're mowing the lawn, working in shop class, or attending a concert—guard your ears with hearing protection devices.

Stuffing cotton in your ears will not do the trick. Good hearing protection is available with a number of devices, the most common and least expensive of which are earplugs.

Earplugs are available at most drug, hardware, music, and sporting goods stores, and custom-made plugs are available through an audiologist.

Made of foam rubber or plastic, earplugs come with a noise reduction rating on the label established by the Environmental Protection Agency.

The Occupational Safety and Health Administration, which regulates hearing safety in the workplace, recommends using earplugs with a rating twice as strong as you need to ensure protection.

For instance, if you're going to be mowing the lawn (90 decibels), you'd need to reduce the noise by about 15 decibels to be in a safe range, so buy earplugs with a 30-decibel rating.

For a rock concert (110 decibels), you'd need 45-decibel plugs. These are usually only available from an audiologist. If you can't get them, buy the strongest rating available in a drugstore (about 30 decibels). The most important thing is that you wear something to block out the sound.

"Most people say that hearing protection devices distort sound," says John Steelnack, an industrial hygienist with OSHA. "They really don't," he says. "They just reduce the intensity."

For those who have already suffered damage, hearing aids can help, but they still cannot restore normal hearing.

People are rarely as satisfied with their hearing aids as with their eyeglasses because many older hearing aids can't clarify sounds. Newer hearing aids are better at picking up certain sound frequencies, screening out much unwanted background noise.

"Basically, a hearing aid is an audio amplifier that provides amplification in the frequency range where the patient has the greatest hearing loss," says Harry Sauberman, chief of the ear, nose and throat division at FDA's Office of Device Evaluation.

"One of the concerns about hearing aids is that many of them amplify ambient [background] noise. That may be the reason people leave them on the dresser. They just don't find them desirable."

Sound Advice

Rock musician Peck cherishes what's left of her hearing. To educate others about noise-induced hearing loss, she helped establish a nonprofit organization called HEAR, for Hearing Education and Awareness for Rockers, with the Haight-Ashbury Free Medical Clinic in San Francisco.

HEAR has garnered a lot of publicity and support in the music industry, including a $10,000 donation from musician Pete Townsend of The Who, who also has hearing loss.

HEAR sponsors free hearing screening in the San Francisco Bay area and has a 24-hour hot line for information about noise-induced hearing loss. For more information, write HEAR at P.O. Box 460847, San Francisco, CA 94146.

For a free pair of 30-decibel earplugs, write to the "Hearing Is Priceless" Program of the House Ear Institute, 2100 West 3rd St., Fifth Floor, Los Angeles, CA 90057.

While Peck doesn't play in a band anymore, she is still a rock music fan. However, now when she goes to concerts, she wears custom-made earplugs. Some are decorated with dangling earring-like ornaments.

She encourages other music fans to take precautions as well. "We're not against music, we're not anti-rock 'n' roll," says Peck. "I just want them to protect their hearing."

—by Rebecca D. Williams

Rebecca D. Williams is a staff writer for FDA Consumer.

Chapter 16

Questions and Answers about Tinnitus

What is tinnitus?

Tinnitus is the subjective experience of hearing noises when there are no external sounds present. Tinnitus is usually described as a ringing, buzzing, roaring, whistling, chirping, whooshing, or hissing noise. It may be heard in one or both ears, may be intermittent or continuous, and the severity (or loudness) may fluctuate.

The word tinnitus comes from the Latin word *tinnire*, which means "to ring or tinkle like a bell."

According to the American Tinnitus Association, 50 million Americans experience tinnitus, and 12 million people have symptoms severe enough to affect their everyday life. Those with severe tinnitus have described the noises as a sharp ringing, a constant din, or cymbals crashing. Some have even likened their tinnitus to an internal siren.

What causes tinnitus?

Tinnitus is not a disease; it is a symptom of an underlying condition. It can arise from a variety of problems of the ear canal, middle ear, inner ear, or the hearing nerve, as well as from other parts of the body.

NICD Publication (547) 8/92-3C 071.

Tinnitus can be caused by something as simple as wax or a foreign body in the ear canal, or by a rare tumor on the hearing nerve. People with Ménière's disease, thought to be caused by an excess of a fluid normally present in the inner ear, experience hearing loss, dizziness, and tinnitus. Otosclerosis, a disease in which the bones in the middle ear are immobilized by bony growth, can also cause tinnitus.

High doses of certain medications, including aspirin and some antibiotics, hypertension (high blood pressure), Temporomandibular Joint Dysfunction (TMJ), and head trauma can all cause tinnitus.

One of the most common causes of tinnitus is exposure to loud sounds such as very loud music, power tools, or firearms used for hunting or target shooting. People often report tinnitus and slight hearing loss following excessive noise exposure. This is usually temporary at first; however, repeated exposure can cause permanent hearing loss and persistent tinnitus. The exact mechanism of tinnitus is yet to be discovered. Advancing age and the accumulative effects of the noisy world in which we live may slowly damage the tiny hair cells in the inner ear and result in a gradual onset of tinnitus.

Is there a connection between tinnitus and hearing loss?

Yes. Although some people with normal hearing experience tinnitus, most people who have tinnitus also have some degree of hearing loss. A plug of wax in the ear, advancing age, certain medications, and noise exposure can all affect a person's hearing as well as cause tinnitus.

What is the treatment for tinnitus?

People with tinnitus should see their physician for a physical examination and an otolaryngologist (an ear, nose, and throat doctor) for an ear exam. They should also have their hearing tested by an audiologist, even if hearing loss is not suspected. Results of audiological tests often help determine what may be causing the tinnitus.

There is no medical or surgical treatment specifically for tinnitus. However, if the possible cause of the tinnitus can be determined, then the treatment of that condition or disease may alleviate the accompanying symptom of tinnitus. For example, surgery to correct a hearing loss associated with otosclerosis may also provide relief from the tinnitus. Many physicians prescribe various drugs in the hope of relieving the tinnitus, and/or tinnitus-associated depression or anxiety.

For many cases of tinnitus, such as those thought to be caused by excessive noise exposure or advancing age, there is no medical or surgical treatment. This does not mean the person with tinnitus must suffer without help. After the examination by the otolaryngologist and the audiological evaluation, the audiologist can describe various methods to help minimize the tinnitus. What works often varies from person to person.

What can be done to relieve tinnitus?

If the person with tinnitus also has a hearing loss, the audiologist may recommend a hearing aid. Many people find that wearing hearing aids reduces or eliminates their tinnitus.

Tinnitus is often worse when the environment is quiet such as when trying to fall sleep. Many people with tinnitus find that listening to a noise generated by something they can control is preferable to listening to their tinnitus. A radio playing soft, pleasant music or even tuned to the "white" noise between stations may provide relief.

Custom tinnitus masking is similar except that the masking sounds are tailored to the individual's particular needs and delivered at ear level with devices that look like hearing aids. They are either called maskers, if they provide only a masking noise, or tinnitus instruments, if they provide amplification and a masking noise. These devices are fitted by audiologists and dispensed in the same way as hearing aids. Many people report that their tinnitus becomes worse in times of tension or stress. Some people use biofeedback to achieve deep relaxation and focus their attention away from the tinnitus. Stress management is also useful for some people who have tinnitus.

Resources

The following list of selected readings and resources will help readers who want more information on the topic or who are trying to locate professionals who are knowledgeable about tinnitus.

Books

Hallam, Richard. *Living with Tinnitus: Dealing with the Ringing in Your Ears*. Wellingborough, England: Thorsons Publishers Limited, 1989. Living With Tinnitus is written by a clinical psychologist and describes ways in which people can learn to tolerate their tinnitus.

Slater, R. and M. Terry. *Tinnitus: A Guide for Sufferers and Professionals*. Dobbs Ferry, NY: Sheridan House. Inc., 1989. A comprehensive text written for both the person with tinnitus and the professional.

Vernon, J. "Tinnitus." In *Gallaudet Encyclopedia of Deaf People and Deafness*. Vol. 3. Edited by J. V. Van Cleve. New York: McGraw-Hill, 1987. Discusses causes and evaluation of tinnitus and describes various approaches to provide relief

Articles

Briner, W. The treatment of tinnitus or... "Can They Do Anything about All Those Crickets in My Head?" *SHHH Journal*, (July/August 1991): 10-12. Describes various treatments professionals may recommend to help lessen tinnitus.

Brown, S.C. *Older Americans and Tinnitus: A Demographic Study and Chartbook*. Monograph Series A, No. 2. Washington, DC: Gallaudet University, Center for Assessment and Demographic Studies, Gallaudet Research Institute, 1990. A 97-page report of studies estimating the prevalence of tinnitus among older Americans.

Delaney, L. "Silence Ringing Ears." *Prevention* (April 1992): 50-54, 122-125. Provides a comprehensive overview of causes of tinnitus and treatments a physician may recommend. The author discusses techniques such as stress reduction and biofeedback which some people use to control their tinnitus. Includes a description of hearing aids and tinnitus maskers.

Gold, V. "Hearing Things." *The Washingtonian*, (February 1991): 37-38. Describes the author's experiences of tinnitus and hearing loss and how he sought help.

Modeland, V. "When Bells Are Ringing (But There Aren't Any Bells)." *FDA Consumer* (April 1989): 9-12. Provides an overview of tinnitus and some of its treatments.

The Hearing Journal, vol. 42, no. 11 (1989). The entire issue focuses on tinnitus, including some technical articles exploring possible causes and treatment of tinnitus, as well as several less technical reviews. Provides background on the American Tinnitus Association, and information on tinnitus maskers.

Consumer and Professional Organizations

American Academy of Otolaryngology—Head and Neck Surgery, Inc.
One Prince Street
Alexandria,VA 22314
(703) 836 4 Voice

A professional organization that publishes an informative and easy-to-read pamphlet on tinnitus. Provides consumers with referrals to otolaryngologists in their local area.

American Speech-Language-Hearing Association (ASHA)
10801 Rockville Pike
Rockville, MD 20852
(800) 638-TALK Voice/TDD

National organization for speech and hearing professionals. ASHA's Consumer Division increases public awareness and acts as a consumer advocate for persons with hearing, speech, and language impairment. Has consumer information on tinnitus.

American Tinnitus Association (ATA)
P.O. Box 5
Portland, OR 97207
(503) 248-9985 Voice

A consumer organization that provides information and education about tinnitus, including telephone counseling. Sponsors local chapters for support and self-help and provides regional referrals for patients seeking help. ATA maintains a bibliography of approximately 1800 writings relating to tinnitus and publishes *Tinnitus Today*, a quarterly magazine for people who have tinnitus.

Ménière's Network
c/o The Ear Foundation
2000 Church Street
Nashville, TN 37236
(615) 329-7807 Voice/TDD
(800) 545-HEAR Voice/TDD

Assists people with Ménière's Disease through education, a quarterly newsletter, support groups and a telephone network. (Tinnitus is a common symptom of Ménière's Disease.)

National Institute on Deafness and Other Communication Disorders
National Institutes of Health
Building 31, Room 3C-35
9000 Rockville Pike
Bethesda, MD 20892
(301) 496-7243 Voice
(301) 402-0252 TDD

Conducts research and provides information on various aspects of hearing, including tinnitus. NIDCD also supports research on taste, balance, smell, speech, language, and voice.

Self Help for Hard of Hearing People, Inc. (SHHH)
7800 Wisconsin Avenue
Bethesda, MD 20814
(301) 657-2248 Voice
(301) 657-2249 TDD

National support and information group for people with hearing loss. Sponsors local chapters and publishes the bimonthly magazine *SHHH Journal* which often includes articles on tinnitus.

The National Information Center on Deafness wishes to thank Maureen McDonald, M.S., CCC-A, who wrote this paper, and Harriet Kaplan, Ph.D., and Gloria Reich, Ph.D., who reviewed the manuscript.

Chapter 17

Update on Tinnitus from the NIDCD

Tinnitus research is important to the National Institute on Deafness and Other Communication Disorders (NIDCD) because of its devastating effects on so many people. For the person who suffers with tinnitus, the sound is often unremitting and extremely distressing.

Tinnitus is a symptom of diseases and disorders of the auditory system as are hearing loss and dizziness. This is true whether tinnitus is accompanied by hearing loss or not. As far as we know, the majority of disease processes and disorders producing tinnitus affect the inner ear although tinnitus arising from involvement of the central auditory pathways undoubtedly occurs.

The mechanisms of tinnitus are largely unknown. Different mechanisms are probably producing tinnitus in the various diseases and disorders of the auditory system. Because the experiences of the individuals who have tinnitus are so varied, all individuals do not and should not be expected to benefit from a single form of treatment.

Tinnitus can be induced by drugs, noise exposure and head trauma as well as by a multitude of diseases of the middle and inner ears. The more that is known about the auditory system, the closer we will be to prevention, amelioration or eradiciation of tinnitus. Study of the normal processes of hearing and the disordered functions of the auditory system are fundamental to understanding and conquering tinnitus. These studies must include structure and function, molecular biology,

---

This document originally appeared in *Tinnitus Today*. Used by permission.

causation and development of the disease process in the auditory system.

The knowledge we have already gained about ototoxicity, damage to the inner ear caused by drugs, has helped prevent some forms of tinnitus. For example, aspirin toxicity causes tinnitus while simultaneously affecting inner-ear hair cell motility in a way that can be measured noninvasively (for otoacoustic emissions). Other groups of drugs or drugs associated with tinnitus include aminoglycoside antibiotics, antidepressants, antihypertensives, nonsteroidal anti-inflammatory agents (which include salicylates such as aspirin as well as others), ergot and ergotamine derivitives, quinidine, atrophine, chloroquine, and cyclobenzaprine. Additionally, caffeine and nicotine and quinine sensitivity can exacerbate tinnitus.

Aminoglycoside antibiotics are used to treat life-threatening bacterial infections, including tuberculosis. Unfortunately, hearing loss and balance deficits are produced in 3 to 18% of the individuals who receive aminoglycoside antibiotics. It is not the antibiotic itself which is ototoxic but rather one of its metabolites, a breakdown product of chemical reactions that make a drug more easily excreted by the body. Recent preliminary evidence suggests that glutathione therapy reduces the ototoxicity of aminoglycosides without affecting the drugs' antibacterial potency. These findings suggest the first potential therapy to reduce the ototoxicity of aminoglycoside antibiotics and possibly the associated tinnitus.

A major area of interest of the NIDCD is the prevention of noise-induced hearing loss. Damaging noise is the cause of hearing loss in approximately 10 million Americans. It results in a hearing loss that is not reversible by any presently available medical or surgical treatment and is often accompanied by tinnitus. Recent research by NIDCD-supported molecular biologists has suggested that heat shock proteins formed in the inner ear in response to moderate levels of sound may provide some protection against intense sound. One million people suffer head injury in the United States each year. Whiplash, cranial and cervical fractures, concussions, temporomandibular joint (TMJ) dysfunction are examples of physical insults that can result in tinnitus. NIDCD is supporting several projects studying sensory hearing loss and tinnitus caused by head injury including a study of high resolution magnetic resonance imaging techniques of the inner ear damage.

Among the strikingly different diseases and disorders with which tinnitus is associated are hyperacusis, Meniere's disease, familial hyperlipidemia, hypertension, hyperthyroidism, anemia, vascular disorders, musculoskeletal problems and presbycusis—the hearing loss associated with aging. In rare cases, unilateral tinnitus can signal cerebellopontine angle tumors including acoustic neurinomas. Objective tinnitus can be associated with vascular problems, such as a glomus tumor, arteriovenous fistula or carotoid artery narrowing as well as venous narrowing. Many of these causes of tinnitus can be cured by present day treatment.

As with hearing loss and dizziness, we have learned that studying symptoms *per se* will not conquer tinnitus. However, progress on each disease of the auditory system is progress toward the conquest of tinnitus. Furthermore, it is unlikely that the pathophysiology related to tinnitus will be solved by any one finding but will be the result of a very long series of findings. The study of tinnitus *per se* does have value in developing therapies for managing the symptom until the understanding of the underlying disease can be accomplished.

Some of these findings are at hand. Many causes of tinnitus lend themselves to relief now, as for example, by reconstructive surgery for chronic otitis media and otosclerosis. The tinnitus of noise-induced hearing loss often disappears after two or three months of avoidance of noise exposure. Prevention of sensorineural hearing loss by vaccination against maternal rubella, measles, mumps, and Haemophilus influenzae type B meningitis also prevents tinnitus.

The NIDCD has as its mission the support of biomedical and behavioral research and research training in both the normal and disordered processes of human communication including hearing, balance, smell, taste, voice, speech and language.

The dollars granted to any area of research are based on competition. Support is not allocated by subject, but through a rigorous, two-tiered peer review process that is designed to identify the highest quality of research. Scientific quality of the application is the decisive criterion in awarding grant monies in order to ensure that well-designed, excellent research is funded.

All of the grants in the hearing program that are supporting studies of normal and disordered mechanisms of hearing and diseases or disorders of the auditory system relate to tinnitus. The NIDCD provided an estimated $85 million dollars for hearing research in FY

1993. Since the conditions that are known to produce tinnitus affect different levels of the auditory system, including both peripheral and central components, research on virtually any aspect of the auditory system is applicable to some forms of tinnitus.

The NIDCD is collaborating with the Department of Veterans Affairs in the evaluation and development of hearing aid technology designed to meet the individual needs of subgroups of consumers, including those who use hearing aids to mask the ringing, buzzing, or roaring of tinnitus. Also, within the hearing section of the extramural research portfolio, the NIDCD supports several grants and contracts on research and development of cochlear implants, which have been found to suppress tinnitus in profoundly hearing-impaired persons.

Other current research supported by the NIDCD includes projects designed to (1) develop a comprehensive database and an understanding of the phenomena of tinnitus that accompany sensorineural hearing loss; (2) study subjective tinnitus and masking devices; (3) understand the role of calcium imbalance in inducing cochlear-type tinnitus; and (4) study of otoacoustic emissions and cochiear functioning.

The Hearing and Hearing Impairment update of the National Strategic Research Plan was released in January 1994. The original plan disseminated in 1989 and this update identify national research priorities and opportunities. Both of these documents call for additional research in tinnitus.

The NIDCD staff recognizes the need to encourage greater activity in tinnitus-related research. In order to address this need, the NIDCD will hold a Workshop on Tinnitus in FY 1995. The workshop will bring together distinguished investigators in many areas of auditory science including recognized tinnitus experts, to analyze the current state of research in tinnitus. This expert group will be asked to suggest important research strategies that can be implemented immediately as well as to formulate a plan for the long term.

We lack, at the present time, promising therapeutic strategies that merit large scale clinical trials for determination of efficacy. Treatment studies should be based on sound hypotheses. Perhaps strategies of this type will evolve from the NIDCD Tinnitus Workshop.

The NIDCD has developed an infrastructure to further research in hearing and balance. The NIDCD has created an Epidemiology, Statistics and Data System Branch that is currently cooperating with the

National Center on Health Statistics on a supplement that will develop new data on the prevalance of tinnitus, hearing impairment and disorders of balance. The Institute is supporting the National Temporal Bone, Hearing and Balance Pathology Resource Registry to promote the study of the histopathology, histochemistry, immuno-histochemistry and molecular biology of the auditory and vestibular systems. Interested individuals can donate their temporal bones for research by contacting Deafness Research Foundation, 9 East 38th Street, New York, NY 10016. These donations are a legacy of great scientific value. Another aspect of the infrastructure is the Hereditary Hearing Impairment Resource Registry. This registry will contribute to the study of hereditary causes of hearing loss that are often associated with tinnitus by allowing families who want to participate in genetic rescarch to do so.

I am pleased to have had this second opportunity to communicate with the readers of *Tinnitus Today*. I hope I have been able to give you a comprehensive view of the multipronged attack on tinnitus by the NIDCD. I am also pleased that Dr. Gloria E. Reich was able to address our National Deafness and Other Communication Disorders Advisory Board meeting on January 7, 1994 and to bring the concerns of the membership of the American Tinnitus Association to this group. Dr. Reich shared your plans for *ATA Mission 2000* with the National Advisory Board. The NIDCD was delighted to have been included as a participant in ATA's research meeting in Dearborn, Michigan and to have been invited to participate in the Fifth International Tinnitus Seminar, July 12-15, 1995, in Portland, Oregon.

The goals for research expressed by the *ATA Mission 2000* plan include mechanisms underlying tinnitus; diagnosis and assessment of tinnitus; treatment of tinnitus; and epidemiology. The NIDCD endorses the statement that areas of mechanism of tinnitus study should include mechanical, chemical, neurogenic, trauma, degeneration, cognitive/psycho-emotional, metabolic, neoplastic, genetic, plasticity, age and epidemiologic correlations. Indeed the major portion of the hearing research portfolio of the NSCD is addressing these topics. I would like to add to the list a major area of study supported by the NIDCD on the regeneration of sensory hair cells from which may come the solutions to tinnitus for many sufferers.

Funding for tinnitus-related research is limited not by the number of scientists who want to study the auditory system but by the amount of funding for hearing research. The success rate of research applications coming to thc NIDCD for funding was 29% in FY 1993 and is estimated to be 28% in FY 1994.

Each of the approaches that have been mentioned are of urgent interest to scientists who are committed to improving knowledge about tinnitus that incapacitates or disrupts the lives of so many Americans. I look forward to a continuing, creative and cooperative dialogue between the ATA and NlDCD. We need and appreciate your support.

—by James B. Snow, Jr., M.D.
Director of the NIDCD

Chapter 18

The Treatment of Tinnitus or "Can They Do Anything About All Those Crickets in My Head?"

Tinnitus, commonly called "ringing in the ears," is better defined as any internally generated sound that a person experiences. The sounds of tinnitus can range from a low hum to the chirp of crickets to the scream of a steam turbine.

Most people with hearing loss hear some sort of sound in their ears but do not consider it troublesome. For other people, the constant intrusion of tinnitus is a major problem. It can complicate sleep, concentration, conversation, or work. Severe tinnitus has been likened to Chinese water torture: it is not especially severe but you cannot escape it.

Cause

Tinnitus is almost always associated with hearing loss of some sort. People with normal hearing and tinnitus are special cases. Tinnitus will not cause your hearing to worsen and does not mean that you will go deaf. However, if you have hearing loss, tinnitus, or both, you should consult a board-certified otologist. Some cases of tinnitus seem to be caused by temporalmandibular joint disorder (TMJ), allergies, otosclerosis, vascular problems, and, in rare cases, tumors. An otologist can determine if any of these conditions cause your

This article originally appeared in *SHHH Journal*, July/August 1991. Used by permission.

tinnitus and recommend treatment. However, many cases of tinnitus are idiopathic, that is, there appears to be no clear cause. These cases are the most difficult to treat.

Testing

The most important test for tinnitus is an audiogram to determine how much hearing loss you have and if it is equal in both ears. Depending on the results of the hearing test and your medical history, your doctor may order an ABR (auditory brainstem response), CT (computerized tomography) scan, or MRI (magnetic resonance imaging).

The CT scan and MRI are special X-ray-like procedures that give your doctor a detailed view of the head and ear and are not painful. The ABR records electrical activity from the parts of your brain involved in hearing. In addition, many doctors will also order a laboratory analysis of your blood. The results of all these tests will help your doctor determine the cause and possible treatment of your tinnitus. One treatment that all doctors will recommend is that the tinnitus patient protect his ears from loud sounds.

Treatment

Treatments for tinnitus fall into three general categories:

- The presentation of sound into the ear through hearing aids or maskers.
- Manipulation of the body, usually through the use of certain prescription or non-prescription drugs.
- So-called "therapies."

Each of these will be discussed in turn.

Hearing Aids or Maskers

Hearing aids help correct tinnitus by giving your ear something else to do besides generating its own sound. The frequencies in which the patients hearing loss occur are often similar to the sounds of tinnitus. By making up for the loss of sound with a hearing aid, the tinnitus can sometimes be suppressed. However, hearing aids do not work for all tinnitus sufferers. So, if you have a significant hearing loss, you should be evaluated for a hearing aid whether or not it helps your tinnitus.

Masking devices help to "cover up" the tinnitus sound. They substitute the sound of the masker for that of the tinnitus. Some people find relief in escaping the tinnitus sound, even if this means replacing it with another sound. Other people use white noise generators for an effect similar to the masker. Still others who do not wish to purchase a white noise generator set their radio between channels to hear the static.

Manipulation of the Body

Usually, this refers to drugs. There are no drugs approved for the treatment of tinnitus by the Food and Drug Administration. Thus, all drugs used to treat tinnitus are investigational, even if they are being used on a routine basis.

Several drugs are routinely used to treat tinnitus. Some of the more commonly prescribed drugs are the antidepressants. These drugs were developed to treat depression but are also prescribed for tinnitus.

Patients typically respond to a prescription for antidepressants with "Doctor, there is nothing wrong with my mind, it's my ears!"

Doctors know this, but antidepressants address two important points related to tinnitus. One is how a person responds to tinnitus is as important as the tinnitus itself. Tinnitus greatly stresses many patients, who may also experience depression-like symptoms but are not aware of them. Tinnitus leads to stress. Stress leads to more tinnitus, which in turn leads to more stress. . . and the cycle goes on. Antidepressants help break the cycle. Using the same reasoning, some doctors recommend counseling, biofeedback, or some other therapy to help break the cycle of stress and tinnitus.

The second point that antidepressants address is that the brain is one of the organs of hearing and it is involved in tinnitus.

Antidepressants may act directly on the brain to alter the tinnitus sound. If your doctor prescribes antidepressants for your tinnitus, do not be offended. These drugs are safe and work for many people.

Some doctors think that tinnitus may be due to poor circulation in the ear. To improve the circulation, they may prescribe niacin, histamine, Persantine, Trental, or another drug. These drugs increase the flow of blood to the ear and brain and work for some people. Still other doctors think tinnitus is similar to a seizure in the auditory cortex of the brain and have used a number of anticonvulsant to treat tinnitus. Tegrerol, Dilantin, and Klonopin have all met with some success. However most of these drugs have significant side effects, including liver damage, and should be used with great care.

Lidocaine is a local anesthetic that reduces the severity of tinnitus for most people. However, Lidocaine must be given by intravenous infusion. The oral forms of lidocaine, Tocainide, are available but can have toxic effects on the heart. Thus, lidocaine and Tocainide are not routinely prescribed for tinnitus.

Furosemide (Lasix) is a diuretic that some doctors now use. Although it is reported to be effective in many people, it does deplete the body of potassium. Patients must undergo regular blood tests to ensure that their blood potassium level does not become dangerously low.

Medical schools and universities are investigating many drugs and other potential treatments for tinnitus. If you are interested in becoming involved in such studies, ask the department of otolaryngology at your local medical school if anyone in your area is working on tinnitus.

Tinnitus "Therapies"

All tinnitus sufferers should be aware of a third treatment category, advertised as tinnitus "therapies." Because many patients with tinnitus begin to despair and will do nearly anything to find relief, unscrupulous companies and persons find willing buyers for these so-called "therapies." Most have no harmful effects, but they amount to a waste of money. Most of these "therapies" are not monitored or approved by the FDA and it is possible some may be dangerous.

There is no magical cure for tinnitus. Although treatments are available, none is guaranteed and some have harmful side effects. Be suspicious of any treatment for tinnitus that claims to be "all natural," without side effects, based on nutritional substances or vitamins, guaranteed, or available by mail order. If you have a question about a treatment for tinnitus, call your doctor or a reputable researcher on tinnitus before you spend your money. If you come across a drug or device that seems questionable, notify the Food and Drug Administration.

Is There Hope?

Tinnitus can be a disturbing disorder. Science and medicine do not yet have sure answers to the causes and treatment of tinnitus. But some treatments are available. Often, the person with tinnitus must be patient and try the treatments offered by their doctor. In this regard also, a self help group and the American Tinnitus Association can offer helpful advice on how to live with tinnitus and can keep you updated on any new advances. The American Tinnitus Association uses its dues to support research on tinnitus.

The most important thing is not to despair. With the efforts of today's doctors and scientists combined, the quest into the causes and treatment of tinnitus continues.

Chapter 19

The Management of Tinnitus: Medical Intervention

Objective Tinnitus

To understand tinnitus, it is best to recall that there are two forms of this perplexing disorder. In the first instance is the condition known as objective tinnitus. Objective tinnitus is best defined as an acoustic-like sensation which can be confirmed by appropriate tests and examination. For example, vascular abnormalities (bruits) can create awareness of the blood flowing through a restricted orifice of arterial or venal systems. This objective tinnitus is reported as an acoustic sensation which is pulsating in nature and coincidental with the heart beat. Also, chronic spasm of the stapedial or tensor tympani muscle creates a "clicking" sensation to which the person will react negatively. Further, spasm of the muscles of the Eustachian tube can create an objective tinnitus that can be very irritating and frustrating to the person experiencing this condition. Temporal mandibular joint (TMJ) dysfunction can produce a tinnitus that is bothersome to the patient.

Fortunately, most objective tinnitus conditions can be treated effectively with appropriate medical, surgical or therapeutic management. For these reasons, objective tinnitus does not constitute a major problem and is of less concern, relative to the frequency of occurrence. Obviously, if the hearing health professional can differentiate between

This article originally appeared in *Audecibel* (Jan/Feb/March 1994). Used by permission.

objective and subjective tinnitus, an appropriate referral can be made and proper counseling or care given.

Subjective Tinnitus

Subjective tinnitus can best be defined as an apparent acoustic sensation for which there is no external cause. That is, the person hears the tinnitus but it can not be heard by others or objectively assessed by existing instrumentation. Subjective tinnitus has been described in many ways.

To some it is a high pitched ringing. To others it is a persistent roar that permeates the very soul of the individual. For many it is a cacophony of sounds. Still others describe their experience as an exposure to music-like sounds that make their presence known 24 hours a day. Some complain that they hear a hissing sound, while others state their tinnitus sounds more like the constant chirping of crickets.

The sensation may be bilateral or unilateral. Several patients will tell you that their tinnitus is louder in one ear than the other. For some, the presence of this subjective tinnitus is intolerable and they would go to any extreme to rid themselves of its constant and irritating presence. Others acknowledge its presence but are not bothered by it and proceed in carrying out their normal daily activities of living without appreciable difficulty. Unfortunately, there are those few who have been so troubled by tinnitus that they have paid the ultimate price—suicide.

Relative to subjective tinnitus, we do know some of the conditions that cause it. For example, noise exposure, various ear pathologies, physical trauma or whiplash injury, excessive use of aspirin, temporal mandibular joint dysfunction and arninoglycocides are thought to be among the rather common causes of tinnitus. For many with tinnitus, the cause is unknown but the symptoms exist, are unrelenting and present a significant problem.

Essentially, two major modes of treatment have emerged over the past several years. The first part of this two-part article will concentrate on the medical model. This is not an exhaustive review of medical intervention but rather an attempt to emphasize some related methods of treatment.

The Medical Model

This model suggests that control of tinnitus (the apparent absence or reduction in subjective loudness) can be achieved through the administration of drugs, application of direct electrical stimulation of the cochlear substance, or surgical procedures which destroy the functional contributions of the ear by sectioning the cochlear branch of the VIII nerve. Sectioning of the VIII nerve for controlling tinnitus is not without considerable risk.

Although procedures based on medical models have had some success in ameliorating the person's response to the presence of tinnitus, none has been sufficiently compelling to gain universal acceptance by the clinician. However, let us examine in somewhat more detail treatment procedures based on medical intervention.

Drug Therapy

Intravenous Lidocaine: This is a local anesthetic that alters central nervous system function and is used frequently in treating those patients having intractable pain. The drug is administered locally and appears to be of limited benefit to the tinnitus sufferer. Its effect is short lived and it is necessary to administer the drug intravenously. Because of these two factors, Lidocaine is not used very often to treat subjective tinnitus. There was a chemical analog of Lidocaine, Tocanide, developed that could be taken orally. However, subsequent controlled studies have revealed that Tocanide provided very limited benefit to those with tinnitus.

Tegretol: This drug is a carbamazephine derivative and its primary use is for the treatment of those with epilepsy, in that it has been demonstrated to have anticonvulsant properties. It is important to remember that most pharmacologists stress that Tegretol is not a simple medication and should not be considered as a proper method of treatment for the relief of minor aches and pains. Somewhat by chance, Tegretol was found to have some positive effect on reducing the apparent loudness of subjective tinnitus. However, this drug must be administered with close medical supervision; especially the monitoring of blood levels. Some of the more dire side effects from the use of Tegretol include aplastic anemia, agranulocytosis (an acute disease characterized by leukopenia, with ulcerative lesions of the throat and other mucous membranes), thrombocytopenia (causing aplastic anemia and hemorrhaging), and leukopenia (a reduction of the number of leukocytes in the blood).

Mysoline: Here, again, this drug is intended for the management of patients with focal epileptic seizures, grand mal, or phychomotor seizures. It does not produce the side effects as does Tegretol, but the physician and the clinician must be aware of the possibility of nausea, anorexia, vomiting, fatigue, hyperirritability, emotional disturbances, sexual impotency, diplopia, nystagmus and drowsiness. Its effect on tinnitus is similar in nature to that of Tegretol. Again, close monitoring of the patient is most important to avoid deleterious side effects.

In general, there is no significant body of evidence to demonstrate the consistent value of either Mysoline or Tegretol. Although the initial indications suggested a positive correlation between these drugs and reduction of tinnitus, later placebo-controlled, double blind studies indicated that neither drug was effective for most. The assumption, of course, was that these anticonvulsant drugs had some effect on neuronal activity of the central auditory system thought to be hyperactive.

Xanax: A recently completed study (Johnson, et. al. 1992) at the Oregon Hearing Research Center investigated Xanax (Alprazolam) as a possible treatment for subjective tinnitus. Xanax is an anti-anxiety drug that has been used successfully for those individuals suffering from depressional episodes. Xanax is a dependent drug and must be prescribed and controlled by the physician. In the Oregon study of Xanax, forty adult patients participated in a double blind experiment. Seventeen of 20 patients in the experimental group (Xanax) and 19 of 20 patients in the placebo (lactose) group completed the study. Of the 17 patients receiving Xanax, 13 (76%) had a reduction in the loudness of their tinnitus when measurements were made using both a tinnitus synthesizer and a visual analog scale. Only one of the 19 patients who received the placebo showed any improvement in the loudness of their tinnitus. No changes were observed in the audiometric data or in tinnitus masking levels for either group. Individuals differed with regard to the dosage required to achieve benefit from the alprazolam and the side effects were minimal for this 12-week study.

Furosemide: Dobie (1992) of the Department of Otolaryngology –Head and Neck Surgery, the University of Texas Health Science Center in San Antonio Texas, first reported his findings on the clinical effects of Furosemide (Lasix). Twenty subjects with subjective tinnitus were involved initially in the study. The mean duration of tinnitus among the experimental group was about 11 years. Each subject was given 80 mg. b.i.d. for the first two weeks. The dosage was increased to 40 mg. t.i.d. for the third and fourth weeks and then to 40 mg. q.i.d. for the fifth and sixth weeks. Several tinnitus scales were used in rating any change in the subjective loudness of the tinnitus during the course of the study.

Of the twenty subjects starting the study, only 12 finished the full course of Furosemide. Only 4 patients of the final 12 answered yes to a global satisfaction question: "Has the drug helped you in any way?" However, two of these mentioned benefits unrelated to tinnitus, (perceived improvement of hearing in one case, and reduction of edema in another). Only 2 of the 12 patients answered yes to a second global question, "Is your tinnitus improved?" It would appear that, although there were some positive statements regarding the benefit of furosemide, the results did not strongly support the value of this drug in reducing or eliminating subjective tinnitus. It was interesting to note that the greatest benefit seemed to be achieved by those who had tinnitus for he shortest period of time.

Guth, et. al. (1991), stated that the clinical administration of Furosemide may indicate that tinnitus is of a peripheral origin if its loudness is reduced. If, on the other hand, Furosemide does not alter the patient's perception of tinnitus, then tinnitus is of a central origin, and Xanax may be the drug of choice.

Dr. Robert Brummet of the Oregon Hearing Research Center states that, *"Because we do not understand the mechanisms by which tinnitus is produced, it is impossible to rationally select a drug that should control tinnitus. However, because so many people are taking a wide variety of drugs for many different reasons, it has been possible to capitalize on some people's spontaneous reports that their tinnitus is relieved when they take certain drugs. These serendipitous discoveries have led to the current armamentarium of drug therapy for tinnitus. At best, though, the current state of knowledge about drug therapy for tinnitus is woefully inadequate. (The Hearing Journal,* November 1988, pp. 34-37.)

According to tinnitus specialist Dr. Robert Johnson (personal communication) there are, nonetheless, those investigators who feel that if a more permanent relief is found for tinnitus patients, it most likely will be in the area of drug therapy. In order to achieve this treatment goal, much more research as needed, using a variety of drugs.

Although drug therapy is still used in the treatment of the tinnitus patient, many practitioners prefer other modalities that do not pose the same degree of compromise and uncertainty as do most drugs.

Direct Electrical Stimulation

The application of an electric stimulus to the ear is not of recent origin. As early as 1800, Volta made the first battery consisting of some 30 separate plates (silver and zinc). Although he did not specifically experiment with relieving tinnitus, it is recorded that attempts to apply a direct current to the ear resulted in an acoustic sensation that was "altogether disagreeable." Shortly thereafter, Grapengiesse applied a direct electrical stimulus to each ear. Although he was hoping to develop a cure or treatment for deafness, he did report the effects of direct current on tinnitus. He simply maintained that some patients responded positively to the stimulus and others did not. He reported, however, that in deaf ears where there was no tinnitus, electrical stimulation produced it. In those deaf ears where there was tinnitus, direct current would often suppress it.

The first use of an alternating current developed by Faraday was that of Duchenne de Boulogne in 1855. He claimed to have cured 8 out of 10 patients through the use of electrical stimulation. What he meant by cure is open to considerable speculation, in view of recent investigations using more sophisticated methods of stimulus control and response assessment.

Based on experiments with cochlear implant devices, it was discovered that for some people, electrical stimulation of neural tissue within the cochlea had an apparent positive effect on eliminating or reducing subjective tinnitus, as long as the stimulus was present. However, some causes of residual inhibition have been reported following electrical stimulation. For example, House (1990) reported the results of transtympanic electrical stimulation on 125 patients with severe tinnitus. A 60 Hz and 16000 Hz current stimulated the promontory. The

160

stimulation time was 20 minutes. Some 20% of the patients stimulated reported some lessening of their tinnitus.

One should point out that success of this magnitude is not statistically significant. Chouard (1982) reported that many of his cochlear implant patients with tinnitus experienced noticeable relief when using the implant device. Again, House, et. al. (1982) reported that about 50% of his implanted patients had some relief from their ongoing tinnitus. It should be noted that 8% of his implanted patients experienced a worsening of their tinnitus while using the implant.

Through the years, various forms of electrical stimulation have been investigated. As with some other forms of treatment, direct electrical stimulation is not without risk. That is, the length, magnitude, and type of electrical stimulus employed will determine the adverse affects on neural and other structures within the cochlea.

In general, studies have demonstrated that the most effective electrical stimulus for the relief of tinnitus is a positive phase direct current. Recall, however, that sinusoidal and bipolar pulses have had positive effects on the reduction of tinnitus for some people. Studies have indicated that the point of electrical stimulation, i.e. extra or intra-tympanic sites, will determine what effect, if any, it has on the elimination or reduction of ongoing, subjective tinnitus. It would appear that the closer the stimulating electrode is to the neural structures of the cochlea the more positive the effect, if indeed there is any alteration of the tinnitus sensation at all. Although there may be significant promise relative to effective management of subjective tinnitus, there is not sufficient data to warrant a great deal of clinical optimism at this time.

Summary

It has been the purpose of the first part of this article to inform the hearing health professional of the complexity of subjective tinnitus. It is not a simple human disorder that is amenable to an "easy fix." Neither has it been the intent of this article to suggest that the hearing aid specialist become involved in some type of management involving the medical model. However, it is important to realize that medical management can be a very significant contribution to the treatment of tinnitus. There is no common consensus as to the causes or cures of tinnitus. There is no single treatment modality, medical or non medical, which has proven sufficiently compelling to have been embraced by all who work with the tinnitus sufferer. In Part II, the role of the hearing health professional in the management of the patient with subjective tinnitus will be stressed.

There is no doubt that the hearing aid specialists can play a very important role in the treatment of tinnitus. However, it is equally as important for the specialist to realize that it is not a simple matter of recommending a hearing aid or a masker device. The management strategy used is of utmost importance, if the individual is to realize lasting benefit. These issues will be discussed in Part II [see Chapter 20].

References

Chouard H. Comments Made at the Symposium of Artificial Auditory Stimulation, Erlangen, September, 1982.

"Cochlear Implants: Progress in Perspective." *Annals of Oto. Rhino and Laryn.* Vol 94, No. 124. W. F. House and K. I. Berliner, ed.

Dobie, R. A. "Furosmide Open Trial for Treatment of Tinnitus. *Tinnitus Today.* Vol. 18. No. 11. (March 1993): 6-9.

Guth, P. S., J. Risey, R. Amedee, C. H. Norris. "A Pharmaceutical Approach to the Treatment of Tinnitus." From the 14th Midwinter Research Meeting of the Association for Research in Otolaryngology in St. Petersburg Beach, Florida. February 3-7, 1991.

House, W. F. "Effects of Electrical Stimulation on Tinnitus." From the Second International Tinnitus Seminar in New York. June 10-11, 1983. Supplement No. 9. *Journal of Laryn. and Oto.*

Johnson, R. M., R. Brummett, and A. Schleuning. "Use of Alprazolam for Relief of Tinnitus." *Arch. Otolaryngol. Head Neck Surg.* Vol. 119. (1993): 842-845.

—*by Robert E. Sandlin, Ph.D.*

Chapter 20

Management of the Tinnitus Patient: Non-Medical Strategies

Part One of this article [see Chapter 19] discussed some management strategies associated with the medical model. It was suggested that the hearing health professional be aware of various management approaches in order to provide more appropriate counseling of the tinnitus patient.

Part Two covers some of the more common non-medical management strategies which have proven effective for some tinnitus patients.

No one treatment modality, medically or non-medically based, has been effective in dealing with all patients having some form of subjective tinnitus. However, almost every patient can be helped to some degree with an effective management program.

As mentioned in Part One, tinnitus is not a simple disorder to deal with. There are many complexities involving not only neurophysiological phenomena but patient behavioral and emotional responses to subjective tinnitus.

For many who work with the tinnitus patient, it is becoming increasingly evident that the psychological state of the individual often determines the effectiveness of any therapeutic modality employed in the treatment of this disorder. One cannot emphasize too strongly the necessity of having some awareness of the psychological status of the individual.

This article originally appeared in *Audecibel*, (April/May/June 1994). Used by permission.

Studies by House (1981) and Reich (1984) regarding personalities of tinnitus patients suggest there are abnormal patterns associated with a number of psychological disorders. Among them are those associated with various forms of depression and neuroses. The presence of such aberrant behavior often interferes with the patient's ability to cope with the disorder.

Following is an actual case history that took place 14 to 15 years ago. The client was a white female in her mid-fifties who was the wife of a naval captain. She had complained of bilateral tinnitus for about two years prior to her visit to our clinic. Her history suggested she was having an extremely difficult time coping with her problem.

She had, on more than one occasion, considered the possibility of ending her life. Further, she stated her social and intimate relationships were affected by the constant presence of the tinnitus. She had been examined by several physicians, none of whom offered treatment or medication which provided relief.

When questioned about those kinds of activities which brought some relief to her, she responded by saying she took 10 to 12 showers a day. This statement was somewhat surprising until it was determined that the water beating down on her head was providing "masking" of her tinnitus. As long as she was in the shower, there was considerable relief.

She was a logical candidate for a masker device. Subsequent clinical testing supported that thinking and she became a very effective user of a tinnitus masker. So successful that she appeared on local radio and TV extolling the virtues of the clinic and exclaiming that her social and interpersonal life were now pleasant experiences.

This euphoria, however, only lasted a few months until the patient said the masker device was no longer effective and her tinnitus had returned to its former, irritating level. She was scheduled for a re-evaluation and it was discovered that her ongoing tinnitus could no longer be masked, regardless of the intensity of the masker signal applied. The audiometric and speech discrimination data were not changed, yet her tinnitus had returned and could not be masked.

This inability to mask her ongoing tinnitus is mentioned because it represents, somewhat, our ignorance as clinicians of the course the disorder will follow and those forces that shape it. After extensive questioning it was determined that her tinnitus became uncontrollable after she was told that she could not accompany her husband to Alaska to a new military post.

Although there is no assurance a correlation existed between her husband's transfer and the inability to mask her tinnitus, it was felt strongly that there was. It is known, for example, there is a positive correlation between stress and an increase in subjective loudness of ongoing tinnitus.

This case history is presented only to underscore clinical problems associated with management of the tinnitus patient. The person's psychological or emotional status can greatly affect the success of any clinical modality used in the treatment program.

There are a number of psychologically oriented programs which have been used in treating the tinnitus patient. Space restrictions do not permit the review of each of the programs; which may range from psychiatric care to other counseling strategies. It is valuable to discuss, however, cognitive therapy as an adjunct treatment for the tinnitus sufferer.

Cognitive Therapy

The primary intent of cognitive therapy is to modify or alter maladaptive behaviors—behaviors which reduce the quality or conduct of life due to the presence of some physical, mental or emotional condition. If, in the application of cognitive therapy, one can modify these unwanted behaviors, then the individual can better cope with the stresses generated by the disorder.

If one is to employ cognitive therapy as a method of treating the tinnitus patient, it would seem logical to design a well-organized and structured set of procedures. Sweetow (1989) suggests three behavioral techniques employing cognitive therapy, which have proven useful in the treatment of the tinnitus patient. They are:

1. Direct modification of overt or covert behaviors through the application of specific behavioral techniques;

2. Manipulation of environmental antecedents or situational demands, and;

3. Manipulation of environmental consequences (Sweetow, p. 38).

What Sweetow refers to is the process by which the patient learns to understand the relationship between his or her maladaptive behaviors caused by the presence of tinnitus. In a sense, one may refer to these behaviors as a type of cognitive distortion. It is the resolution of these distortions that provides positive relief from tinnitus. Relief does not imply that the tinnitus is absent, but rather that one's behavior to it has been significantly modified. Some distortions are:

1. Mental filter—dwelling on a negative event so that all reality becomes clouded. (This kind of behavior is seen often in tinnitus patients. They often feel that the tinnitus will never go away and any comment or suggestion to the contrary is automatically denied.)

2. "Should" statements—e.g., creating guilt by believing you "should" have done something differently. (This is a common behavior seen in tinnitus patients. Many feel they should have done something different, or should have been more solicitous to their health or should have been kinder to others, etc. Some feel they are being punished because they should have done something else and failed to do so. This kind of behavior is seen more often in those patients for whom the tinnitus was of violent and sudden onset.)

3. Disqualifying the positive—e.g., positive experiences don't count. (There are those patients who will discredit any positive experience relating to tinnitus. For example, the tinnitus may be greatly reduced or even absent for a period of time. However, these positive experiences don't count because the patient is certain the tinnitus will return and they will be as miserable as ever.)

There are a number of other cognitive distortions of which the reader should be aware. See Sweetow (1989) for a more in-depth analysis. Suffice it to say that one of the effective management strategies for subjective tinnitus is cognitive therapy.

Biofeedback

Biofeedback is not new to the medical or applied sciences. It stemmed from the practice of Eastern religions and was adapted to other pursuits such as meditation and physiological processes involving the heart and its function as well as the physiology of other body organs (Grossman 1976).

It is well documented that through meditation one is able to alter physiological states. We know, for example, that such ailments as migraine headaches, abnormal muscle tension, and anxiety can be effectively modified through conscious effort and appropriate mental focusing.

It has been generally accepted among practitioners working with tinnitus patients, that stress can exacerbate the subjective loudness. Although the mechanism for this phenomenon is unknown, it is apparent that stress can create a number of physiological disturbances that may have negative consequences. Therefore, it seems rather straightforward to employ some treatment modality which would eliminate or reduce stress contributing to increased loudness of the tinnitus.

Biofeedback has been most instrumental in providing a means by which the patient can control his or her stress level. Apparently it makes little difference what the stressor is, or the environment in which it is generated. Biofeedback, if properly managed, can be effective in teaching the patient a means of relaxation. When in a relaxed state it becomes an easier task for the patient to visualize that part of the body to be relaxed. Relaxation through biofeedback intervention not only provides a means by which muscle relaxation is possible, but provides a means of visualizing other sensory sensations such as warmth and coolness.

Relative to tinnitus, it has been suggested by Grossman (1989, Section 9, p. 2), that:

> "...tinnitus is measured before treatment as to tonal content and subjective loudness. The same assessment is repeated after treatment. Even though the patient may feel better and be appreciative of having been improved when the actual measurement of tinnitus is made it is usually still there. What has been removed is that portion of the symptom caused by anxiety reinforcement. As a matter of fact if the patient has

no element of anxiety reinforcing his tinnitus biofeedback may not be particularly beneficial."

Biofeedback is often coupled to other methods of patient management such as counseling or other forms of psychologically-based intervention. This is not to suggest that biofeedback must be coupled to other treatment modalities, but rather that for some a multi-disciplinary approach is more productive.

Biofeedback, as with all other current forms of treatment, is not a panacea. It does not promise an absolute resolution of the problem. It is, however, a method which has proven beneficial to some. To that extent it is important the hearing instrument dispenser be aware of its contribution to the treatment of tinnitus.

Tinnitus Maskers and Combination Devices

The application of a controlled noise to the offending ear(s) to reduce tinnitus loudness is well known and has an extended history. Johnson and his colleagues (1989) tell us that "...Aristotle in the 3rd century B.C. reported that the buzzing in his ears ceased when he was in the presence of other sounds." Since this time, others have reported the effects of a masking noise on the reduction of tinnitus loudness Jones and Knudsen, 1928; Feldmann, H., 1987 and vernon, 1977).

Such observations and subsequent practices are of great importance to the hearing health professional. Although commercially available masker devices do not work for all individuals, the frequency of success is such that it plays a major role in the clinical management of tinnitus.

A masker device produces a controlled narrow or broad band of noise. Often, these devices have a potentiometer controlling frequency shaping of the output response as well as the volume. Such devices are selected on the basis of a tinnitus evaluation to determine whether the patient can be masked by a noise band and whether there is a period of residual inhibition following the withdrawal of the noise to the offending ear.

Residual inhibition is best defined as the absence or reduction of tinnitus loudness following a specified period of exposure to a noise source. In general, residual inhibition is greater the longer the patient is exposed to the masking signal. Although many patients report some degree of residual inhibition following masker use, the neurophysiological mechanisms are not understood entirely. Parenthetically, it is interesting to note that hearing aid devices alone do not promote significant residual inhibition.

A combination device is simply a masker signal and a hearing aid in the same physical housing. The patient has independent control over the output of the hearing aid and the masking signal. Johnson and his coresearchers (1989) report that a combination device is more effective than just a masker device alone.

Success underlying the use of a masker or combination device is most probably a psychological phenomenon. Most individuals with tinnitus complain of the constant presence of an unwanted sound in their head or at their ear(s). For the majority, subjective tinnitus is present 24 hours a day. Although it may vary in intensity and frequency composition, it is ever-present. It can interfere with social interaction, concentration, sleep and emotional stability. There is no way for the individual to ignore the tinnitus. With the introduction of an external noise (via a masker or combination device) sufficient to mask the ongoing tinnitus, the noise is "external" to the head. That is, the noise is outside the head and part of the acoustic environment. It is a much easier task for one to ignore an external stimulus than an internally generated one.

All of us experience noises of our external acoustic environment and, normally, are not bothered by them. We are psychologically able to ignore environmental sounds unless they have immediate significance to us. For example, a young mother is exposed to a number of everyday sounds in the home and is oblivious to them. Yet, when the baby cries, she is immediately alerted and takes appropriate action. This ability to ignore one's acoustic environment makes it possible for the tinnitus masker to be effective as a method of treatment.

There is no doubt that the use of a masker or combination device has been beneficial to many. Unfortunately, not all who have tinnitus can benefit from masker use (Johnson et al. 1969, Johnson and Agnew, 1993). There is no general consensus among serious investigators why masker devices are effective for some and of no value to others. The etiology of subjective tinnitus is most likely multicausal. That is, the site of lesion (neurogenerating site) causing tinnitus can occur at any point along the auditory pathway; from the cochlea to the auditory cortex.

There is even some evidence to suggest that sensory systems, other than auditory, can cause subjective tinnitus. It may be that masker devices are effective for those who have the same or similar etiological factors creating tinnitus. If such is the case, then it is logical to assume that masker device effectiveness is restricted to that group having common causal factors.

Regardless of the percent of individuals helped by masker or combination devices, the hearing health professional should evaluate the person's response to the administration of a controlled masking signal.

However, when so doing, it is important to realize that maximum effectiveness may be achieved after an extended period of use. The person should be counseled relative to reasonable expectations from a masker device and a structured follow up evaluation should be formulated.

The intent of this two-part article has been to present rather basic information about tinnitus and its management. It was not the intent to offer exhaustive commentary or extensive review of therapeutic practices, but rather to present an overview of major considerations in dealing with people with subjective tinnitus.

There is a clinical responsibility that hearing health professionals can exercise when working with those having subjective tinnitus. It is hoped that this article has added to the information needed to effectively deal with the tinnitus patient.

References

Feldmann, H. "Historical Remarks." Proceedings III International Tinnitus Seminar in Munster, Germany. Harsch Verlag, Karlsruhe, 1987: 210-213.

Grossan, M. "Treatment of Subjective Tinnitus with Biofeedback." *Ear, Nose & Throat.* 55. (1976): 314-318.

Grossan, M. "The Biofeedback Program." In *The Understanding and Treatment of Tinnitus*, ed. R Sandlin. Portland, Oregon: American Tinnitus Association. 1989.

House, P. "Personality of the Tinnitus Patient." In *Tinnitus, Ciba Foundation Symposium 85*, ed. D. Everest and G. Lawrenson. London: Pitman. 1981.

Johnson, R., L. Press, S. Griest, K. Sorter, and B. Lentz. "A Tinnitus Masking Program: Efficacy and Safety." *Hear. Jour.* (November 1989): 18-21.

Johnson, R. and J. Agnew. "New Tinnitus Masking Devices Allow Patient Clinician Tuning." *Hear. Instrum.* Vol. 44, No. 1. (1993): 25-26.

Jones, I. and V. Knudsen. "Certain Aspects of Tinnitus, Particularly Treatment." *Laryngoscope*. 1928.

Reich, G. and R. Johnson. "Personality Characteristics of Tinnitus Patients." From the Proceedings of the II International Tinnitus Seminar. Supplement 9, *Jour. Laryng. & Oto.* (1984).

Sweetow, R. "Cognitive Aspects of Tinnitus Patient Management." *Ear & Hear*. Vol. 7, No. 6. (1986): 390-396.

Sweetow, R. "Adjunctive Approaches to the Tinnitus—Patient Management." *Hear. Jour.* (November 1989): 38-43.

—by Robert E. Sandlin, Ph.D.

Chapter 21

Recent Advances in Tinnitus: Management and Therapy

Hearing Aids and Tinnitus Maskers

It is well established that an external stimulus, such as a broad-band noise, can mask tinnitus in some patients (Feldmann, 1971; Vernon, 1977). Several wearable and nonwearable devices are available to provide a masking noise for tinnitus relief. Tinnitus maskers are available in which the spectral shape of the noise can be adjusted.

Most patients with tinnitus also have a hearing loss and are therefore candidates for a hearing aid. A hearing aid could mask tinnitus either by amplifying noise or by producing its own internal noise. Some hearing aids combine the amplification of sounds and a tinnitus masking noise in the same unit. By improving communication, hearing aids can also reduce stress, which in turn may reduce the tinnitus.

Several reviews are available on the fitting of tinnitus maskers (Coles, 1987; Hazell et al., 1985; Sheldrake, Wood, and Cooper, 1985: Tyler and Bentler, 1987). There is no way to determine if a patient will benefit from a tinnitus masker without actually trying it. Furthermore, it seems appropriate to try unilateral fittings for the right and left ears, as well as a binaural fining. A one-month trial period, keeping a daily record of different configurations, is probably the best approach. The tinnitus does not have to be completely masked to be effective. Many patients are satisfied with partial masking.

This excerpt originally appeared as part of "Recent Advances in Tinnitus" in the *American Journal of Audiology*, November 1992. Used by permission.

The actual number of people who benefit from tinnitus maskers is somewhat controversial. High success rates have been reported by some groups (Hazell et al., 1985; Schleuning, Johnson, and Vernon, 1980; Shulman and Goldstein, 1987). Other reports have been less optimistic (Stephens and Corcoran, 1985). The success rate depends on the population studied and the definition of success. Previous reviews of this area are provided by McFadden (1982) and Tyler and Bentler (1987).

A recent study attempted to separate the placebo effect in tinnitus masker treatment. It might be expected that some patients would feel they had benefited from the masker, when in fact they were benefiting from the attention and counseling that they received from the masker fining and rehabilitation sessions.

Erlandsson, Ringdahl, Hutchins, and Carlsson (1987) compared the effectiveness of a programmable tinnitus masker and a placebo device. The placebo was allegedly supposed to produce an electrical reduction of tinnitus, but no electrical current passed from a wearable processor unit (with flashing lights) and an ear canal electrode. Of 17 patients, 7 reported a reduction during the masker trial, but 5 also reported a reduction during the placebo trial.

Sheldrake and Hazell (1992) studied 204 tinnitus patients who used hearings aids or tinnitus maskers. They reported that 37% of the tinnitus patients stopped using their maskers during a 10-year period. Several reasons might account for such findings: (a) the tinnitus resolved: (b) the individuals found other, more effective, ways of managing their tinnitus; (c) the masker lost its effectiveness in masking a stable tinnitus; (d) the tinnitus increased in magnitude and the masker lost its effectiveness; or (e) the masker was never really effective, and the patient stopped using it after a "placebo" effect wore off.

Given that there is no widely accepted successful treatment for tinnitus, it important to have maskers available to help those people who respond favorably. Although the number of patients for whom this is effective may be small and placebo effects may influence results, tinnitus maskers are able to help some patients cope.

Medications

The search for a pharmacological treatment for tinnitus continues. Lidocaine has been shown to reduce tinnitus in many patients in controlled studies (e.g., Duckert and Rees, 1983; Martin and Coleman,

1980). However, it must be administered intravenously and has some undesirable side effects. Unfortunately, although investigations continue (Murai, Tyler, Harker, and Stouffer, 1992), the number of promising drugs is very limited. These investigations are hampered by the lack of an animal model and the fact that tinnitus is a general symptom, and the mechanism responsible for it is likely different in different patients.

Behavior Modification for Tinnitus Treatment

Counseling and psychological treatments are potentially one of the most important forms of tinnitus treatment. Fortunately, there are now several groups carefully examining different psychological protocols and the relative merits of these different approaches (Hallam and Jakes, 1987; Lindberg, Scott, Lyttkens, and Melin, 1987; Wilson, Bowen, and Farag, 1992) using control groups. These groups are exploring the effectiveness of cognitive therapy, relaxation training, biofeedback, and coping techniques. Although a consensus has not been reached, preliminary results are encouraging. For example, Wilson, Bowen, and Farag reported that a combined cognitive-therapy/relaxation-training approach was beneficial. Their cognitive therapy consisted of attempts to reduce negative appraisals and to "implement distraction and attention-diversion techniques." The relaxation training involved standard techniques of tensing and relaxing various body muscles.

Electrical Suppression

The sensory effects of electrical current applied to the ear were reponed very early, and particularly so for tinnitus (Field, 1893). The specific effects of positive and negative direct current have been identified specifically. A negative direct current induces sound sensations but is relatively ineffective at reducing tinnitus. A positive direct current can suppress tinnitus without producing additional sound perception (Aran and Cazals, 1981). This effect was most pronounced when the site of the tinnitus, as well as the site of the original lesion, could be clearly identified to the test ear. Positive direct current is known to inhibit activity on auditory-nerve fibers and negative current is excitatory (Konishi, Teas, and Wernick, 1970).

175

There is interest in using alternating current to reduce tinnitus, and its effectiveness in some patients has been reported (Vernon, 1977). A recent study has shown that an eardrum electrode site can be effective for reducing tinnitus in some patients (Kuk, Tyler, Rustad, Harker, and Tye-Murray, 1989). Studies are in progress comparing the relative effectiveness of stimulating from the eardrum and from the medial wall of the middle-ear cavity adjacent to the round window.

With the development of cochlear implants for the profoundly deaf, who often experience strong tinnitus sensations, several reports have noted the reduction of tinnitus in patients with electrical prosthesis (Berliner, Cunningham, and House, 1987; Hazell, Meerton, and Conway, 1989; Tyler and Kelsay, 1990). One should distinguish among (a) the effects of surgical implantation itself (without electrical stimulation); (b) the specific effect of the electrical current on tinnitus (with the device turned on, with and without test stimuli); and (c) when the device is used for speech perception. A recent study by Gibson (1992) on patients with a multichannel cochlear implant reported that a reduction of tinnitus was reported in 38%, 26%, and 61% of the patients, respectively, using the three criteria noted above.

Implantation specifically for tinnitus suppression has occasionally been attempted with alternating current (Hazell et al. 1989) and direct current (Cazals, Rouanet, Negrevergne, and Lagourgue, 1984). However, it is well known that unbalanced charges can provoke tissue damage. and the direct currents cannot be used on a long-term basis.

There is hope of finding the appropriate waveform of electrical stimulation that would be charge balanced and effective at suppressing the tinnitus.

References

Aran, J. M. and Y. Cazals. "Electrical Supression of Tinnitus." In *Tinnitus: Ciba Foundation Symposium 85*, ed. D. Evered. London: Pitman Books, 1981.

Berliner, K. I., J. K. Cunningham, and W. F. House. "Effect of the Cochlear Implant on Tinnitus in Profoundly Deaf Patients." In *Proceedings of the III International Tinnitus Seminar*, Karlsruhe, Germany: Harsch Verlag. 1987.

Cazals, Y., J. F. Rouanet, M. Negrevergne, and P. Lagourgue. "First Results of Electrical Stimulation with a Round-Window Electrode in Totally Deaf Parents." *Archives of Oto-Rhino-Laryngology*. Vol. 239. (1984).

Coles, R. R. A. "Tinnitus and Its Management." In *Scott-Brown's Otolaryngology*, ed. S. D. G. Stevens and A. G. Kerr. Guildford: Butterworth, 1987.

Duckert, L. and T. Rees. "Treatment of Tinnitus with Intravenous Lidocaine: A Double-Blind Randomized Trial." *Otolaryngology—Head and Neck Surgery*. Vol. 91. (1993): 550-555.

Erlandsson, S., A. Ringdahl, T. Hutchins, and S. G. Carlsson. "Treatment of Tinnitus: A Controlled Comparison of Masking and Placebo." *British Journal of Audiology*. Vol. 21. (1987): 168-179.

Feldmann, H., "Homolateral and Contralateral Masking of Tinnitus by Noisebands and by Pure Tones." *Audiology.* Vol. 10. (1971): 138-144.

Field, G. P. *A Manual of Diseases of the Ear*. London: Balliere, Tindall and Cox. 1893.

Gibson, W. P. R. "The Effect of Electrical Stimulation and Cochlear Implantation on Tinnitus." In *Tinnitus 91, Proceedings of the IV International Tinnitus Seminar*. ed. J. M. Aran and R. Dauman. Amsterdam: Kugler and Ghedini. 1992.

Hallam, R. S. and S. C. Jakes. "An Evaluation of Relaxation Training in Chronic Tinnitus Sufferers."

Hazell, J. W. P. *Tinnitus*. London: Churchill Livingstone. 1987.

Hazell, W. P. J., L. J. Meerton, and J. J. Conway. "Electrical Tinnitus Supression (ETS) with a Single Channel Cochlear Implant." *Journal of Laryngology and Otology.* Supplement 18. (1989): 39-44.

Konishi, T., D. C. Teas, and J. S. Wernick. "Effects of Electrical Currents Applied to Cochlear Partition on Discharges in Individual Auditory-Nerve Fibers. I. Prolonged Direct-Current Polarization." *Journal of the Acoustical Society of America*. Vol. 47. (1970): 1519-1526.

Kuk, F. K., R. S. Tyler, N. Rustad, L. A. Harker, and N. Tye-Murray. "Alternating Current at the Eardrum for Tinnitus Reduction." *Journal of Speech and Hearing Research*. Vol. 32. (1989): 393-400.

Lindberg, P., B. Scott, L. Lyttkens, and L. Melin "The Effects of Behavioral Treatment on Tinnitus in an Experimental Group Study and as an Approach in Clinical Management of Tinnitus." In *Proceedings of the III International Tinnitus Seminal*. Karlsruhe, Germany: Harsch Verlag. 1987.

Martin, F. W. and B. H. Coleman. "Tinnitus: A Doubleblind Crossover Controlled Trial to Evaluate the Use of Lignocaine." *Clinical Otolaryngology*. Vol. 5, No. 3. (1980).

McFadden, D. *Tinnitus: Facts, Theories, and Treatments.* Washington D. C.: National Academy Press. 1982.

Murai, K., R. S. Tyler, L. A. Harker, and J. L. Stouffer. "Pharmacological Treatment of Tinnitus." *American Journal of Otolaryngology.* 1992.

Schleuning, A. M., R. M. Johnson, and J. A. Vernon. "Evaluation of a Tinnitus Masking Program: A Follow-up Study of 598 Paatients." *Ear and Hearing*. Vol. 1. (1980): 71-74.

Sheldrake, J. B., S. M. Wood, and H. R. Cooper. "Practical Aspects of the Instrumental Management of Tinnitus." *British Journal of Audiology*. Vol. 19. (1985): 147-150.

Shulman, A. and B. Goldstein. *Proceedings of the III International Tinnitus Seminar*. Karlsruhe, Germany: Harsch Verlag. 1987

Stephens, S. D. G. and A. L. Corcoran. "A Controlled Study of Tinnitus Masking." *British Journal of Audiology*. Vol. 19. (1985): 159-167.

Tyler, R. S. and R. W. Bentler. "Tinnitus Maskers and Hearing Aids for Tinnitus." In *Seminars in Hearing*. Vol. 8, No. 1. (1987): 49-61.

Tyler, R. S. and D. Kelsay. "Advantages and Disadvantages Perceived by Some of the Better Cochlear-Implant Patients." *American Journal of Otolaryngology*. Vol. 11. (1990).

Vernon, "Attempts to Releive Tinnitus." *Journal of the American Auditory Society*. Vol. 2. (1977): 124-131.

Wilson, P. H., M. Bowen, and P. Farag, "Cognitive and Relaxation Techniques in the Management of Tinnitus." In *Tinnitus 91, Proceedings of the IV International Tinnitus Seminar*. ed. J. M. Aran and R. Dauman. Amsterdam: Kugler and Ghedini. 1992.

—by Richard S. Tyler,
The University of Iowa;
Jean-Marie Aran
and René Dauman,
Hospital Pellegrin,
Bordeaux Cedex, France.

Chapter 22

Hearing and Older People

Introduction

It is easy to take good hearing for granted. For people with hearing impairments, words in a conversation may be misunderstood, musical notes might be missed, and a ringing doorbell may go unanswered. Hearing impairment ranges from having difficulty understanding words or hearing certain sounds to total deafness.

Because of fear, misinformation, or vanity, some people will not admit to themselves or anyone else that they have a hearing problem. It has been estimated, however, that about 30 percent of adults age 65 through 74 and about 50 percent of those age 75 through 79 suffer some degree of hearing loss. In the United States alone, more than 10 million older people are hearing impaired.

If ignored and untreated, hearing problems can grow worse, hindering communication with others, limiting social activities, and reducing the choices of leisure time activities. People with hearing impairments often withdraw socially to avoid the frustration and embarrassment of not being able to understand what is being said. In addition, hearing-impaired people may become suspicious of relatives and friends who "mumble" or "don't speak up."

Hearing loss may cause an older person to be wrongly labeled as "confused," "unresponsive," or "uncooperative." At times a person's

National Institute on Aging; National Institute on Deafness and Other Communication Disorders.

feelings of powerlessness and frustration in trying to communicate with others result in depression and withdrawal.

Older people today more often demand greater satisfaction from life, but those with hearing impairments can find the quality of their lives reduced. Fortunately, help is available in the form of treatment with medicines, special training, a hearing aid or an alternate listening device, and surgery.

Some Common Signs of Hearing Impairment

- Words are difficult to understand.
- Another person's speech sounds slurred or mumbled, worsening when there is background noise.
- Speech can be hard or impossible to understand, depending on the kind of hearing impairment.
- Certain sounds are overly loud or annoying.
- A hissing or ringing background noise may be heard constantly or the sound may be interrupted.
- TV shows, concerts, or social gatherings are less enjoyable because much goes unheard.

Diagnosis of Hearing Problems

If you have trouble hearing, see your doctor for treatment or a referral to an ear specialist. By ignoring the problem, you may be overlooking a serious medical condition. Hearing impairments may be caused by exposure to very loud noises over a long period of time, viral infections, vascular disorders (such as heart conditions or stroke), head injuries, tumors, heredity, certain medications, or age-related changes in the ear.

In some cases, the diagnosis and treatment of a hearing problem may take place in the family doctor's office. More complicated cases may require the help of specialists known as otologists, otolaryngologists, or otorhinolaryngologists—all of whom are trained to perform surgery on the head and neck. These specialists are doctors of medicine or doctors of osteopathy with extensive training in ear problems. They will take a medical history, ask about problems affecting family members, conduct a thorough exam, and order any needed tests.

An audiologist is another health professional who is trained to identify and measure hearing loss and to help with rehabilitation. However, audiologists do not prescribe drugs or perform surgery. To measure hearing they use a device that produces sounds of different pitches and loudness (an audiometer), as well as other electronic devices. These hearing measurements test a person's ability to understand speech. The tests are painless and can quickly locate a hearing problem, allowing the doctor to recommend a course of treatment.

Types of Hearing Loss

Conductive hearing loss occurs in some older people. It involves the blocking of sounds that are carried from the ear drums (tympanic membrane) to the inner ear. This may be caused by ear wax in the ear canal, fluid in the middle ear, or abnormal bone growth or infection in the middle ear.

Sensorineural hearing loss involves damage to parts of the inner ear or auditory nerve. When sensorineural hearing loss occurs in older people, it is called presbycusis (pronounced prez-bee-KU-sis). Changes in the delicate workings of the inner ear lead to difficulties understanding speech and possibly an intolerance for loud sounds, but not total deafness. Thus, "don't shout—I'm not deaf!" is often said by older people with this type of hearing impairment.

Every year after age 50 we are likely to lose some of our hearing ability. The decline is gradual, but by age 60 or 70 as many as 25 percent of older people are noticeably hearing impaired. Just as the graying of hair occurs at different rates, presbycusis may develop differently from person to person.

Although presbycusis is usually attributed to aging, it does not affect everyone. In fact, some researchers view it as a disease. Environmental noise, certain medicines, improper diet, and genetic makeup may contribute to this disorder. The condition is permanent, but there is much a person can do to function well.

Central auditory dysfunction is a third type of hearing loss that occurs in older people, although it is quite rare. It is caused by damage to the nerve centers within the brain. Sound levels are not affected, but understanding language usually is. The causes include extended illness with a high fever, head injuries, vascular problems, or tumors. A central auditory dysfunction cannot be treated medically or surgically; but for some, special training by an audiologist or speech pathologist can help.

Treatment

Examination and test results from the family doctor, ear specialist, and audiologist will determine the best treatment for a specific hearing problem. In some cases, medical treatment such as cleansing the ear canal to remove ear wax or surgery may restore some or all hearing ability.

At other times a hearing aid may be recommended. A hearing aid is a small device designed to make sounds louder. Before you can buy a hearing aid, you must either obtain a written statement from your doctor (saying that your hearing impairment has been medically evaluated and that you might benefit from a hearing aid) or sign a waiver stating that you do not desire medical evaluation.

Many hearing aids are on the market, each offering different kinds of help for different problems. Professional advice is needed regarding the design, model, and brand of the hearing aid best for you. This advice, which is part of your hearing aid evaluation, is given by the audiologist who considers your hearing level, your understanding of speech in each ear, your ability to handle the aid and its controls, and your concern about appearance and comfort.

Remember that you are buying a product and specific services, including any necessary adjustments, counseling in the use of the aid, maintenance, and repairs throughout the warranty period. Before deciding where to buy your aid, consider the quality of service as well as the quality of the product.

Buy an aid with only those features you need. The most costly hearing aid may not be the best for you while the one selling for less may offer more satisfaction. Also, be aware that the controls for many of the special features are tiny and may be difficult to adjust. Practice will make operating the aid easier. Your hearing aid dealer (usually called a "dispenser") should have the patience and skill to help you through the adjustment period. It is a good idea to take advantage of his or her help since it often takes at least a month to become comfortable with a new hearing aid.

People with certain types of hearing impairments may need special help. Speech reading allows people to receive visual cues from lip movements as well as facial expressions, body posture and gestures, and the environment. Auditory training may include hearing aid orientation, but it is also designed to help hearing-impaired persons identify and better handle their specific communication problems. Both speech reading and auditory training can reduce the handicapping effects of the hearing loss. If needed, counseling is also available so that people with hearing impairments can understand their communication abilities and limitations while maintaining a positive image.

If You Have Problems Hearing

If you suspect there may be a problem with your hearing, visit your doctor as soon as possible. Medicare will pay for the doctor's exam and hearing tests that are ordered by the doctor. Medicare will not pay for the hearing aid.

How to Help Yourself

- Ask your doctor to explain the cause of your hearing problem and if you should see a specialist.
- Don't hesitate to ask people to repeat what they have just said.
- Try to reduce background noise (stereo, television, or radio).
- Tell people that you have a hearing problem and what they can do to make communication easier.

If You Know Someone Who Has a Hearing Problem

- Speak at your normal rate, but not too rapidly. Do not over articulate. This distorts the sounds of speech and makes visual clues more difficult. Shouting will not make the message any clearer and may distort it.

- Speak to the person at a distance of 3 to 6 feet. Position yourself near good light so that your lip movements, facial expressions, and gestures may be seen clearly. Wait until you are visible to the hearing impaired person before speaking. Avoid chewing, eating, or covering your mouth while speaking.

- Never speak directly into the person's ear. This prevents the listener from making use of visual cues.

- If the listener does not understand what was said, rephrase the idea in short, simple sentences.

- Arrange living rooms or meeting rooms so that no one is more than 6 feet apart and all are completely visible. In meetings or group activities where there is a speaker presenting information, ask the speaker to use the public address system.

- Treat the hearing-impaired person with respect. Include the person in all discussions about him or her. This helps relieve the feelings of isolation common in hearing-impaired people.

For More Information

If you would like further information about hearing problems, contact the organizations listed below. Please be sure to state clearly what type of information you would like to receive.

The American Academy of Otolaryngology, Head and Neck Surgery, Inc., is a professional society of medical doctors specializing in diseases of the ear, nose, and throat. They can provide information on hearing, balance, and other disorders affecting the ear, nose, and throat. Write to One Prince Street, Alexandria, VA 22314.

The American Speech-Language-Hearing Association and the National Association of Hearing and Speech Action can both answer questions or mail information on hearing aids or hearing loss and communication problems in older people. They can also provide a list of certified audiologists and speech language pathologists. Write to the American Speech-Language-Hearing Association at 10801 Rockville Pike, Dept. AP, Rockville, MD 20852; or call the National Association of Hearing & Speech Action at (800) 638-8255.

Self Help for Hard of Hearing People, Inc., is a national self-help organization for those who are hard of hearing. SHHH can help with information on coping with a hearing loss and new hearing aids and technology, and they publish the *Shhh Journal* bimonthly. Write to SHHH, 7800 Wisconsin Avenue, Bethesda, MD 20892.

The National Information Center on Deafness at Gallaudet University provides information on all areas related to deafness and hearing loss including educational programs, vocational training, sign language programs, law, technology, and barrier-free design. Write to the NICD, 800 Florida Avenue, NE., Washington, DC 20002.

The National Institute on Deafness and Other Communication Disorders at the National Institutes of Health provides information on research on hearing, balance, smell, taste, voice, speech, and language. Write to the NIDCD, Building 31, Room 1B62, Bethesda, MD 20892.

Their National Information Clearinghouse also provides information to health professionals, patients, industry, and the public. Write to the NIDCD Clearinghouse, P.O. Box 37777, Washington, DC 20013-7777.

The National Institute on Aging offers information on a range of health issues that concern older people. Write to the NIA Information Center, P.O. Box 8057, Gaithersburg, MD 20898-8057.

Chapter 23

Hearing Loss: Information for Professionals in the Aging Network

The over-65 population is growing rapidly. In 1989, 29 million men and women were 65 years of age or older. The U.S. Bureau of the Census (1983) projects that by the year 2000, the number of people in this age range will be more than 35 million (one in every 7.5 people).

As a professional in the aging network, you are probably well acquainted with these statistics. Yet, you may not be aware of a problem that confronts a large number of older people: hearing loss.

According to the National Health Interview Survey of 1984, about 24 percent of the population between the ages of 65 and 74 have a hearing loss, nearly twice the percentage for people between the ages of 45 and 64. In the 75 and older age group, the prevalence jumps from 24 to approximately 36 percent.

The World of Reduced Sound

Those of us who have good hearing usually take it for granted. Untouched by hearing loss, we do not realize the impact it can have on everyday life. Try imagining a life without sound, a world devoid of

---

This publication is one of a series produced by the National Information Center on Deafness and the American Speech-Language-Hearing Association. The series focuses on understanding the realities of hearing loss and suggests practical adjustments for people with hearing loss, their families, friends, and the professionals who serve them. Series Editor: Loraine DiPietro, Director, National Information Center on Deafness, Gallaudet University.

music, voices, and laughter. Now imagine hearing only *partial* sounds: This is the world of the person who is hard of hearing. Normal hearing allows full participation in all types of communication. Consider how much information we receive daily from conversations, and from radio and television. Without thinking, we rely on our hearing for the signals that shape daily life (the sounds of door bells, telephones, alarm clocks, car horns, and fire alarms) and for the most important link to others—the ability to express ideas and feelings in conversation.

Research has shown that the ability to communicate is so vital to both the psychological and physical independence of the aging person that when the *quality* of communication is impaired, so is the quality of life. For many older people in our society, hearing loss prevents complete participation in, enjoyment of, and benefiting from the sounds and voices surrounding them. The impact of hearing loss is potentially devastating—simply trying to understand what is being said becomes frustrating, exhausting, and depressing. Add these realities of hearing loss to the social realities of reduced communication outlets for many older adults, and the outcome is a situation fraught with emotional trauma.

Further, unlike other physical disabilities, hearing loss isn't visible and often goes unnoticed. Eyeglasses signal a loss of vision, and a cane warns of mobility problems, but deteriorating hearing often goes undetected or—even worse—misunderstood.

The older individual, not realizing a hearing loss exists, may assume that others are whispering when, in fact, the hearing loss is distorting the sound of voices. It's not difficult to imagine the potential for communication problems when it seems as though everyone is whispering. At the same time, it's easy to imagine how quickly *you* might find someone "peculiar" who insisted you were whispering when you knew you were not. Unfortunately, by the time the hearing loss is identified, personal relationships are often damaged and the person who is hard of hearing has withdrawn from communication attempts.

Because of the increased incidence of hearing loss among older people, its effects on the quality of the older adult's life, and its invisibility, it is important to have both a sensitivity to the potential for hearing loss and an awareness of how to facilitate communication with a person who has a hearing loss. Fortunately, the majority of people with hearing losses can be helped. Understanding the ear and how it works is helpful to understanding hearing losses and ways to improve communication.

How We Hear

The ear has three major parts: outer, middle, and inner. The **outer ear** is the part we're most familiar with; it can be seen and touched. The outer ear canal (or tunnel), about 2.54 cm to 3.81 cm (approximately 1 inch to 1 1/2 inches) in length, ends at the **tympanic membrane**, or eardrum. This thin, tough, elastic, tissue divides the outer ear from the middle ear.

The middle ear is a small air-filled space containing a chain of three tiny bones—the **malleus**, **incus**, and **stapes**. The bones lead from the tympanic membrane (eardrum) to the inner ear.

The **inner ear** is the end organ for hearing and balance. It is here that the **cochlea** is found. Coiled, resembling a snail's shell, the cochlea is so small that a few drops of the special fluids necessary for hearing fill it completely. Within the cochlea are thousands of tiny cells that look like hairs and are called, not surprisingly, **hair cells**. These are connected to the **auditory** nerve, the nerve of hearing. The auditory nerve relays signals from the ear to the brain.

How do these components work together to let us "hear"? Sound enters the external ear canal striking the eardrum. This causes the eardrum and the three chained bones in the middle ear to move back and forth. The movement (or vibration) produces small waves that ripple the cochlea's special inner ear fluid. (Imagine the ripples caused by a rock thrown into a still pond.) The tiny hair cells respond to the ripples by producing nerve impulses that travel along the auditory nerve to the brain. In the brain the "sounds" are actually "heard" or perceived and understood.

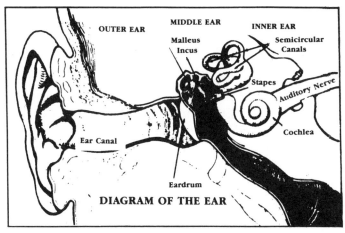

DIAGRAM OF THE EAR

What Causes Hearing Loss?

Disorders of the outer, middle, or inner ear, the auditory nerve, or the brain can result in hearing losses. For example, ear wax impacted in the outer ear canal (a common occurrence in the aging ear), holes in the eardrum, fluid inside the middle ear, or interference with the movements of the middle ear bones can cause hearing loss. Disorders such as these, occurring in the outer or middle ear, are called **conductive**. Generally, conductive disorders can be medically or surgically treated.

Disorders of the inner ear or auditory nerve are called **sensorineural**. Loss of hair cells in the inner ear (from constant exposure to loud noises or aging) and tumors on the auditory nerve are examples of sensorineural disorders. Sometimes hearing loss results from problems within the brain. These are known as **central auditory disorders**. Usually, neither sensorineural nor central auditory disorders can be medically or surgically treated.

What Hearing Loss Sounds Like

Think back to your image of a world of partial sound. When someone, especially an older person, becomes "hard of hearing" we tend to think we understand the consequences. Sounds become fainter and distant. We assume that our older acquaintances simply need more volume. Just shout loud enough and they'll understand.

Unfortunately, our assumption may be very wrong. The effects of hearing losses are as varied as their causes. *Reduction in the loudness of sounds* is, indeed, one effect of hearing loss. An older person with such a hearing loss may not be able to make out a name shouted across a room or hear the warning honk of a car horn.

But hearing losses may cause problems other than reduced sound. Some hearing losses result in a *distortion of sound*. An older person with this type of loss may complain, "I can hear you, but I can't understand you." Sounds filter through like an old, scratchy recording of a song or a static-filled radio broadcast. With a distortion problem, the person may not be able to differentiate between many of the sounds of speech. For example, words with similar sounds, like *fit* and *sit*, or *math* and *mass* may be easily confused. Shouting at a person with this type of loss does not help. An increase in volume does not improve the *quality* of the sound or make words any clearer.

190

A third possible effect of hearing loss is something called *recruitment*. Recruitment is an abnormal growth in the loudness of a sound. Recruitment sufferers have a narrow range between when a sound is loud enough to hear and when it becomes too loud, which is painful. For example, normally, when you listen to TV or radio there is quite a range (distance) between a comfortable listening level and a level that hurts your ears. With recruitment that range (distance) becomes very small. This means that often people with a recruitment problem cannot tolerate loud voices or sounds. Shouting at them may result in complaints that "you're talking too loudly" or "you're hurting my ears." Some might even say, "Don't shout at me, I'm not deaf!"

Finally, any overview of hearing and older adults is incomplete without a discussion of *presbycusis*, a hearing loss specifically linked with aging.

What is Presbycusis?

In the process of aging, the ear and its structures—like other parts of the body—undergo changes. **Presbycusis** (the name comes from the Greek words *presbys*, meaning "old man," and *akousis*, meaning "hearing") is a communication disorder characterized by progressive degeneration of the auditory function.

The catchall term, presbycusis, includes many types of auditory deterioration. For example, it may mean the simple loss of hearing sensitivity through chemical and mechanical changes in the inner ear and breakdown of the inner ear structures. More often, however, it refers to complex degenerative changes occurring along the nerve pathways leading to the brain. These complex changes, in turn, may result in a slowing down of the signals traveling from ear to the brain.

Although presbycusis-linked breakdowns happen to some degree in the outer and middle ear, the most significant changes are those occurring in the inner ear. As disorders affecting the inner ear (sensorineural) cannot be medically or surgically treated, these breakdowns cause permanent hearing loss.

Most often presbycusis occurs in both ears—affecting them equally. Just as some people turn gray more slowly than others, some individuals may feel the effects of presbycusis later and less severely than others. However, if you live long enough, the fact remains that, sooner or later, presbycusis will affect you.

How Hearing Loss Affects Communication

As mentioned earlier, hearing loss causes a reduction of loudness and a lack of clarity which results in difficulty hearing and understanding speech. Problems in hearing and understanding the spoken word often leave the older hard of hearing person feeling defeated, frustrated, angry, embarrassed, anxious, and withdrawn. When coupled with the other losses often experienced by older adults in our society—the loss of a steady income, loss of a spouse, loss of easy access to transportation, and a less active social life—the loss of the ability to hear and understand what others are saying can be the last straw. Hearing loss of any sort can help barricade the older individual behind a terrible wall of isolation.

No matter what the cause of hearing loss, the effect on communication is the same. Sentences need to be repeated, the speaker's frustration becomes apparent, and, in turn, the person with the hearing loss feels pressured to understand the words the first time and not ask questions. Anxiety builds. Soon the older listener's frustration equals the speaker's. Sometimes the result is anger—"Why don't you talk more plainly!" After enough of these experiences, the older person begins to withdraw from these situations that are so fraught with frustration. The chain reaction is in motion: anxiety breeds failure; failure breeds frustration; and frustration leads to further failure, ending in a move toward isolation.

To further complicate matters, the individual's hearing loss may go unnoticed because it is not *visible*. When the older person doesn't respond to a question, or can't seem to follow a conversation, the assumption may be that his/her attention is wandering. Hearing loss may not be identified as the real problem until the older person erupts in frustration. Not recognizing that a hearing loss may be behind the person's communication problems and/or being intolerant of and insensitive to the deaf or hard of hearing person's communication needs can serve to further frustrate, anger, and isolate the older individual.

What Can Be Done?

As a professional in the aging network, you should be aware that people with hearing losses can be helped. Even when hearing loss is permanent, communication can be made easier and less stressful. And

192

just as important, you need to know how older adults with hearing losses can find the help they need. Professional assistance from a certified audiologist is usually the first step toward audiologic rehabilitation.

The Audiologist's Role

An audiologist specializes in preventing, identifying, and assessing hearing loss; fitting hearing aids and assistive listening devices; training individuals in their use; and other rehabilitative services.

When hearing loss is suspected, it is important that the individual consult an audiologist to determine if a hearing loss exists, and if so:

- the type of hearing loss;
- communication problems associated with the loss; and
- the necessity for audiologic rehabilitation.

If the client's hearing can be improved through the use of a hearing aid or another assistive listening device, the audiologist selects an appropriate instrument, fits it, shows how to care for and maintain it, and provides an individualized program of audiologic rehabilitation to develop maximum communication skills.

What To Expect From Audiologic Rehabilitation

Audiologic rehabilitation refers to the audiologist's nonmedical efforts to develop and improve a client's communication skills. Typically, a rehabilitation program consists of the hearing aid evaluation and orientation; recommendations of personal listening systems or assistive devices for the individual's living environment; auditory training; training in speechreading and speech conservation; and counseling for the family as well as the person with the hearing loss.

Hearing Aid Evaluation

First the audiologist conducts a complete hearing evaluation, determines if a hearing aid may be useful, and counsels the individual about communication abilities with and without the use of an aid. Then the audiologist conducts tests to find an appropriate aid, and selects one that maximizes the client's hearing and understanding of speech while best meeting additional listening needs.

In working with an older client, the audiologist takes some special considerations into account. They include the client's:

- self-image
- motivation
- adaptability
- attitude toward hearing aids
- hand and finger mobility
- eyesight.

All of these factors help determine whether the older adult client will be a successful hearing aid user. Also, they may reveal the need for assistance from such support people as family, friends, or institutional staff. If appropriate, these people may then be included in counseling sessions with the audiologist.

Most older adults with hearing losses can benefit from using a hearing aid. Some, however, are able to benefit only partially, while others are unable to benefit at all. Without a comprehensive hearing evaluation by an audiologist, it is possible that an older consumer may waste money on an inappropriate instrument or end up with a device that may further damage hearing and create a negative attitude toward any future hearing aid and rehabilitative procedure.

Hearing Aid Orientation

During the hearing aid orientation, the older client and any involved support individuals learn what the hearing aid can and cannot do to improve communication, what the user's communication abilities are with use of the aid, what new communication adjustments the aid itself will require, what communication problems will remain, and how to minimize them.

Auditory Training

Special listening sessions are an example of one type of auditory training. During these, the client wears an amplification device and practices listening to speech and other environmental sounds. This practice helps the person with a hearing loss learn to listen in a new way and to adjust to amplified sounds.

Speechreading

Speechreading, often taken to mean lipreading, actually involves receiving visual cues from all lip movements, facial expressions, body postures and gestures, and the surrounding environment. Everyone has developed some speechreading skill. When hearing loss occurs, it becomes necessary to develop these skills as fully as possible. Since success in speechreading is often linked to eyesight, an older person with diminished vision will have more trouble distinguishing lip movements, facial expressions, and gestures.

While hearing aid orientation, auditory training, and speech-reading do not improve damaged hearing, they do reduce the handi-capping effects of the hearing loss.

In addition to hearing aids, there are numerous other devices and systems that improve communication, alert people to environmental signals, or make hearing loss less isolating. Included are signal lights or vibrators to replace auditory signals such as doorbells, alarms, or even a crying infant. There are also telephone aids ranging from am-plifiers to make the signals louder, to Telecommunication Devices for the Deaf (TDDs) which send typed messages through the telephone. Small and large group listening systems, used with and without hear-ing aids, can make church or the theater more pleasurable for a per-son with a hearing loss. The audiologist is familiar with the range of assistive listening devices and can demonstrate to older clients how such devices may help them cope with their hearing loss.

Counseling

Counseling is an ongoing process that may involve not only the deaf or hard of hearing person, but others who live or work with the client. For example, counseling sessions may focus on helping the cli-ent maintain a positive self-image. In counseling sessions:

- the person with a hearing loss learns to understand how ag-ing affects hearing and how hearing loss, in turn, affects com-munication

195

- family members learn about the problems associated with hearing loss

- both may learn some simple ways to improve communication.

Periodic follow-up appointments with the audiologist are necessary to ensure consistent use and independent care of the hearing aid; to monitor changes in the client's communication abilities; and to monitor social, emotional, and psychological factors related to hearing loss and hearing aid use. If indicated, an audiologist may refer the client for further counseling support in therapy sessions conducted by a psychiatrist, psychologist, or trained social worker.

Communication Tips

Having learned what the audiologist can do to improve communication for the older client with a hearing loss, how can you help? There are no mysterious strategies or magical techniques involved in helping the older person with a hearing loss communicate more efficiently and comfortably in one-to-one situations. The following list of tips includes many things that seem too obvious to mention, but are easily overlooked. They should make communicating easier and less stressful.

When talking to a person with a hearing loss:

- Wait until the person can see you before speaking. If necessary, touch the person to get attention.

- Never speak directly into the person's ear. This may distort your message and hide all visual cues (i.e., your facial expressions).

- Try to position yourself about 3 to 6 feet from the person when speaking, not up too close.

- Speak slightly louder than normal, but don't shout. Remember that shouting won't make your message any clearer, and may distort it.

- Speak at your normal rate.

- Avoid chewing, eating, or covering your mouth with your hands while speaking.

- Do not exaggerate sounds when speaking. This distorts the message and makes it hard to "read" visual cues from your facial expression.

- Clue the hard of hearing person about the conversation topic whenever possible.

- Rephrase your statement into shorter, simpler sentences if you suspect you are not being understood. Don't keep repeating the same statement if it's not getting through.

Consider the communication environment:

- Arrange the room so that the speaker's face and body can be easily seen.

- Be aware of lighting. Good lighting on the face of the speaker is important. It allows the deaf or hard of hearing person to monitor the facial expressions, gestures, and lip and body movements that provide communication clues.

- Try to reduce any competing or background noises. They hinder communication.

- Encourage the person with a hearing loss to participate in group activities and expand social communication.

- Be sensitive to the fact that hearing loss in older people often affects the higher frequencies. It may be more difficult for your client to understand the higher-pitched voices of women and children.

Finally, be aware of assistive devices.

- If you know that someone has a hearing aid and is not using it, encourage its use.

- If the hearing aid isn't working, refer the person to an audiologist.

- Encourage routine audiological evaluations.

- If appropriate, attend audiologic rehabilitation classes with the older hard of hearing person.

- If needed, assist the person with the hearing aid or other assistive device by learning to change the battery, clean the earpiece, and help with other maintenance procedures.

- Encourage the person to have an assistive devices evaluation at an assistive devices center.

Summary

Hearing loss is a common disorder associated with aging. We can expect hearing loss to be a prominent problem in the future as the number of older adults increases. People working with this population must understand how to identify symptoms of hearing loss, how to get help for deaf or hard of hearing individuals, what options are available to improve the person's environment and communication events, and how to provide support and understanding to increase the quality of the person's life and foster independent living.

Some Thoughts on Communication and the Older Person With a Hearing Loss

In our society, the older person experiences serious reductions in communication. Consider the older person living in a nursing home environment. According to one study of spoken communication conducted in a nursing home, 83 percent of the residents felt that they talked very little with other residents, yet 80 percent indicated that they enjoyed talking, especially with friendly, intelligent partners (Lubinski, Morrison, and Rigrodsky, 1981). Reseachers commonly heard residents say, "But there's no one like me here to talk to."

The research went on to show that language usage is influenced by the environment in which it occurs. In the nursing home environment, the residents perceived many implicit and explicit "rules" about communication. For example, they felt that the staff were "too busy to talk." While they indicated talking most often in public places like auditoriums, halls, and movies, they also said they avoided talking in those places because, "A lot of things get around here to the supervisors" or "The best thing is to keep quiet and keep out of trouble."

But it is not only the older person in the nursing home environment who experiences serious reductions in communication. Many barriers to effective communication exist for the aging person in the community. Researchers have found that, like the nursing home staff, community members give the impression that they are "too busy too talk" (Waugh, Thomas, and Fozard, 1978; Eysenck, 1975). These reductions in communication mean a reduction in the quality of life for the older person.

The older adult with a hearing loss is hit by a double whammy— the typical lack of communication experienced by older adults plus the communication breakdown from hearing loss. Most people, even if they take the time to communicate with an older friend or neighbor, do not know how to improve communication through gestures, repetition, and similar strategies.

While in recent years society has made some environmental adjustments to improve the quality of life for older people with disabilities, relatively little attention has been given to the speech and language needs of the hard of hearing members of the community. The "invisibility" of hearing loss helps contribute both to a deepening lack of communication for the older person and to a lack of attention to the possibilities for enhancing communication. Unlike many physical handicaps, unless an individual is wearing a hearing aid, a hearing loss may go unnoticed. (And remember, in some cases, hearing aids are of no benefit to particular individuals.) As a result, reactions of the general public to the older person with a hearing loss may be insensitive. For example, you would probably readily assist a physically disabled person across a busy street, or read the fine print of a bus schedule aloud to a visually impaired person. However, when communicating with someone whom you do not "see" as disabled—someone whose hearing loss is unknown to you—you may tend toward being impatient or intolerant. Continually meeting with this sort of communication rebuff can, understandably, lead the older person with a hearing loss toward further isolation. Further exacerbated by repeated misunderstanding and the growing perception of being excluded from communication, the individual's isolation may progress to a state of complete withdrawal and a lack of desire for continued living.

The implications of reduced communication extend to areas other than the psychological, since effective communication is necessary for older people to maintain physical independence. Research has shown that the aged individuals most likely to be placed in nursing homes and chronic disease institutions are "not the incontinent or bedridden . . . but the older family member with a hearing or speech deficit of proportion sufficient to make communication decidedly difficult," (Howell, 1971). If the older person needs physical assistance, some workable communication system must exist to allow the person to obtain the needed help. Even if support networks exist to monitor and assist the older person living in the noninstitutional setting, the older person must be able to provide information on how others can assist with everyday functioning in such areas as self-care, mobility, safety, and pain control.

It is important to consider in this context those devices that have broadened communication opportunities for deaf and hard of hearing people in our society and which may enhance both the psychological and physical independence of older adults with hearing loss. Such relatively recent innovations as TDDs (telecommunications devices for deaf people), amplified telephones, and captioned TV, for example, make possible access to various communication resources. However, these devices, when they are available, assist only a small segment of the population with hearing loss: those who are deaf and those who can benefit from the use of a hearing aid.

The remainder of people with hearing loss—both in the community and in the institutional setting—must fend for themselves at meetings, movies, church services, and other social situations. As more assistive listening devices and systems enter the market, and as more people become aware of their availability and potential, the hope is that the number of people benefiting will also increase.

The ability to communicate is vital to the psychological and physical independence of older adults. Helping to maintain that ability in adults with hearing loss will be an important goal for everyone who is involved in working with this population.

References

Eysenck, M.W. (1975). "Retrieval from Semantic Memory as a Function of Age." *Journal of Gerontology*, 30, 174–180.

Howell, S. (1971). "Advocates for the Elderly: A Contribution to the Reshaping of the Professional Image." *Hearing and Speech News*, 39(6), 7–9.

Lubinski, R., Morrison, E.B., & Rigrodsky, S. (1981). "Perception of Spoken Communication by Elderly Chronically Ill Patients in an Institutional Setting." *Journal of Speech and Hearing Disorders*, 46, 405–412.

U.S. Bureau of the Census. (1983). "Provisional Projections of the Population of States, by Age and Sex: 1980 to 2000." *Current Population Reports Series P-25 No. 937*. Washington, DC: U.S. Government Printing Office.

Waugh, N.D., Thomas, J.C., & Fozard, J.L. (1978). "Retrieval Time from Different Memory Stores." *Journal of Gerontology*, 33, 718-724

Suggested Readings

American Speech-Language-Hearing Association. (1979). "Communication Problems and Behaviors of the Older American." Rockville, MD.

American Speech-Language-Hearing Association. (1985) *Gerontology and Communication Disorders*. Rockville, MD.

American Speech-Language-Hearing Association/Gallaudet University. (1989). *When Hearing Fades: Community Health Center Responses to Hearing Loss in Elderly Clients*. Rockville, MD.

Lubinski, R.B. (1978-1979). "Why So Little Interest in Whether or Not Old People Talk: A Review of Recent Research on Verbal Communication among the Elderly." *International Journal of Aging and Human Development*, 9, 237-245.

Mueller, H.G. & Geoffrey, V.C., (Eds.) (1987). *Communication Disorders in Aging*. Washington, DC: Gallaudet University Press.

National Institute of Neurological Disease and Stroke. (1982). *Hearing Loss: Hope Through Research* (NIH Publication No. 82-157). Washington, DC: U.S. Government Printing Office.

Rupp, R. (1977). "The Roles of the Audiologist." *Journal of the Academy of Rehabilitation Audiology*, 10(1), 10-17.

U.S. Congress, Office of Technology Assessment. (1986). *Hearing Impairment and Elderly People: A Background Paper* (OTABP-A-30). Washington, DC: U.S. Government Printing Office.

Additional Resources

American Speech-Language-Hearing Association (ASHA)
10801 Rockville Pike
Rockville, MD 20852
(301) 897-5700 Voice/TDD
(800) 638-8255 Voice/TDD HELPLINE

ASHA provides public information about communication disorders, including deafness, and the role of speech and hearing professionals in rehabilitation. Information about local direct services is also available through this organization.

National Information Center on Deafness
Gallaudet University
800 Florida Avenue NE
Washington, DC 20002-3695
(202) 651-5051 Voice
(202) 651-5052 TDD

NICD serves as a centralized source of up-to-date, objective information on topics dealing with deafness and hearing loss. NICD collects, develops, and disseminates information about all aspects of hearing loss and services offered to deaf and hard of hearing people across the nation. It also provides information about Gallaudet University.

—by Peggy S. Williams, Ph.D.
Deputy Executive Director
American Speech-Language-Hearing Association
with the assistance of Joanne J. Weiner, M.A.
Director, Member/Staff Information Division
American Speech-Language-Hearing Association
Rockville, MD

Chapter 24

Cholesteatoma:
A Serious Ear Condition

- What is a cholesteatoma?
- Why did it occur in the ear?
- How does it occur?
- How is it dangerous?
- When should something be done about it?
- If nothing is done, what can happen?
- Will I always have this problem?
- Can it be removed or cured?

What is a cholesteatoma?

A cholesteatoma is a skin growth that occurs in an abnormal location, the middle ear behind the eardrum. It is usually due to repeated infection which causes an ingrowth of the skin of the eardrum. Cholesteatomas often take the form of a cyst or pouch which sheds layers of old skin that builds up inside the ear. Over time, the cholesteatoma can increase in size and destroy the surrounding delicate bones of the middle ear. Hearing loss, dizziness, and facial muscle paralysis are rare but can result from continued cholesteatoma growth.

How does it occur?

A cholesteatoma usually occurs because of poor eustachian tube function as well as infection in the middle ear. The eustachian tube conveys air from the back of the nose into the middle ear to equalize ear pressure ("clear the ears"). When the eustachian tubes work poorly, perhaps due to allergy, a cold or sinusitis, the air in the middle ear is absorbed by the body, and a partial vacuum results in the ear. The vacuum pressure sucks in a pouch or sac by stretching the eardrum, especially areas weakened by previous infections. This sac often becomes a cholesteatoma. A rare congenital form of cholesteatoma (one present at birth) can occur in the middle ear and elsewhere, such as in the nearby skull bones. However, the type of cholesteatoma associated with ear infections is most common.

What are the symptoms?

Initially, the ear may drain, sometimes with a foul odor. As the cholesteatoma pouch or sac enlarges, it can cause *a full feeling or pressure* in the ear, along with *hearing loss*. (An ache *behind or in* the ear, especially at night, may cause significant discomfort.) Dizziness, or muscle weakness on one side of the face (the side of the infected ear) can also occur. Any, or all, of these symptoms are good reasons to seek medical evaluation.

Is it dangerous?

Ear cholesteatomas can be dangerous and should never be ignored. Bone erosion can cause the infection to spread into the surrounding areas, including the inner ear and brain. If untreated, deafness, brain abscess, meningitis, and rarely death can occur.

What treatment can be provided?

An examination by an otolaryngologist–head and neck surgeon can confirm the presence of a cholesteatoma. Initial treatment may consist of a careful cleaning of the ear, antibiotics, and ear drops. Therapy aims to stop drainage in the ear by controlling the infection.

The extent or growth characteristics of a cholesteatoma must also be evaluated.

Large or complicated cholesteatomas usually require surgical treatment to protect the patient from serious complications. Hearing and balance tests, x-rays of the mastoid (the skull bone next to the ear), and CAT scans (3-D x-rays) of the mastoid may be necessary. These tests are performed to determine the hearing level remaining in the ear and the extent of destruction the cholesteatoma has caused.

Surgery is performed under general anesthesia in most cases. The primary purpose of the surgery is to remove the cholesteatoma and infection and achieve an infection-free, dry ear. Hearing preservation or restoration is the second goal of surgery. In cases of severe ear destruction, reconstruction may not be possible. Facial nerve repair or procedures to control dizziness are rarely required. Reconstruction of the middle ear is not always possible in one operation; and therefore, a second operation may be performed six to twelve months later. The second operation will attempt to restore hearing and, at the same time, inspect the middle ear space and mastoid for residual cholesteatoma. Admission to the hospital is usually done the morning of surgery, and if the surgery is performed early in the morning, discharge may be the same day. For some patients, an overnight stay is necessary. In rare cases of serious infection, prolonged hospitalization for antibiotic treatment may be necessary. Time off from work is typically one to two weeks.

Follow-up office visits after surgical treatment are necessary and important, because cholesteatoma sometimes recurs. In cases where an open mastoidectomy cavity has been created, office visits every few months are needed in order to clean out the mastoid cavity and prevent new infections. In some patients, there must be lifelong periodic ear examinations.

Summary

Cholesteatoma is a serious but treatable ear condition which can only be diagnosed by medical examination. Persisting earache, ear drainage, ear pressure, hearing loss, dizziness, or facial muscle weakness signals the need for evaluation by an otolaryngologist–head and neck surgeon.

What Is Otolaryngology–Head and Neck Surgery?

Otolaryngology–head and neck surgery is a specialty concerned with medical treatment and surgery of the ear, nose, throat and related structures of the head and neck. The specialty encompasses cosmetic facial reconstruction, surgery of benign and malignant tumors of the head and neck, management of patients with loss of hearing and balance, endoscopic examination of air and food passages and treatment of allergic, sinus, laryngeal, thyroid and esophageal disorders.

To qualify for the American Board of Otolaryngology certification examination, a physician must complete five or more years of post–M.D. (or D.O.) specialty training.

Chapter 25

Perforated Eardrum

Causes of Eardrum Perforation

The causes of perforated eardrum are usually from trauma or infection. Some circumstances in which a perforated eardrum can occur include:

- if the ear is struck squarely with an open hand
- with a skull fracture
- after a sudden explosion
- if an object (such as a bobby pin, Q-tip, or stick) is pushed too far into the ear canal
- as a result of hot slag (from welding) or acid entering the ear canal.

Middle ear infections may cause pain, hearing loss and spontaneous rupture (tear) of the eardrum resulting in a perforation. In this circumstance, there may be infected or bloody drainage from the ear. In medical terms, this is called otitis media with perforation.

On rare occasions a small hole may remain in the eardrum after a previously placed PE tube (pressure equalizing) either falls out or is removed by the physician.

Most eardrum perforations heal spontaneously within weeks after rupture, although some may take up to several months. During the healing process the ear must be protected from water and trauma. Those eardrum perforations which do not heal on their own may require surgery.

Effects on Hearing from Perforated Eardrum

Usually, the larger the perforation, the greater the loss of hearing. The location of the hole (perforation) in the eardrum also effects the degree of hearing loss. If severe trauma (e.g. skull fracture) disrupts the bones in the middle ear which transmit sound or causes injury to the inner ear structures, the loss of hearing may be quite severe.

If the perforated eardrum is due to a sudden traumatic or explosive event, the loss of hearing can be great and ringing in the ear (tinnitus) may be severe. In this case the hearing usually returns partially, and the ringing diminishes in a few days. Chronic infection as a result of the perforation can cause major hearing loss.

Treatment of the Perforated Eardrum

Before attempting any correction of the perforation, a hearing test should be performed. The benefits of closing a perforation include prevention of water entering the ear while showering, bathing or swimming (which could cause ear infection), improved hearing, and diminished tinnitus. It also may prevent the development of cholesteatoma (skin cyst in the middle ear), which can cause chronic infection and destruction of ear structures.

If the perforation is very small, otolaryngologists may choose to observe the perforation over time to see if it will close spontaneously. They also might try to patch a cooperative patient's eardrum in the office. Working with a microscope, your doctor may touch the edges of the eardrum with a chemical to stimulate growth and then place a thin paper patch on the eardrum. Usually with closure of the tympanic membrane improvement in hearing is noted. Several applications of a patch (up to three or four) may be required before the perforation closes completely. If your physician feels that a paper patch will not provide prompt or adequate closure of the hole in the eardrum, or attempts with paper patching do not promote healing, surgery is considered.

There are a variety of surgical techniques, but all basically place tissue across the perforation allowing healing. The name of this procedure is called tympanoplasty. Surgery is typically quite successful in closing the perforation permanently, and improving hearing. It is usually done on an outpatient basis.

Your doctor will advise you regarding the proper management of a perforated eardrum.

What Is Otolaryngology–Head and Neck Surgery?

Otolaryngology–head and neck surgery is a specialty concerned with the medical and surgical treatment of the ears, nose, throat and related structures of the head and neck. The specialty encompasses cosmetic facial reconstruction, surgery of benign and malignant tumors of the head and neck, management of patients with loss of hearing and balance, endoscopic examination of air and food passages and treatment of allergic, sinus, laryngeal, thyroid and esophageal disorders.

To qualify for the American Board of Otolaryngology certification examination, a physician must complete five or more years of post–M.D. (or D.O.) specialty training.

Chapter 26

Barotrauma

Barotrauma, also referred to as aero-otitis, is the result of injury to the middle ear caused by a significant difference between air pressure in the middle ear and the atmospheric pressure surrounding it. This difference can occur during high diving or skin diving, during travel on airplanes or submarines, while working in tunnels, and at high altitudes in the mountains.

Barotrauma occurs when the Eustachian tube (the tube that connects the middle ear to the back of the throat) does not open and close freely during changes in air pressure, usually in the presence of a cold. Colds inflame the tissue at the mouth of the Eustachian tube and prevent it from opening and closing properly. At higher altitudes, the middle ear contains less air than at lower altitudes where the surrounding outside pressure is greater and the air is more dense. Under normal circumstances, as the atmospheric pressure increases during descent, more air enters the middle ear through the Eustachian tube and equalizes the air pressure in the middle ear to atmospheric pressure. If air does not enter, the difference in pressure between the outside and the middle ear builds up, forces the eardrum inward, and results in pain. Sometimes, clear fluid collects in the middle ear.

Depending on the amount and location of damage, hearing loss may be temporary or permanent, greater in the high or low frequencies, may fluctuate or remain stable, and range in severity. Some

This article was originally published by the American Speech-Language-Hearing Association in *Let's Talk*, No. 45. Used by permission.

people also experience dizziness and tinnitus (ringing, humming, or buzzing sounds).

The best way to avoid barotrauma is to avoid activities that may result in significant air pressure changes when you have a cold. If you cannot avoid such activity, try to open and close your Eustachian tube as often as possible during pressure changes. Continuous swallowing, chewing gum, drinking, yawning, moving the jaw around, and pinching the nostrils closed while blowing will force the Eustachian tube open. Referral to a physician may be needed for medication such as inhalants, antihistamines, or decongestants to reduce inflammation around the Eustachian tube and fluid in the middle ear space.

Chapter 27

Questions and Answers: Otosclerosis

What is otosclerosis?

Otosclerosis is a disorder of the middle ear that causes conductive progressive hearing loss, found in approximately one of every 200 persons. It occurs when bony deposits cause the stapes footplate (the innermost bone of the middle ear) to become fixed or immobilized. When this happens, sound vibrations cannot be passed to the inner ear, resulting in conductive hearing loss. In addition, the bone around the stapes becomes spongy. Some sensorineural deafness caused by damage spreading to the inner ear may eventually occur. It is common for both ears to be affected.

What is the cause?

Despite a great amount of research, otosclerosis is not yet fully understood. We do know that more than 50% of patients have a family history of the disorder. It is most often seen in Whites, found less frequently among Chinese, and is very rare among Blacks. More common among females, otosclerosis symptoms may begin, or be worsened by pregnancy.

Along with these factors, other plausible theories as to the cause include an alkaline phosphatase or an enzyme deficiency. A study at

This article was originally published in the House Ear Institute's *Review*, Summer 1993.

HEI suggests a connection between viral infection and otosclerosis, which is interesting, since the numbers of patients with otosclerosis have declined.

What are the symptoms of otosclerosis?

Patients may complain of ear discomfort or tinnitus, a sensation of sound in the affected ear that occurs in about 80% of patients. The onset of otosclerosis frequently begins in a person's third to fifth decade.

How is the diagnosis made?

The otologist begins with a thorough history to review ear disease, history of head injury, hearing loss among family members, and exposure to noise. Secondly, an examination of the ear, along with simple tests, determines whether the hearing loss is conductive or sensorineural. A complete audiometric evaluation is performed by an audiologist to determine the degree of hearing loss.

What forms of treatment are available?

The majority of patients with conductive deafness caused by otosclerosis can be treated with a stapedectomy, an outpatient procedure performed under local anesthesia. This surgery has a success rate of 90 to 95%. The surgery involves removal of the stapes bone and reconstruction of that sound-conducting mechanism with a prosthesis. If the hearing loss is severe and involves the hearing nerve, the surgery may not completely restore hearing, but does improve it so that the patient may gain better use of a hearing aid. Patients usually return to work about a week after the stapedectomy.

Patients who are not candidates for stapes surgery may be helped with a properly fitted hearing aid. The patient should be evaluated by an audiologist to determine how much benefit will be derived from amplification.

To prevent further nerve loss due to otosclerosis, sodium fluoride and calcium therapy may be prescribed. This medication causes the disorder to go into an "inactive" phase.

What current research work at HEI will add to our knowledge about otosclerosis?

Thanks to the foresight of Howard House, M.D., and our past patients who thought enough of future generations, we have been able to establish our temporal bone histopathology collection. Many of those patients had otosclerosis. By looking at their clinical records, surgical reports and audiograms, we are able to determine what factors were present that allowed them to benefit or not benefit from surgery. Many of the advances in otosclerosis treatment have been the direct result of this ongoing research. With new techniques in analyzing temporal bones, such as immunohistochemistry, we can go back to the bones and re-evaluate them based on new knowledge.

An example of this type of research is work that was done by one of our fellows, Mike McKenna, M.D. He was able to identify some viral particles in the otosclerotic focus. This research has led to the theory of a virus as the possible cause of otosclerosis. We are also learning more about the genetics of otosclerosis and will attempt to identify the gene responsible for it.

Our major advances and research have been in the surgical management of otosclerosis. The focus is on improving technique in order to reduce the incidence of further hearing loss or dizziness as a result of surgery. Now the techniques are refined to the point that patients are going home on the day of surgery and the success rate of improving hearing is greater than 90%. In order to continue to make these advances, it is important for the physicians of the House Ear Clinic to work closely with the researchers at the House Ear Institute.

—by John House, M.D.
HEI President and Medical Advisor

Chapter 28

Cochlear Implants

Since the development of cochlear implants in the 1960s, more than 3,000 persons—children and adults—have been implanted with a variety of these devices. Controversy exists on several issues, including determination of appropriate candidates, selection of a single-channel or multichannel device, suitable preimplantation and post-implantation assessments, and rehabilitation procedures.

Some reports have claimed a spectacular return of hearing in deaf persons with cochlear implants. Unfortunately, to date, no person can be documented to have had normal hearing restored by this device. On the other hand, the cochlear implant does provide significant benefits for some in a variety of ways.

Currently, we do not have the degree of understanding of disease mechanisms and disorders of function for hearing disorders that is common to other human organs and functions. This is partly because the organ of hearing is encased in bone and cannot be visualized during life. In addition, there are only limited numbers of qualified laboratories and scientists to prepare and evaluate specimens obtained after death. These methods are the essentials by which great strides have been made for disorders of other organs and systems.

Further, in our efforts regarding disorders of communication, particularly those related to language, we must not discount possibilities of new medical, surgical, and technological methods.

National Institutes of Health Consensus Development Conference Statement; Volume 7, Number 2; May 4, 1988.

The charge of this panel, however, is appropriately restricted to the development of a consensus regarding five questions related to cochlear implants. These are addressed separately for adults and children because of special considerations necessary for the developing child. (A section on special considerations for children follows the fourth question.)

- Who is a suitable candidate for a cochlear implant?
- What are the advantages and disadvantages of the different types of cochlear implants?
- How effective are cochlear implants?
- What are the risks and limitations of cochlear implantation?
- What are the special considerations for children?
- What are the important directions for future research?

To address these questions the National Institute of Neurological and Communicative Disorders and Stroke and the Office of Medical Applications of Research of the National Institutes of Health convened a Consensus Development Conference on Cochlear Implants on May 24, 1988. Cosponsors of the conference were the National Institute on Aging and the National Institute of Child Health and Human Development of the National Institutes of Health, the Food and Drug Administration, and the Veterans Administration. After a day and a half of presentations by experts and discussion by the audience, a consensus panel drawn from specialists and generalists from the medical profession and related scientific disciplines, clinical investigators, and public representatives considered the evidence and came to the following conclusions.

1. Who Is a Suitable Candidate for a Cochlear Implant?

Of the 15 million persons in the United States with significant hearing impairment, less than 1 percent are potential candidates for a cochlear implant. The selection of a specific person for a cochlear implant is not straightforward. There are no strict standardized criteria for accepting or rejecting a candidate. Traditionally, the cochlear implant subject has been a postlingually deafened adult who met certain audiological, medical, and psychological criteria, which differed partially from one implant team to the next. In general, it was considered crucial that the subject show no residual hearing (total hearing loss) and no significant benefit from a conventional hearing aid. These seemingly straightforward criteria did not always work well in practice, and there emerged different definitions of "residual hearing" and "significant benefit from a hearing aid." Needs and wishes of individual subjects are also significant variables for implant candidacy. Finally, the issue of candidacy is further complicated because it has not been possible, preoperatively, to predict success with a cochlear implant in a specific person.

Recognizing the uncertainty about the operational meaning of "residual hearing" and "successful hearing aid use," potential conflicts between subjects' wishes and objective criteria, and the absence of prognostic tools with regard to specific implants, the following discussion attempts to specify characteristics of adults who are potential users of cochlear implants. Because of the lack of data predicting the success of implants, the following stringent criteria are suggested:

- **Audiological Criteria.** Indications in favor of an implant are a profound sensorineural hearing loss bilaterally, aided thresholds greater than 60 dB HL, 0 percent correct on open-set speech recognition, and a lack of substantial increase in lipreading with an appropriately fitted hearing aid.

- **Electrophysiological Criteria.** Measurement of electrical auditory brainstem responses as well as of middle and long-latency evoked potentials should be a basic component in candidate selection. The absence of neural responses to electrical stimulation may or may not prove to be a contraindication.

- **Medical Surgical Criteria.** The usual candidate is a healthy, postlingually deafened adult. The medical history, physical examination, and laboratory tests are used to include or exclude candidates and to assist the implant team in planning a total program, including auditory training.

  There are a number of possible complicating factors, including anatomical features, that affect implantation of the device: previous stapedectomy, temporal bone fractures, ossification of the cochlea, and congenital anomalies such as absence of the cochlea or auditory nerve. The question of

219

candidacy should be reevaluated after preexisting ear problems such as eustachian tube dysfunction, chronic ear disease, and cholesteatoma have been treated.

- **Psychophysical Criteria.** Although a number of psychophysical data are available on implant subjects (temporal integration, gap detection, forward masking, pitch, loudness), none are considered critical in the candidacy issue. Rather, psychophysical data are critical to issues of efficacy and implant design. To date, preoperative psychophysical performance has not been a good predictor of speech recognition performance.

- **Psychological and Linguistic Criteria.** With respect to candidacy, most psychological testing is done for exclusionary reasons, usually mental retardation and psychiatric disorders.

The Issue of New Criteria for Cochlear Implant Candidacy

The field of cochlear implantation is changing rapidly, particularly technology, assessment procedures, and the significant firsthand experience by several groups of dedicated clinical investigators. One major result, which seems particularly noticeable as multichannel implants become more common, is exceptional performance by a small percentage of implantees on open-set tests of speech recognition. These results are truly encouraging and raise theoretical and practical questions. One theoretical question is "What is the upper limit on performance by cochlear implantees on open-set tests of speech recognition?" A practical question concerns the possibility for revising the criteria for candidacy.

Consider the following example. A subject obtains open-set performance of 10 percent with a conventional hearing aid, and the expected (mean or median) performance for similar subjects with a particular implant is 38 percent. Is the subject a suitable implant candidate? This question has several important ramifications. Revision of current criteria should be considered only after a rigorously controlled trial with a small, select group of persons has been completed. Such rigor is required because of the unpredictability of success with an implant and the possibility of decreased performance in persons who have measurable preoperative open-set speech recognition.

2. What are the advantages and disadvantages of the different types of cochlear implants?

Cochlear implants can be categorized in at least three important ways. Electrodes may be inserted either within the cochlea **(intracochlear)** or placed outside the cochlea **(extracochlear)**; the signals may be transmitted through either one channel **(single channel)** or several independent channels (multichannel); and only certain features of the speech signal may be transmitted **(feature extraction)**, or the input signal may be transmitted to the electrodes without extracting specific speech cues **(non-feature specific)**. These methods of categorization are the most important.

Cochlear implants also may be categorized according to the types of electrodes used (e.g., monopolar, bipolar), method of stimulation (e.g., pulsatile, continuous), or signal transmission through the skin by wires (using a percutaneous plug) or by electromagnetic means.

In an extracochlear implant, the electrodes may be attached to the round window niche or, in some cases, to the promontory. Single-channel stimulation is more common in this form of implant. In an intracochlear implant, an electrode or electrode array is inserted into the cochlea. For multichannel operation, the electrode array is usually inserted quite deeply into the cochlea (toward the apex), whereas for single-channel operation, a short single-channel electrode that does not extend beyond the first bend in the cochlea can be used. Multiple electrode arrays have been developed with as many as 22 electrodes that can be stimulated independently. Speech-feature processing typically involves extraction of the voice-fundamental frequency, format frequencies, and determination of whether the speech sound is voiced or voiceless. In non-feature-specific processing, the signals are usually transmitted directly to the electrodes without radical transformation. In a multichannel system of this type, known as a filter-bank system, signals in different frequency bands are transmitted separately to different electrodes.

Extracochlear stimulation, in contrast to intracochlear stimulation, has the advantage that the procedure does not invade the cochlea and is reversible. The disadvantages of extracochlear stimulation are narrower dynamic range, higher current density, and, concomitantly, a greater potential for stimulating other neural tissue, possibly resulting in facial nerve stimulation or vertigo. An additional concern is maintaining long-term contact between the external electrode and the round window or promontory.

The major advantages of intracochlear stimulation are relative ease of placement (particularly for short electrodes), closer proximity to neural structures, potential for lower current density, wider dynamic range, and more convenient tonotopic stimulation. The potential disadvantages of intracochlear stimulation include the usual hazards of surgery, insertion trauma, the possibility of mechanical damage to the cochlea, osteoneogenesis, possible release of ototoxic corrosion products, and the difficulty of replacing the device, should the need arise.

Several of the above disadvantages are reduced by the use of a short, single-channel electrode. There is, however, no general agreement as to the relative advantages of using short electrodes.

Multichannel stimulation has the advantage that information can be transmitted in a form that is easier for the user to understand. Because of interactions between the stimuli of electrodes activated simultaneously, the number of effective independent channels may be reduced. Feature-extraction systems are predicated on the assumption that certain aspects of the speech signal can be identified as being especially important and that these features can be transmitted effectively to the electrode array. Feature-extraction systems have the advantages of reducing interelectrode interference and, if the preceding assumption is correct, simplifying the understanding of signals received from the implant. A disadvantage of feature-extraction systems is that of possible errors in the estimation of speech parameters.

The current evidence suggests that multichannel intracochlear stimulation produces superior speech-recognition performance compared with single-channel stimulation. However, interpretation of the present data is complicated by differences in subject selection procedures among research groups and the lack of a common body of standardized tests. Speech-recognition performance is similar for single-channel intracochlear implants in comparison with single-channel extracochlear implants, and for multichannel feature-extraction implants in comparison with non-feature-specific filter-bank-type implants.

3. How effective are cochlear implants?

Few medical interventions yield outcomes as varied as those for cochlear implantation. Though no persons with implants can be said to have their hearing fully restored, some communicate face-to-face with comparative ease, and even a few (about 5 percent) can carry on normal conversation without lipreading. The most common outcome is some improvement in speechreading ability. On the other hand, some persons with implants can barely distinguish between simple environmental sounds such as car traffic and the doorbell. Different studies report an appreciable number of persons with implants (2 to 15 percent) who may choose to discontinue the use of their prostheses. Despite the variability of these results, a large majority of persons welcome their implants, a reaction that is understandable and testifies to their strong desire to maintain or achieve some awareness of sound stimulation.

Variability in results arises partly because of differences among the implanted persons. Although all suffer profound hearing difficulties, the medical, linguistic, and psychological histories, as well as general cognitive skills, differ widely among them. In addition to these factors, the condition of the peripheral and central auditory system, both before and after surgery, is often impossible to assess with any accuracy. Finally, the efficacy of implantation is difficult to assess because of the variety of different procedures and tests used for this purpose. There are simply no standardized procedures presently available for such evaluation, although their presence would materially increase research progress in this field.

All of these reasons make it impossible to predict with any degree of accuracy the outcome for a particular person. However, despite these uncertainties, the available evidence suggests the following broad generalizations:

- Speechreading is nearly always facilitated when using the implant, either of the single-channel or multichannel variety.

- Persons who have previously acquired language skills and have experienced hearing seem to benefit more from the implant than those without these characteristics.

- The bulk of the evidence from the United States suggests that speech recognition performance is superior in multichannel implants compared with single-channel implants. This generalization needs to be qualified somewhat. (See Question 2 on

223

Advantages and Disadvantages of Different Types of Cochlear Implants.)

- The process of cochlear implantation represents a major change in the person's life. A strong interdisciplinary rehabilitation team provides a prudent support system to aid in this difficult transition. Consulting and counseling the person with an implant and his or her family, coupled with a training program of aural rehabilitation, facilitates the maximal use of the implant.

- There is convincing evidence of improved speech production in some implanted persons.

4. What are the risks and limitations of cochlear implantation?

Risks

Medical complications include all of the risks associated with surgery conducted under general anesthesia. These are small but finite for persons in good general health but increase with age and other confounding conditions.

The surgery for placement of the implant may traumatize the cochlear endosteum and initiate new bone growth, which has the potential for damaging surviving neural elements and for complicating any replacements of the device. There is no present evidence to suggest that there is an increase in the spread of infection from the middle ear to the inner ear caused by implanting the device. There is, however, a risk of postsurgical infection at the site of the skin flap behind the ear and of a failure of the flap to heal normally, which could necessitate removal of the device. The operation also may damage the facial nerve or the vestibular system. Most cases of postimplant facial nerve paralysis and vestibular symptoms appear to have been transient. However, data on vestibular effects of implants have only been obtained from individuals with intact visual and proprioceptive systems. More data are necessary to evaluate risks of total incapacitation that could potentially result from complications of implantation in a unilaterally functioning labyrinth in a person with other sensory deficits. Passage of current through the implant at levels necessary for auditory stimulation may cause stimulation of the facial nerve. Data suggest that current in the implant is unlikely to produce vestibular symptoms. Placement of the implant may cause a reduction in tinnitus in some individuals but also may cause an increase in a smaller percentage of persons with implants.

Use of the implant may interfere with the use of residual hearing cues from the other ear or other modalities. The need for replacement surgery after equipment failure or for upgrading to another device exposes the person with an implant to the same risks and has the potential to cause the same damage as the initial operation.

Although there are encouraging data suggesting that corrosion of platinum electrodes used for 3 years was minimal, the effects of current passage and solubilization of metal from the electrode tip in the fluid medium of the scala tympani of the cochlea have the potential for deleterious effects on surviving neural elements. More data are necessary to evaluate these risks. Similarly, more data are needed to evaluate the potential deleterious effects of low currents used over long time periods or of local heating effects due to high current densities as could be generated by alternative implant designs.

Finally, there is a possibility of psychological problems developing for the person with an implant and/or his or her family because of unrealistic expectations about improvements related to implant use.

Limitations

The effective use of cochlear implants is limited by a number of considerations. Some disease processes associated with hearing loss cause changes in the temporal bone that may prevent or compromise the appropriate insertion of the device. Chief among these are congenital malformations, whose anatomy increases the difficulty of inserting the electrode array in proximity to the neural elements to be stimulated, and osteoneogenesis secondary to meningitis, suppurative otitis media, and obliterative otosclerosis, which may obscure the round window niche and make it difficult to insert the electrode. Previous otologic trauma or surgery may result in fibrosis and osteoneogenesis, which produce the same difficulties. Another concern with hearing loss caused by meningitis is the small number of patients who spontaneously recover hearing. Because implantation may destroy cochlear structures necessary for normal hearing, there is a need to balance waiting a suitable interval to ensure that spontaneous recovery does not occur and placing an implant before osteoneogenesis has obliterated the cochlea.

Some candidates for implantation with congenital malformations may not be suitable because of increased difficulty of accurate electrode placement and increased likelihood of damage to the neural elements, the facial nerve, and endosteum. Some congenitally deaf adults also may be inappropriate candidates for implants because of psychological commitments to the deaf world and nonauditory communication modes.

Placement of an implant also limits the ability of the implantee in several activities. All persons with implants need to avoid activities that could physically damage or displace the implant (e.g., boxing or contact sports). Several medical tests and treatments are incompatible with preservation of implant function, including the use of magnetic resonance imaging (MRI), electrocautery near the implant, and diathermy and radiation therapy of the implant area.

It is not yet clear what minimum neural elements must be present for effective transmission of the electrical signal, although absence of all spiral ganglion cells and all auditory nerve fibers precludes success.

Special Considerations for Children

At the present time, cochlear implants for children are classified by the FDA as investigational devices. A minimal age limit of 2 years may be appropriate for cochlear implant candidacy for anatomic and neurodevelopmental reasons. In principle, the same criteria that apply to adults apply to children, whenever possible. It is recommended that hearing loss in children be corroborated with both behavioral and electrophysiological techniques. Indications in favor of an implant are profound sensorineural hearing loss bilaterally and aided thresholds greater than 60 dB HL, with confirmation of test/retest reliability.

A minimum of a 6-month trial with appropriate amplification and rehabilitation is recommended, with the addition of a trial for a tactile aid. The latter is recommended so that children may learn stimulus/response associations that will be useful in the later evaluation of a cochlear implant. It is suggested that the criterion for lack of success with a hearing aid in younger children be the failure to improve on a closed-set task of simple pattern perception. This observation should be corroborated with subjective reports from parents and others for younger children. Adult criteria may be applied to older children. As with the adult subjects, the a priori prediction of success with a cochlear implant for a particular child does not appear possible at this time.

The loss of even minimal residual hearing has far more serious consequences for a child in the language and speech acquisition process than it has for an adult. For this reason, greater caution is recommended in the implantation of children with measurable thresholds at 4000 and 8000 Hz. Any change in guidelines for the implantation of children should follow additional trials for adults.

Children have received both intracochlear and extracochlear and single-channel and multichannel devices. Presently, it is not possible to determine which type of device—single-channel or multichannel— is superior based on the available evidence. Even fewer data exist for specific speech perception tasks with multichannel extracochlear devices. It is advisable that children receive an implant in only one ear.

Children with implants still must be regarded as hearing impaired, even with improved detection thresholds in the range of conversational speech. These children will continue to require educational, audiological, and speech and language support services for long periods of time.

Efficacy measures, comparing preimplant and postimplant performance, are complicated by the continuing development of the children, particularly in speech and language skills. There are no studies that adequately separate the effect of the implant from improvement due to maturation and training. The interaction of cochlear implants with training approaches, such as Total Communication and Cued Speech, should be studied.

The long-term changes due to prosthesis-tissue interactions are currently unknown. Further, it is not known how the implant would affect the developing auditory pathways. In considering cochlear implantation in children, the potential and possibly long-term effects of the implant, either beneficial or deleterious, are unknown.

5. What are the important directions for future research?

There are numerous research issues in connection with candidate selection. One is the criteria for candidacy for prelingually deafened adults and the possible need for novel preimplant and postimplant training programs. A second issue is special populations, including visually impaired, learning-disabled, and retarded persons. The third involves the ear to be implanted, either the ear with "better hearing" or the ear with "poorer hearing." A fourth issue involves the use of a hearing aid in one ear and an implant in the other. A related issue is the efficacy of vibrotactile devices; such devices may have significant utility as a supplement to an implant, as a preimplant training device, or possibly as an alternative to a cochlear implant in some persons. Finally, data on high-frequency hearing (>4kHz) are needed on implant candidates because part of the variance in the performance of implantees may reflect differences in preimplant capability at high frequencies. Improved methods for predicting success with a cochlear implant need to be developed, possibly with tests using data from new imaging techniques such as positron emission tomography (PET) and electromagnetic recordings of auditory cortex activity (SQUID).

Standardized methods should be developed for the evaluation of implant effectiveness. This would then permit comparative study of single-channel and multichannel implants and investigation of alternative methods of signal coding. Improved networking among research groups is recommended and would clearly help in developing a common body of standardized tests and standardized selection criteria.

There should be continued study of presently implanted and yet-to-be-implanted adults to assess long-term effectiveness of cochlear implants.

The inability to predict who will be able to use implants or which signal components are critical for language comprehension reflects our lack of information about basic auditory mechanisms. To address this, we need information about many aspects of audition, including the perception of speech and other auditory signals. Appropriate measures of the integrity of the central auditory pathways need to be developed.

More work is needed on the effects of long-term electrical stimulation at varying levels of intensity, and the effects of new implant procedures and reimplantation in animals.

Further information is needed to identify the mechanisms leading to surgically obtained or spontaneous return of hearing following losses due to meningitis and other pathologic processes.

To further our understanding of basic mechanisms, there is a critical need for correlated histopathological evaluation of the temporal bones and brains of implanted persons and others with documented hearing losses from a variety of causes.

It is important to develop methods to assess the efficacy of the cochlear implant in improving the wearer's quality of life and daily functioning.

There is a clear need for standardized tests for young children, both for the selection of cochlear implant candidates and for the measurement of implant efficacy. These tests need to be based on tasks appropriate for younger, prelinguistic children. More research is required on effective aural rehabilitation procedures. In addition, research is necessary to determine effective ways to educate professionals in the new technology of cochlear implants and its effects on implanted children. Research on the plasticity of the nervous system should be encouraged in both animal and human studies.

The preliminary findings of some benefit and the confounding effects of maturation and training indicate the need for well-controlled, prospective studies in children. Ideally, these studies should be small, randomized trials with precisely defined endpoints and should include appropriate audiological, behavioral, and biostatistical input into the design, analysis, and interpretation. These studies should not only control for maturation and training, but should compare the effect of cochlear implants with alternative methods of treatment.

Conclusion

The cochlear implant is an important step in our long-range goal of understanding, preventing, and treating hearing impairment and resulting language disorders.

There are candidates for whom a cochlear prosthesis implant is appropriate. The specific type of implant chosen for a given person depends upon many variables. It appears that multichannel implants may have some superior features in adults when compared with the single-channel type.

In some persons there is a substantial improvement in speech recognition after implantation, although, more typically, there is improvement in speechreading.

The risks are few but definite. The limitations are many. Foremost of these is that implantation does not restore normal hearing.

There are very special needs concerning the evaluation and treatment of children.

Finally, future research goals should include not only improvements in cochlear implants and methods of testing, but, more importantly, a search for the understanding of mechanisms of disorders and diseases of the ear.

Chapter 29

Cochlear Implants in Adults and Children

Introduction

Cochlear implants are now firmly established as effective options in the habilitation and rehabilitation of individuals with profound hearing impairment. Worldwide, more than 12,000 people have attained some degree of sound perception with cochlear implants, and the multichannel cochlear implant has become a widely accepted auditory prosthesis for both adults and children. The vast majority of adults who are deaf and have cochlear implants derive substantial benefit from them when they are used in conjunction with speechreading. Many of these individuals are able to understand some speech without speechreading, and some of these individuals are able to communicate by telephone. Benefits have also been observed in children, including those who lost their hearing prelingually; moreover, there is evidence that the benefits derived improve with continued use. New speech-sound processing techniques have improved the effectiveness of cochlear implants, increasing user performance levels to ones previously unseen.

The NIH sponsored a Consensus Development Conference on Cochlear Implants in 1988. Since then, implant technology has been continually improved. Questions unanswered at that time have now been resolved. New issues have emerged that must be addressed.

This NIH publication is an unnumbered consensus statement from the Consensus Development Conference held on May 15-17, 1995.

231

For example, the performance of some severely to profoundly hearing-impaired adults using hearing aids is poorer than that of even more severely hearing-impaired individuals using cochlear implants with advanced speech-processing strategies. It is possible that cochlear implants could be beneficial for some of these individuals. Therefore, the criteria for implantation should be re-examined. The ability to predict preoperatively the level of performance at which an individual implant recipient will function is highly desirable. Currently, the limited prediction of implant efficacy in a specific individual remains a pressing problem. Agreement does not exist on the definition of a successful implant user. What are the appropriate expectations for individuals using cochlear implants? How is benefit defined and measured? What are the audiological, educational, and psychosocial impacts of this intervention and is it cost-effective? Advancing technology will allow for the modification of existing devices or the development of new devices. It is therefore important to know what risks and benefits are associated with device explantation/reimplantation. Surgical and other risks and possible long-term effects of cochlear implants require evaluation.

Implantation of individuals with multiple disabilities, the elderly, and children, particularly children who are prelingually deaf, engenders special questions. Longitudinal studies are providing information on the development of auditory speech perception and production and language skills in children who are deaf and have a cochlear implant. What educational setting is best for the development of speech and language in these children? Are cochlear implants efficacious in children who are prelingually deaf?

To address these new issues since the 1988 Consensus Development Conference (CDC) on Cochlear Implants, the National Institute on Deafness and Other Communication Disorders, together with the NIH Office of Medical Applications of Research, convened a Consensus Development Conference on Cochlear Implants in Adults and Children, May 15-17, 1995. The conference was cosponsored by the National Institute on Aging, the National Institute of Child Health and Human Development, the National Institute of Neurological Disorders and Stroke, and the Department of Veterans Affairs.

The conference was convened to summarize current knowledge about the range of benefits and limitations of cochlear implantation that have accrued to date. Such knowledge is an important basis for informed choices for individuals and their families whose philosophy of communication is dedicated to spoken discourse. Issues related to the acquisition of sign language were not directly addressed by the panel, because the focus of the conference was to synthesize thoughtfully the new information on cochlear implant technology and its use. The panel acknowledges the value and contributions of bilingual-bicultural approaches to deafness.

This conference brought together specialists in auditory anatomy and physiology, otolaryngology, audiology, aural rehabilitation, education, speech-language pathology, bioengineering, and other related disciplines as well as representatives from the public. After 1-1/2 days of presentations and audience discussion, an independent, non-Federal consensus panel weighed the scientific evidence and developed a draft statement that addressed the following five questions:

1. What Factors Affect the Auditory Performance of Cochlear Implant Recipients?

Subject Factors

Auditory performance, defined as the ability to detect, discriminate, recognize, or identify acoustic signals, including speech, is highly variable among individuals using cochlear implants. Since the 1988 CDC on Cochlear Implants, however, some factors associated with outcome variability are now better understood.

Etiology

Because of a larger subject sample, the effects of etiology can now be distinguished from other factors such as the duration of deafness and the age of onset. Meningitic deafness does not necessarily limit the benefit of cochlear implantation in the absence of central nervous system complications, cochlear ossification, or cochlear occlusion. Children with congenital deafness and children with prelingually acquired meningitic deafness, for example, achieve similar auditory performance if the cochlear implant is received before age 6 years. In general, etiology does not appear to impact auditory performance in either children or adults.

Age of Onset of Deafness

The age of onset continues to have important implications for cochlear implantation, depending on whether the hearing impairment occurred before (prelingual), during (perilingual), or after (postlingual) learning speech and language. At the time of the last CDC, data on cochlear implantation suggested that children or adults with post-lingual onset of deafness had better auditory performance than children or adults with prelingual or perilingual onsets. On average, current data following auditory performance in children over a longer period of time support this finding. However, the difference between children with postlingual and prelingual-perilingual onsets appears to lessen with time. Large individual differences remain within each group.

Age at Implantation

Previous data suggested that prelingually or perilingually deaf-ened persons who were implanted in adolescence or adulthood did not achieve as good auditory performance as those implanted during childhood, although individual differences were recognized. Current data continue to support the importance of early detection of hearing loss and implantation for maximal auditory performance. However, it is still unclear whether implantation at age 2, for example, ultimately results in better auditory performance than implantation at age 3.

Duration of Deafness

As deafness endures, even in postlingually deafened individuals, some acquired skills and knowledge may decline and some behaviors that work against successful adaptation to a sensory device may de-velop. Individuals with shorter durations of auditory deprivation tend to achieve better auditory performance from any type of sensory aid, including cochlear implants, than individuals with longer durations of auditory deprivation.

Residual Hearing

Cochlear implants tend to give people with profound deafness a level of auditory performance that is similar to, or better than, the performance of people with severe hearing impairment who use hearing aids. These data raise the issue of whether cochlear implants might give persons with severe hearing impairment and some residual hearing even better auditory performance than they can attain with a hearing aid. No residual hearing is typically defined as profound hearing loss and no open-set speech recognition. However, the degree of preimplantation residual hearing does not predict postimplantation auditory performance. Research is now addressing the critical distinction between the importance of residual pure tone sensitivity compared with that of overall residual auditory capacities and functional communication status.

Electrophysiological Factors

Some surviving spiral ganglion cells are necessary for auditory performance with a cochlear implant. Degenerative changes occur in both ganglion cells and central auditory neurons following sensorineural deafening. Although a relationship between the number of surviving ganglion cells and psychophysical performance has been demonstrated in animals, a direct relationship between ganglion cell survival and level of auditory performance in humans has not been shown. Animal studies also suggest that electrical stimulation increases ganglion cell survival and also modifies the functional organization of the central auditory system. The implications of these new findings remain to be determined.

Device Factors

The task of representing speech stimuli as electrical stimuli is central to the design of cochlear implants. Designs vary according to (1) the placement, number, and relationship among the electrodes; (2) the way in which stimulus information is conveyed from an external processor to the electrodes; and (3) how the electrical stimuli are derived from the speech input (and other signals). Changes in cochlear implant design/processing strategies and their effects on auditory performance are discussed in Section 3.

2. What Are the Benefits and Limitations of Cochlear Implantation?

Impact on Speech Perception in Adults

Cochlear implantation has a profound impact on hearing and speech reception in postlingually deafened adults. Most individuals demonstrate significantly enhanced speechreading capabilities, attaining scores of 90-100 percent correct on everyday sentence materials. Speech recognition afforded by the cochlear implant effectively supplements the information least favorably cued through speechreading. A majority of those individuals with the latest speech processors for their implants will score above 80 percent correct on high-context sentences without visual cues. Performance on single-word testing in these individuals is notably poorer, although even these scores have been significantly improved with newer speech-processing strategies. Recognition of environmental sounds and even appreciation of music have been repeatedly observed in adult implant recipients. Noisy environments remain a problem for cochlear-implanted adults, significantly detracting from speech-perception abilities. Prelingually deafened adults have generally shown little improvement in speech perception scores after cochlear implantation, but many of these individuals derive satisfaction from hearing environmental sounds and continue to use their implants.

Speech Perception, Speech Production. and Language Acquisition in Children

Improvements in the speech perception and speech production of children following cochlear implantation are often reported as primary benefits. Variability across children is substantial. Factors such as age of onset, age of implantation, the nature and intensity of (re)habilitation, and mode of communication contribute to this variability. Using tests commonly applied to children and adults with hearing impairments (e.g., pattern perception, closed-set word identification, and open-set perception), perceptual performance increases on average with each succeeding year post implantation. Shortly after implantation, performance may be broadly comparable to that of some children with hearing aids and over time may improve to match that of children who are highly successful hearing aid users. Children implanted at younger ages are on average more accurate in their production of consonants, vowels, intonation, and rhythm. Speech produced by children with implants is more accurate than speech produced by children with comparable hearing losses using vibro-tactile or hearing aids. One year after implantation, speech intelligibility is twice that typically reported for children with profound hearing impairments and continues to improve. Oral-aural communication training appears to result in substantially greater speech intelligibility than manually based total communication.

The language outcomes in children with cochlear implants have received less attention. Reports involving small numbers of children suggest that implantation in conjunction with education plus habilitation leads to advances in oral language acquisition. The nature and pace of language acquisition may be influenced by the age of onset, age at implantation, nature and intensity of habilitation, and mode of communication.

One current limitation is that children are typically implanted at no earlier than age 2 years, which is beyond what may be critical periods of auditory input for the acquisition of oral language. Benefits are not realized immediately, but rather are manifested over time, with some children continuing to show improvement over several years few studies have used language as an outcome measure. The assessment of speech perception, language production, and language comprehension in young children is particularly challenging. Furthermore, all results in children have been reported for single-channel or feature-based devices only, despite the relatively rapid evolution of alternatives in speech-coding strategies. Oral language development in deaf children, including those with cochlear implants, remains a slow, training-intensive process, and results will typically be delayed in comparison with normally hearing peers.

Psychologic and Social Issues in Adults and Children

Although psychological evaluation has previously been a part of the preimplant evaluation process, comparatively little research has been conducted on the long-term psychological and social effects of electing for implantation. Still, the psychological and social impact for adults is generally quite positive, and there appears to be agreement between preimplantation expectations and later benefit. This benefit is expressed as a decline in loneliness, depression and social isolation and an increase in self-esteem, independence, social integration, and vocational prospects.

Many adults report being able to function socially or vocationally in ways comparable to those with moderate hearing loss. Furthermore, they describe a new or renewed curiosity about the experience of hearing and the phenomena of sound. In some cases the experience of implantation becomes an integral part of the individual's identity, leading implant users to participate and share experiences in self-interest and advocacy groups.

Negative psychological and social impact is less frequently observed and is often related to concerns about the maintenance and/or malfunction of the implant and external hardware. Other social insecurities may result from the difficulty of hearing amidst background noise, and from unreasonable expectations of the aural-only benefit on the part of the implant user or his/her family and friends.

The assessment of psychological impact in children with implants lags behind that for the adult population, in part because psychological outcome is a factor of audiological benefit, which is realized more slowly in children. Additionally, such assessment must consider the child's family setting. Because language acquisition is closely associated with identity, social development, and social integration, the impact of implantation on a child's development in these areas deserves more study in order to produce useful indicators that can bear upon parental decision-making processes.

Rehabilitation and Educational Issues

Although a cochlear implant can provide dramatic augmentation of the auditory information perceived by deaf children and adults, it is clear that training and educational intervention play a fundamental role in optimizing postimplant benefit. Access to postimplant rehabilitation involving professionals familiar with cochlear implants must be provided to ensure successful outcomes for implant recipients.

Rehabilitation efforts must be tailored to meet individual needs, and protocols should be developed to reflect therapies effective for various types of individuals receiving implants. Therapeutic intervention with prelingually deaf adults may differ significantly in both time and content from that of postlingually deaf recipients.

Pediatric cochlear implantation requires a multidisciplinary team composed of physicians, audiologists, speech-language pathologists, rehabilitation specialists, and educators familiar with cochlear implants. These professionals must work together in a long-term relationship to support the child's auditory and oral development. Although the effects of communication mode in implantation habilitation have not been sufficiently documented, it is clear that the educational programs for children with cochlear implants must include auditory and speech instruction using the auditory information offered by the implant.

Cost-Utility

The cost-benefit or cost-utility of cochlear implantation must be calculated for children and adults separately. For adults, the cost of cochlear implantation includes the initial costs of assessment, the device, implantation, rehabilitation, system overhead, and maintenance. The benefit or utility is estimated as a function of quality of life over time. On this basis, cochlear implantation whether at age 45 years or 70 years compares quite favorably to many medical procedures now commonly in use (e.g., implantable defibrillator insertion).

Although it appears that the cost-utility estimates for children are also quite favorable, we are still in the early stages of cochlear implant application and cannot yet estimate the cost or potential cost savings that will accrue in the area of (re)habilitation and education.

3. What Are the Technical and Safety Considerations of Cochlear Implantation?

Cochlear Implant Design Issues

A cochlear implant works by providing direct electrical stimulation to the auditory nerve, bypassing the usual transducer cells that are absent or nonfunctional in a deaf cochlea. Over the past 10 years, significant improvements have been made in the technology used to accomplish auditory stimulation.

The best performance in speech recognition occurs with intracochlear electrodes that are close to the nerves to be stimulated, thus minimizing undesirable side effects.

Early implants used only a single electrode; it has been found that these single-channel implants rarely provide open-set speech perception. Most recent implants have used multielectrode arrays that provide a number of independent channels of stimulation. Such devices provide more information about the acoustic signal and give better performance on speech recognition. No agreement exists on the optimum number of channels, although at least 4-6 channels seem to be necessary.

Much of the recent progress in implant performance has involved improvements in the speech processors, which convert sound into the electrical stimulus. The best performance comes with speech processors that attempt to preserve the normal frequency code or spectral representation of the cochlea. These are distinguished from feature-based processors, which attempt to analyze certain features known to be important to speech perception and present only those features through the electrodes. A major problem in multichannel implants is channel interaction, in which two electrodes stimulate overlapping populations of nerves. Channel interaction has now been minimized with speech processors that activate the electrodes in a nonsimultaneous or interleaved fashion, which has been shown to improve speech recognition significantly.

A final design issue is the means by which the stimulus information is passed through the skin from the speech processor to the electrodes. In a transcutaneous system, the skin is intact and the coupling is done electromagnetically to an implanted antenna. In a percutaneous system, the leads are passed directly through the skin. The two systems have slightly different surgical complications, which are discussed below. The percutaneous system (1) provides a more flexible connection to the electrodes in case a change in speech processor is desired, (2) is easier to troubleshoot in case of electrode problems, and (3) is magnetic resonance imaging (MRI) compatible. Currently, percutaneous systems are not commercially available.

Issues Related to Magnetic Resonance Imaging

Magnetic Resonance Imaging (MRI) is increasingly the diagnostic tool of choice for a variety of medical conditions. Implants that use transcutaneous connectors contain an implanted magnet and some ferrous materials that are incompatible with the high magnetic fields of an MRI scanner. Implant manufacturers are redesigning their devices to circumvent this problem. Potential MRI risks should be part of the informed consent procedure for persons considering an implant. The external speech processor cannot be made MRI compatible and should not be taken into the scanner.

Surgical Issues

Cochlear implantation entails risks common to most surgical procedures, e.g., general anesthetic exposure, as well as unique risks that are influenced by device design, individual anatomy and pathology, and surgical technique. Comparative data of major complications incurred in adult implantation show a halving of the complication rate to approximately 5 percent in 1993. The complication rate in pediatric implantation is less than that currently seen in adults. Overall, the complication rate compares favorably to the 10 percent rate seen with pacemaker/defibrillator implantation. Major complications, i.e., those requiring revision surgery, include flap problems, device migration or extrusion, and device failure. Facial palsy is also considered a major complication but is distinctly uncommon and rarely permanent. Notably, no mortalities have been attributed to cochlear implantation.

Alterations in surgical technique, especially flap design, have led to a considerable reduction in the flap complication rate, which is particularly relevant to transcutaneous devices. Alterations in surgical technique, particularly in methods used to anchor the device, have contributed to a decrease in device migration/extrusion.

All implants are potentially prone to failure—either because of manufacturing defects or use-related trauma. Pedestal fracture is a problem unique to the percutaneous device, but occurs rarely. Manufacturer redesign has produced electrode arrays that are smaller but sturdier. For the most commonly implanted device, 95 percent of implants are still functioning after 9 years. Most current implants with transcutaneous connectors do not provide self-test capability for the implanted portion, making it cumbersome to test for simple electrode failure, such as open and short circuits. Failure detection is particularly problematic in young children. Device manufacturers should include self-test circuity in future implant designs.

Minor complications are those that resolve without surgical intervention. The most common is unwanted facial nerve stimulation with electrode activation, which is readily rectified by device reprogramming. In percutaneous devices, pedestal infections are uncommon and can be treated successfully with antibiotics, but on rare occasions may require explantation.

Reimplantation is necessary in approximately 5 percent of cases because of improper electrode insertion or migration, device failure, serious flap complication, or loss of manufacturer support. In general, reimplantation in the same ear is usually possible, and thus far individual auditory performance after reimplantation equals or exceeds that seen with the original implant.

Long-term complications of implantation relate to flap breakdown, electrode migration and receiver/stimulator migration. Particularly in the child, the potential consequences of otitis media have been of concern, but as the implanted electrode becomes ensheathed in a fibrous envelope, it appears protected from the consequences of local infection.

4. Who Is a Candidate for Cochlear Implantation?

Adults

Cochlear implants are often highly successful in postlingually deafened adults with severe/profound hearing loss with no speech perception benefit from hearing aids. Previously, individuals receiving marginal benefit from hearing aids were not considered implant candidates. Ironically, such individuals often have less speech perception than more severely deafened persons who receive implants. Recent data show that most marginally successful hearing aid users implanted with a cochlear implant will have improved speech perception performance. It is therefore reasonable to extend cochlear implants to postlingually deafened adult individuals currently obtaining marginal benefit from other amplification systems. Prelingually deafened adults may also be suitable for implantation, although these candidates must be counseled regarding realistic expectations. Existing data indicate that these individuals achieve minimal improvement in speech recognition skills. However, there may be other basic benefits such as improved sound awareness that correlate with psychological satisfaction and safety needs.

Because of the wide variability in speech perception and recognition in persons with similar hearing impairments, all candidates require in-depth counseling of the surgery, its risks and benefits, rehabilitation, and alternatives to cochlear implantation. To give adequate informed consent, adult candidates should understand that large variability in individual audiologic performance precludes preoperative prediction of success. Determining implant candidacy requires consideration of both objective audiological variables as well as the subjective needs and wishes of individual candidates. Specific characteristics of potential adult cochlear implant recipients are provided below.

Audiologic Criteria

Indications in favor of an implant are a severe-to-profound sensorineural hearing loss bilaterally and open-set sentence recognition scores less than or equal to 30 percent under best aided conditions. Duration of deafness and age of onset have been shown to influence auditory performance with cochlear implants and should be discussed with potential candidates.

In general, when there is no residual hearing in either ear, the ear with better closed-set performance, more sensitive electrical thresholds, shorter period of auditory deprivation, or better radiologic characteristics is implanted. However, when there is residual hearing, the poorer ear should be chosen, provided that there is radiologic evidence of cochlear patency.

Medical and Surgical Criteria

Traditionally, implantation candidacy was limited to healthy persons. Although there may be specific medical contraindications to surgery and implantation such as poor anesthetic risk, severe mental retardation, severe psychiatric disorders, and organic brain syndromes, cochlear implantation should be offered to a wider population of individuals. In some circumstances, such as in individuals with low vision, implantation may be a tool to promote independence and other quality-of-life goals.

The medical history, physical examination, and laboratory tests are important tools in candidacy evaluation. Individuals with active ear pathology require treatment and re-evaluation prior to implantation. The standard evaluation includes high-resolution computed tomography (CT) scans that serve to detect mixed fibrous and bony occlusions and anatomical abnormalities. MRI provides better resolution of soft tissue structures and should supplement the CT scan when indicated. These imaging techniques should be used to identify abnormalities that may compromise or impede implant surgery or device use.

The results of electrophysiologic tests do not predict implant success. However, in selected individuals, such as those with cochlear obliteration or in decisions regarding ear of implantation, the results of promontory stimulation may be useful.

Children

Cochlear implants have also been shown to result in successful speech perception in children. Currently, the earliest age of implantation is 24 months, but there are reasons to reassess this age threshold. A younger age of implantation may limit the negative consequences of auditory deprivation and may allow more efficient acquisition of speech and language. Determining whether cochlear implant benefits are greater in children implanted at age 2-3 years as compared to those implanted at age 4-5 years might resolve this issue, but sufficient data are unavailable. It is also not clear that the benefits of implantation before age 2 years would offset potential liabilities associated with the increased difficulty in obtaining reliable and valid characterization of hearing and functional communication status at the younger age. A number of children under age 2 years have received implants, both internationally and in the United States, when it was thought that bone growth associated with meningitis would preclude implantation at a later date. Speech/language data obtained on such children will be helpful in determining the potential benefits of early implantation and therefore may help to guide future policy.

Audiologic Criteria

Children age 2 years or older with profound (>90 dBHL) sensorineural hearing loss bilaterally and minimal speech perception under best aided conditions may be considered for cochlear implantation. In the young child, auditory brainstem response, stapedial reflex testing, and/or otoacoustic emission testing may be useful when combined with auditory behavioral responses to determine hearing status. Prior to implantation, a trial period with appropriate amplification combined with intensive auditory training should have been attempted to ensure that maximal benefit has been achieved. When the validity of behavioral test results is compromised by maturational factors, the above criteria should be applied in the most stringent manner (i.e., worse hearing sensitivity, longer trial periods, and so on). Current research may broaden audiometric criteria for candidacy to better reflect functional auditory capacity.

Medical and Surgical Criteria

Children should undergo a complete medical evaluation to rule out the presence of active disease, which would be a contraindication to surgery. The child must be otologically stable and free of active middle ear disease prior to cochlear implantation. The radiologic imaging criteria used in adult candidates can be applied to children.

Psychosocial Criteria

Preoperative assessment should entail evaluation of the child in the context of the home and social and educational milieu to assure that implantation is the proper intervention. In some instances psychosocial factors may be used as exclusionary criteria; however, in most cases it should serve only as baseline data for tracking cochlear implant outcomes.

Informed Consent

The parents of a deaf child are responsible for deciding whether to elect cochlear implantation. The informed consent process should be used to empower parents in their decision-making. The parents must understand that cochlear implants do not restore normal hearing and that auditory and speech outcomes are highly variable and unpredictable. They must be informed of the advantages, disadvantages, and risks associated with implantation to establish realistic expectations. Furthermore, the importance of long-term rehabilitation to success with cochlear implants must be stressed. As part of the process of informed consent, parents must be told that alternative approaches to habilitation are available. All children should be included in the informed consent process to the extent that they are able, as their active participation is crucial to (re)habilitative success.

5. What Are the Directions for Future Research on Cochlear Implantation?

1. Research must attempt to explain the wide variation in performance across individual cochlear implant users. New tools, such as functional imaging of the brain, might be

applied to unexplored variables such as the ability of the implant to activate the central auditory system. Investigations of the role of higher level cognitive processes in cochlear implant performance are needed.

2. The strides that have been made in improving speech perception of cochlear implant users should continue through improvements in electrode design and signal processing strategies. Noise-reduction technologies and enhancement of performance using binaural implants are promising areas.

3. Studies of the effects of cochlear stimulation on auditory neurons have provided clear evidence of plasticity in both the survival of neural elements and in receptive field organization. Comparisons of neural plasticity in animal experiments and of adaptation to cochlear implant electrical stimulation by humans provide a unique opportunity to study the relationships between neural activity and auditory perception.

4. Comparative research on language development in children with normal hearing, children with hearing impairment who use hearing aids, deaf children with cochlear implants, and deaf children using American Sign Language should be conducted. These studies should be longitudinal and reflect current theoretical and empirical advances in neurolinguistics and psycholinguistics.

5. Studies of the relationship between the development of speech perception and speech production in cochlear implant users must continue. Implanted deaf children provide a unique opportunity to examine these developmental processes and their relationship to the acquisition of aural/oral language. Such information is crucial to understanding and enhancing the performance of implanted prelingual children and may help define optimal age for implantation.

6. Adequate tools for the assessment of nonspeech benefits of implantation should be applied to gain a better understanding of the full effects of implantation on the quality of life of

246

implant recipients. This may be particularly useful for implant recipients who do not realize significant speech-perception benefit. Such data will help in evaluating the cost-utility of cochlear implantation.

7. Identifying the components of successful (re)habilitation approaches will facilitate extension of these services to all children and adults receiving cochlear implants, as will comparison of model and routine service programs.

Conclusions

1. Cochlear implantation improves communication ability in most adults with deafness and frequently leads to positive psychological and social benefits as well. The greatest benefits seen to date have occurred in postlingually deafened adults. Cochlear implantation in prelingually deafened adults provides more limited improvement in speech perception, but offers important environmental sound awareness. Cochlear implantation outcomes are more variable in children. Nonetheless, gradual, steady improvement in speech perception, speech production, and language does occur. There is substantial unexplained variability in the performance of implant users of all ages, and implants are not appropriate for all individuals.

2. Currently children at least 2 years old and adults with profound deafness are candidates for implantation. Cochlear implant candidacy should be extended to adults with severe hearing impairment and poor open-set sentence discrimination, i.e., less than or equal to 30 percent in the best aided condition. Although there are theoretical reasons to lower the age of implantation in children data are too scarce to justify a change in criteria. Additional data may justify a change in age and audiologic criteria.

3. Auditory performance with a cochlear implant varies among individuals. The data indicate that performance is better in individuals who (1) have shorter durations of deafness, (2)

were implanted before age 6 years, and (3) acquired language before their hearing loss occurred. Auditory performance is not affected by etiology of hearing loss.

4. Access to optimal educational and (re)habilitation services is important to adults and is critical to children to maximize the benefits available from cochlear implantation.

5. The current generation of intracochlear, multichannel implants with spectrally based speech processors provides a substantial improvement over the previous generation of devices, especially when nonsimultaneous electrode activation is used.

6. The low complication rate and high reliability for cochlear implants compares favorably with other implanted electronic devices, and continues to improve.

7. Current devices are not MRI compatible, and users and physicians should be acutely aware of this problem. Implant manufacturers should include MRI compatibility and internal self-test systems in future devices.

8. Percutaneous connectors offer many research and clinical opportunities, including MRI compatibility, ease of electrode testing, and processor upgrades, and they should not be abandoned.

About the NIH Consensus Development Program

NIH Consensus Statements are prepared by a nonadvocate, non-Federal panel of experts, based on (1) presentations by investigators working in areas relevant to the consensus questions during a 2-day public session, (2) questions and statements from conference attendees during open discussion periods that are part of the public session, and (3) closed deliberations by the panel during the remainder of the second day and morning of the third. This statement is an independent report of the panel and is not a policy statement of the NIH or the Federal Government.

Statement Availability

Preparation and distribution of this statement is the responsibility of the Office of Medical Applications of Research of the National Institutes of Health. Free copies of this statement as well as all other available NIH Consensus Statements and NIH Technology Assessment Statements may be obtained from the following resources:

NIH Consensus Program Information Service
P.O. Box 2577
Kensington, MD 20891
Telephone 1-800-NIH-OMAR (644-6627)
Fax (301) 816-2494

NIH Office of Medical Applications of Research
Federal Building, Room 618
7550 Wisconsin Avenue MSC 9120
Bethesda, MD 20892-9120

Full-text versions of statements are also available online through an electronic bulletin board system and through the Internet:

NIH Information Center BBS
(301) 480-5144

Internet

Gopher
gopher://gopher.nih.gov/Health and Clinical Information

World Wide Web
http://text.nlm.nih.gov

ftp
ftp://public.nlm.nih.gov/hstat/nihcdcs

Chapter 30

Questions and Answers about Cochlear Implants

What is a cochlear implant?

A cochlear implant is a device that provides the sensation of hearing to individuals with profound hearing loss. A receiver/stimulator and an electrode array are surgically implanted and a microphone, speech processor, and transmitting coil are worn externally. The external parts are easily removed by the user when the implant is not being used.

How is a cochlear implant different from a hearing aid?

Worn externally, a hearing aid makes incoming sounds louder. For some people with very profound hearing impairment, these louder signals are not useful because of the degree of damage in the inner ear. A cochlear implant bypasses the damaged hair cells in the inner ear and directly stimulates the auditory (hearing) nerve. Parts of the implant are surgically implanted and several components are worn externally.

Who can benefit from a cochlear implant?

Cochlear implants can help people who have profound hearing loss in both ears, and who receive very little or no benefit from hearing

Gallaudet University publication (288) 8/92-3C 070. Used by permission.

aids. These people should be in good general health and have desire, motivation, and realistic expectations for the implant. Cochlear implants have been approved by the Food and Drug Administration (FDA) for adults who lost their hearing after learning language and for children older than two years of age.

How much hearing does a cochlear implant provide?

Most cochlear implant users can detect (hear) medium to loud sounds, including normally loud speech. Many can learn to recognize some environmental sounds. This awareness of sound and its rhythms often helps to improve speechreading (lipreading) ability. Some cochlear implant users can understand words or sentences without the use of speechreading. This is especially true if a multichannel implant is used. A few of these people can use the phone.

Clearly, the results differ from person to person, and it is important to understand that a cochlear implant does not restore an individual's hearing to normal levels. Unfortunately, it is difficult to predict how much speech understanding any one individual will receive, although it is known that, as a group, individuals who lost their hearing after learning language (that is, who are post-lingually deafened) will do better than those deafened before they developed language.

What is the process of getting a cochlear implant?

There are three principal examinations preliminary to getting a cochlear implant. The first step is an evaluation by an audiologist. This includes various hearing tests and a trial period with a hearing aid or, in some cases, a vibrotactile device. It is important for the potential cochlear implant candidate to try a hearing aid (or vibrotactile device) to determine if these devices can provide any significant help. The otolaryngologist (ear, nose, and throat doctor) who will perform the surgery completes a thorough examination, and x-rays are taken of the inner ear. Some programs also require a psychological evaluation. Candidates for cochlear implant surgery have a physical exam before the surgery.

[There are two sets of components in a cochlear implant: external and internal. The external parts include the speech processor, a directional microphone, and a cable and transmitter. The internal components, which are surgically implanted, include: a magnet, a receiver/stimulator, and an electrode array that extends from the receiver/stimulator into the cochlea.]

About four to six weeks after surgery, the implantee receives the external part of the implant, and the device is "tuned" or adjusted for the individual user. Then the implantee begins intensive training to learn to use the implant and interpret the sounds that the implant provides. Regular training sessions follow for several months after the fitting. During these sessions the audiologist continues adjusting or "tuning" the device and leads the implantee in exercises to develop listening and speechreading skills. Given the importance of these intensive training sessions, anyone considering such surgery must determine the availability of follow-up training from the cochlear implant team performing the surgery.

What is involved with cochlear implant surgery?

Surgery is performed under general anesthesia and takes approximately two to five hours. The internal parts of the device are implanted under the skin behind the ear and into the inner portion of the ear. The hospital stay is usually 24 to 48 hours, and the implant patient will require three to five weeks to heal. The otolaryngologist discusses the risks of surgery with all candidates prior to the operation.

What are the limitations of the cochlear implant?

The cochlear implant cannot help all people with profound hearing loss, and it helps some people more than others. The full benefit of the cochlear implant is not seen overnight—it takes time, training, and experience.

The "electrode array" of the implant is located within the cochlea during surgery. These electrodes stimulate the nerve fibers within the inner ear.

Can a cochlear implant user participate in sports?

Cochlear implants require special care. They can be worn when playing most sports, as long as the external parts are protected from moisture and damage from being hit. The external parts must be removed for swimming, but normal perspiration is usually not a

problem. Playing rough contact sports such as football is not recommended, and implant users should not scuba dive.

How much does a cochlear implant cost?

In general, the total cost for the pre-implant evaluations, surgery,
the implant itself, hospital expenses, and fitting, tuning, and follow-up
ranges from $32,000 to $40,000. Many insurance companies and some
Medicare and Medicaid programs provide full or partial coverage. Potential candidates should check with their insurance company regarding insurance coverage.

What about cochlear implants for children?

Children as young as two years of age are potential candidates
for cochlear implants. Children who use cochlear implants require consistent daily auditory stimulation. Thus, supportive educational and
home environments are absolutely necessary for a successful cochlear
implant outcome with a child. The child and the family must be committed to intensive training both at school and at the cochlear implant
center. Teachers and other personnel who work with the child in the
school are also important participants in this process.

Although few would argue the benefit of a cochlear implant for
adults deafened after years of hearing, some people in the deaf community raise questions regarding the appropriateness of cochlear implants for children with profound hearing loss. The concerns go beyond
medical considerations. Some believe that providing cochlear implants
to deaf children undermines the cultural integrity of the deaf community and furthers the perspective that hearing loss is a disease to be
"fixed" rather than a cultural difference. Some members of the deaf
community advocate the use of sign language and identification with
other people with hearing loss rather than implantation and auditory/
oral communication for deaf children.

Is a cochlear implant right for me (or my child)?

Only the potential cochlear implant candidate (or a child's parents) can answer this question. Getting a cochlear implant is a serious
matter, to be undertaken only after lengthy consideration. Medical,
social, time, and financial issues must be addressed. The potential

candidate must consider that surgery is involved and that a significant time commitment for follow-up is necessary. (When the potential candidate is a child who is old enough to be involved in the decision-making process, his or her wishes relative to a cochlear implant must be considered.) For some individuals and families, cultural issues also play a part in the decision.

Ultimately, the decision to get or forego a cochlear implant is a very personal one.

How can cochlear implant users and family members find support groups?

Locating and getting to know other people with cochlear implants can be a source of support for users and family members. Such support and opportunities for networking are available through Cochlear Implant Club International and from implant users who are members of Alexander Graham Bell Association of the Deaf, Self Help for Hard of Hearing People, and the Association of Late-Deafened Adults.

The National Information Center on Deafness wishes to thank Maureen McDonald, M.S., CCC-A, who wrote this paper, and Larry E. Dalzell, Ph.D., Harriet Kaplan, Ph.D., and William H. McFarland, Ph.D., who reviewed the manuscript.

Resources

The following resources are starting points in gathering information about cochlear implants. They may help clarify the various issues involved, and can identify appropriate professionals who provide cochlear implant services.

Publications

Clickener, P.A. "How Can I Keep from Singing? A Story about a Cochlear Implant." *SHHH Journal* (July/August 1989): 3-7. A cochlear implant user recalls the implant surgery, hook-up, and initial experiences with a cochlear implant.

Clickener, P.A. "Taking the Mystery Out of Cochlear Implants." *SHHH Journal* (January/ February 1991): 11-14. The author addresses common questions and misperceptions about cochlear implants and shares experiences from several years of cochlear implant use.

Cochlear Corporation. *Issues and Answers*. Cochlear Corporation, 1990; 1992. An information booklet presented in question-and-answer format. Two versions are available, one for adults (1990) and one for parents considering a cochlear implant for their child (1992). Available from:

Cochlear Corporation
61 Inverness Drive East, Suite 200
Englewood, CO 80112
(800) 458-4999 Voice/TDD (outside Colorado)
(303) 790-9010 Voice/TDD (inside Colorado)

Greater Los Angeles Council on Deafness, Inc. "Cochlear Implant Surgery." Position Paper, Ad Hoc Committee on Ear Surgery, 1985. An older resource. However, it provides a discussion of some of the cultural issues surrounding cochlear implant use. Available from:

Greater Los Angeles Council on Deafness, Inc.
616 S. Westmoreland Ave.
Los Angeles, CA 90005
(213) 383-2220 Voice/TDD

Horn,R.M., R. J. Nozza, and J. N. Dolitsky. "Audiological and Medical Considerations for Children with Cochlear Implants." *American Annals of the Deaf* 13, no. 2, (1991): 82-86. The authors discuss the audiological, medical, and educational considerations of cochlear implant use by children. They describe the surgical procedure and postoperative management.

Moora, C.R. "Funding a Cochlear Implant." *SHHH Journal*, (March/April 1992): 35-36. An informative article in which the author describes how to work with health insurance companies to maximize coverage of cochlear implants. Moora also describes additional sources of funding for implants and follow-up rehabilitation services.

National Association of the Deaf. *Cochlear Implants*. National Association of the Deaf, 1987.

National Association of the Deaf. *Cochlear Implants in Children*. National Association of the Deaf, 1991. These position papers reflect the view of some people in the deaf community regarding cochlear implants. Available from:

The National Association of the Deaf
814 Thayer Ave.
Silver Spring, MD 20910
(301) 587-1788 Voice
(301) 587-1789 TDD

National Institutes of Health. *Cochlear Implants—National Institutes of Health Consensus Development Conference Statement*, 7, no. 2 (1988). Report of the National Institutes of Health Consensus Development Conference on Cochlear Implants which included presentations by members of the medical profession and related disciplines, clinical researchers, and public representatives. The report addresses criteria for candidate selection, different types of implants, effectiveness and risks of implantation, and special considerations for children. Information is slightly dated but still useful. Available from:

The U.S. Department Health and Human Services
Public Health Service Office of Medical Applications of Research
Building 1, Room 216
Bethesda, MD 20892

Tye-Murray, N., ed. *Cochlear Implants and Children: A Handbook for Parents, Teachers, and Speech and Hearing Professionals*. Washington, DC: Alexander Graham Bell Association, 1992. Provides an overview of cochlear implants for parents and teachers of cochlear implant recipients. Describes multichannel cochlear implant designs, how to maintain the device, techniques for helping the child adjust to the implant at home and school, and the importance of the interaction between parent, teacher, and speech professional in the child's habilitation.

Consumer and Professional Organizations

Alexander Graham Bell Association for the Deaf, Inc.
3417 Volta Place NW
Washington, DC 20007
(202) 337-5220 Voice/TDD

Member organization that disseminates information on hearing loss to all interested individuals.

American Academy of Otolaryngology—Head-and-Neck Surgery, Inc.
One Prince St.
Alexandria, VA 22314
(703) 836-1411 Voice

A professional organization that publishes an informative and easy-to-read pamphlet on cochlear implant surgery. Provides consumers with referrals to otolaryngologists in their local area.

American Speech-Language-Hearing Association (ASHA)
10801 Rockville Pike
Rockville, MD 20852
(800) 638-TALK Voice/TDD

National organization for speech and hearing professionals. ASHA's Consumer Division increases public awareness and acts as a consumer advocate for persons with hearing, speech, and language impairment. Has consumer information on cochlear implants.

Cochlear Implant Club International (CICI)
P.O. Box 464
Buffalo, NY 14223

CICI's local chapters throughout the U.S. provide information and support for those considering surgery as well as cochlear implant users and their families.

HASBRO National Cochlear Implant Training Institute (CITI)
New York League for the Hard of Hearing
71 West 23rd St.
New York, NY 10010
(212) 741-7698

The HASBRO CITI is a national resource center to assist profession-als and families in designing and implementing rehabilitation services for children with cochlear implants. Staff will generate an individual-ized rehabilitation plan focusing on improving the listening/speaking skills of the child with a cochlear implant and will also provide on-site rehabilitation planning at schools to help the teacher meet the indi-vidual needs of each child.

Hear Now
4001 South Magnolia Way,
Suite 100
Denver, CO 80237
(800) 648-HEAR (Voice/TDD)

Provides assistance programs for cochlear implants and hearing aids for people who cannot afford to buy them.

Self Help for Hard of Hearing People, Inc. (SHHH)
7800 Wisconsin Avenue
Bethesda,MD 20814
(301) 657-2248 Voice
(301) 657-2249 TDD

National support and information group for people with hearing loss. Provides articles and information on cochlear implants.

National Rehabilitation Information Center (NARIC)
8455 Colesville Road, Suite 935
Silver Spring, MD 20910
(301) 588-9284 Voice/TDD
(800) 34-NARIC Voice/TDD

An information service and research library that provides infor-mation and conducts custom database searches on issues related to rehabilitation. NARIC has a listing of publications on cochlear im-plants.

Chapter 31

Health Technology Review: Cochlear Implantation in Outpatient Settings

This review examines the appropriateness of performing cochlear implant procedures in outpatient clinical settings including ambulatory surgical centers. A cochlear implant is a prosthetic device used to produce the sensation of sound through the generation of electrical signals, which are perceived as an analog of environmental sound waves.[1] Most patients with profound sensorineural deafness (no useful hearing) have lost the hair cells that transduce acoustic vibrations into electrical activity in the auditory nerve. Of the 15 million persons in the United States with significant hearing impairment, fewer than 1% are considered potential candidates for a cochlear implant.[2] Cochlear implant systems employ an externally worn microphone, signal (speech) processor, and transmitter to receive sound and produce electrical signals.[3] The prosthesis includes a surgically implanted receiver and electrode to excite the remaining auditory nerve fibers electrically according to a speech-processing algorithm that is driven by the signals picked up by the external microphone, thus inducing sensations of sound in the patient.

A multichannel device with as many as 22 electrodes (electrode arrays), each of which can be stimulated independently, has been developed. Two multichannel devices are approved for marketing by the Food and Drug Administration: the 3M Company device (for adults

U.S. Department of Health and Human Services; Publication PB92-221290; AHCPR Pub. No. 92-0072; Health Technology Review, No. 3, August 1992.

only) and the Nucleus device from Cochlear Corporation (for children and adults). Only the Nucleus device is currently being implanted.

Approximately 300 to 500 cochlear implant procedures are performed each year in the United States. A small but growing number are being performed as outpatient procedures, and Medicare has recently added cochlear implantation to its list of covered surgical services provided at ambulatory surgical centers. There is no evidence that any cochlear implant operation has been performed in an ambulatory surgical center.

The implantation procedure, considered delicate but not complex or risky, enables the surgeon to fasten an electrode array in the vicinity of auditory nerve fibers while maintaining the integrity of both the inner and middle ears. The operation is performed under strictly aseptic conditions, and a general anesthetic is used. The surgical procedure includes the creation of a large scalp flap; a mastoidectomy is then performed utilizing an approach through the facial recess to the middle ear that exposes the round window of the cochlear base. A seat (bed) is formed in the mastoid, parietal, and/or occipital bones to retain the signal-receiving and stimulation device, which is from 1.5 to 2.5 cm in diameter and about 0.5 cm thick. The electrode array is inserted into the scala tympani via the round window, and the receiving coil is fastened in its surgically formed recess. This procedure usually takes from 1.5 to 3 hours.[1,3] The surgical implant operation for children is similar but requires modifications of the surgical technique.[4] A transorbital radiograph of the patient, to document and ensure electrode position, is taken immediately after the surgery. In most cases patients are hospitalized (observed) for 24 to 48 hours after surgery.

Possible medical complications include all those associated with general anesthesia. Published data regarding inhospital cochlear implantation indicate few postoperative complications.[1,5] Major complications are usually related to surgical technique, and they include flap necrosis, improper electrode placement, and rare facial nerve problems. Minor complications include dehiscence, infection, facial nerve stimulation, and dizziness.[5]

According to Kveton and Balkany,[1] clinical trials with two cochlear implant devices in almost 500 children produced significant complications in 2.4% in the 3M series and 3.5% in the Nucleus series. Complications included infection and extrusion, pain and inflammation, delayed wound healing and extrusion, skin flap complications, transient drainage, electrode displacement or misplacement, and fa-

262

cial nerve damage. Complications were successfully resolved, except in one patient with an unresolved but improved facial palsy.

The recent review by Cohen and Hoffman[5] of the surgical experience of 696 adults and 309 children in the United States found that there have been no deaths attributable to implantation of these devices, few serious major complications, and relatively few minor complications. (Major medical-surgical complications are those that require additional surgery and/or hospitalization, and minor complications are those that are treated with medication alone.) Complications were less frequent in children than in adults but were more likely to occur in younger children than in those older than 7 years of age.

A review of 459 implants with the Nucleus device in adults[5] found 23 (5%) major complications and 32 (7%) minor complications. Major complications included scalp breakdown requiring implant removal; compressed or incorrect electrode position; perilymph fistula; severe seventh nerve stimulation leading to implant removal; and one life-threatening case of meningitis, which resolved under treatment. Minor complications included flap problems; seventh nerve weakness or stimulation; and transient dizziness.

There are no published data that specifically address the operative morbidity or clinical effectiveness of cochlear implantation in outpatient settings. Opinions from acknowledged leaders in the field of cochlear implantation were sought in lieu of the data needed to compare the safety and clinical effectiveness of inpatient and outpatient procedures. According to Maureen Hannley, Director of Research, American Academy of Otolaryngology—Head and Neck Surgery, cochlear implantations can be performed safely and effectively in outpatient settings, including ambulatory surgical centers. The procedure is considered not especially difficult nor more complicated than other procedures presently performed by otolaryngologists in outpatient settings. Professional judgment on the part of the clinician should determine which patients are not suitable for outpatient surgery. Some patients may require an inpatient procedure because of coexisting morbidity (e.g., diabetes or epilepsy).

Some of the leading otolaryngologists performing cochlear implantation in the United States believe that the safety of the patient as well as the clinical effectiveness of the procedure are not diminished by implantation in an outpatient setting when protocols and guidelines are established to maintain safe and effective surgical outcomes (personal communications, Juliana Gulya, Georgetown University; Thomas Balkany, University of Miami; Noel Cohen, New York University; and Richard Miyamota, University of Indiana).

Adequate training in cochlear implantation, regardless of the setting, is essential. An overnight stay is considered a minimal requirement for appropriate care and observation and to allow for recovery from anesthesia and any dizziness that may occur, the detection of infection, and the removal of drains. A Public Health Service official at the National Institutes of Health, who is recognized as a national expert in the field of deafness, was consulted. In his opinion, cochlear implantation can be performed safely and effectively in an outpatient setting and should include an overnight stay to provide proper patient management and observation.

In regard to outpatient cochlear implantation, there is no evidence, based on the information obtained by this Office, that the safety of the patient and effectiveness of the procedure would be compromised as long as the same protocols and guidelines utilized for inpatient procedures are practiced. Such practices would also include allowing the patient to remain in a medical facility overnight for postoperative observation and treatment deemed clinically necessary, as well as providing for additional observation time or hospitalization as required.

—by Martin Erlichman, M.S.
and Thomas V. Holohan, M.D.

References

1. Kveton J, Balkany TH. Status of cochlear implantation in children. J Pediatr 1991;118:1-7.

2. Consensus Development Panel. National Institutes of Health Consensus Development Conference Statement on Cochlear Implants. Arch Otolaryngol Head Neck Surg 1989; 115:31-36.

3. Cochlear Implant Devices for the Profoundly Hearing Impaired. Health Technology Assessment Report, 1986, No. 2. Rockville, MD: National Center for Health Services Research and Health Care Technology Assessment.

4. Clark GM, Cohen NL, Shepherd RK. Surgical and safety considerations of multichannel cochlear implants in children. Ear Hear 1991;12(4):155-245.

5. Cohen NL, Hoffman RA. Complications of cochlear implant surgery in adults and children. Ann Otol Rhinol Laryngol 1991:100:708-711.

Technology Reviews are brief evaluations of health technologies prepared by the Office of Health Technology Assessment, Agency for Health Care Policy and Research (OHTA/AHCPR) of the Public Health Service. Reviews may be composed in lieu of a technology assessment because: the medical or scientific questions are limited and do not warrant the resources required for a full assessment; the available evidence is limited and the published medical or scientific literature is insufficient in quality or quantity for an assessment; or the time frame available precludes utilization of the full, formal assessment process.

This review was prepared in response to a request from the Civilian Health and Medical Program of the Uniformed Services.

Part Two

Speech and Language Disorders

Chapter 32

Language and Language Impairments

Overview

Language is the expression of human communication through which knowledge, belief and behavior can be experienced, explained and shared. The ability to manipulate language to satisfy needs and desires and to express thoughts, observations and values is an important human pursuit that directly influences the quality of life for any individual.

The broad goals of research on language are to understand the nature of normal language function, including the underlying bases and mechanisms involved. One goal of this work is to build the foundation necessary to develop and evaluate intervention and rehabilitation strategies to improve and enhance the communication process for individuals with language disorders. The understanding of normal language (whether spoken, signed or written) provides a basis for comparison in investigations of language disorders. It is critical to understand how language is produced and understood, what its biological and neural substrates and organizing principles are, how it is learned by children and how it is processed.

This document is a portion of the National Strategic Research Plan for Balance and the Vestibular System and Language and Language Impairments, compiled by the National Institute on Deafness and Other Communication Disorders, a division of the National Institutes of Health.

For an adequate understanding of language functioning in children and adults, research efforts must include all of the diverse groups that make up contemporary United States society. These populations include racial and ethnic minority groups and groups categorized in terms of gender, age, geographic region and social and economic status.

In the United States, there may be as many as one half million persons who were born deaf or who lost their hearing before they acquired spoken language. In the world at large the number may approach 10 million. A large proportion of these individuals use a form of signed language as their primary mode of communication. Some use spoken English exclusively. Many use both. Research and services related to deafness must be concerned with the impairment of auditory language and with the status of and access to signed or spoken languages which are perceived visually.

There exists another group of at least one million people whose hearing impairment is less severe but was acquired during childhood. Most of these individuals use spoken language as their primary mode of communication, although some also use a signed language. Despite the substantial benefit of auditory input to such people, their language acquisition is often characterized by difficulties not faced by normal hearing people.

Individuals with normal hearing, as well as those with a hearing impairment, may exhibit a disorder of language, that is, a deficit of language comprehension, production or use sufficient to impair interpersonal communication. In young children, these disorders frequently involve difficulty in the acquisition of the ambient spoken or signed language and may also lead to impairment in reading and writing. In adults and older children, impaired persons include aphasic individuals who have lost their previous levels of language competence as a result of brain injury.

Language impairments impede economic self-sufficiency, academic performance and employment opportunities. It is estimated that between six and eight million individuals in the United States have some form of language impairment. In addition to loss of livelihood, these disorders impose social isolation and personal suffering on the affected individuals and place an enormous emotional and economic burden on their families and on society as a whole. These disorders have a life-long impact on the ability of those affected to make their way or even to survive in our technologically advanced society.

Disorders of language affect children and adults differently. For the child who does not use language normally from birth or who acquires the impairment in childhood, the disorder occurs in the context of a language system that is not fully developed or acquired. In contrast, damage to the language apparatus in adults disrupts a system that is less malleable in the face of neural damage. Adults with aphasia commonly have highly-selective deficits and more highly-developed compensatory mechanisms. Neurologic, physiologic and metabolic differences between children and adults provide particular problems and challenges to the study of language disorders in these populations. As a result, while the broad goals of research on language disorders are similar for children and adults, the research agendas for these two groups are considered separately.

Recent Accomplishments

Multicultural Issues

The majority of children from all cultures acquire language with little difficulty, including those who are reared in multicultural environments. However, the assessment of disorders within multicultural groups can be complicated by a variety of factors. For example, individuals who are members of multicultural populations such as African-, Asian- and Hispanic-Americans may be incorrectly identified as language impaired due to the use of culturally-inappropriate language assessment instruments. On the other hand, such groups are more likely to live in conditions of poverty, which give rise to various health and social conditions that are linked to increased risk of communication disorders.

There are likely to be pertinent differences in prevalence, causes and manifestations of language disorders among diverse cultural populations. For example, sickle cell anemia, a condition associated with an increased prevalence of sensorineural hearing loss and neurological impairment, is estimated to occur in one in every 500 African-American children. To the extent that these complications directly influence language learning, such children are at considerable risk. Current data also show a very high prevalence of chronic middle ear disease among Pacific Rim, Alaskan Native and Native American populations. The prevalence of hypertension and diabetes, two of the primary risk factors for stroke, may be higher among low socioeconomic groups. Thus, there is likely to be an increased occurrence of aphasia in these groups

Language disorders have been found to occur in children with elevated blood lead levels. The highest blood lead levels have been found in children living in low-income households within the inner cities of large urban areas.

Language Among Deaf Children and Adults

Language acquisition takes place naturally for most children; those who have normal hearing and those who are deaf with signing deaf parents. Many deaf children use a natural sign language, American Sign Language (ASL), which shares an underlying organization with spoken language. Recent electrophysiological findings show that, in spite of the very different input/output systems employed, the same areas in the left hemisphere of the brain are involved in language tasks in native signers and speakers of English. However, despite the ease with which they acquire ASL, many deaf children of deaf parents have inordinate difficulty learning to read and write.

Studies of the acquisition of ASL suggest that signers acquiring the language at a later age demonstrate grammatical deviations from more standard ASL. These deviations persist even four or five decades after acquisition has taken place. This finding suggests the existence of critical periods for acquiring signed language that parallel those documented for spoken language.

Studies of deaf children of hearing or oral deaf parents indicate that, with intensive oral training, their acquisition of spoken language and reading tends to be superior to that of deaf children with equivalent levels of hearing impairment who do not have such training. However, deaf children of hearing or oral deaf parents often display substantial delays learning to read and write.

The dominant pedagogical methodology employed currently in the United States in teaching language to deaf children involves the exposure to artificial signing systems, which are intended to represent and model English and to promote the natural acquisition of English grammar. Recent research suggests that deaf children of hearing parents, when exposed only to artificial signing systems, develop some idiosyncratic grammatical patterns that may not reflect the structure of English or of ASL.

Another methodology currently employed emphasizes the development of spoken language exclusively. Some deaf children exposed to this method throughout their educational program achieve English language competence without the knowledge of sign language.

Cued Speech, a system of communication which uses simple hand cues in conjunction with the natural mouth movements of speech, emphasizes the natural development of spoken language. Many deaf people exposed to this system throughout their educational history achieve English language competence.

Just as speech is one of the basic building blocks of language for hearing people, signing is one of the basic building blocks of language for some deaf people. Thus, the study of sign language perception is as critical to an understanding of the language of many deaf people as the study of speech perception is to understanding the language of hearing people and deaf people who use auditory and/or visual means for perceiving spoken language. Such studies will provide insight into the nature of language processing in deaf people and will lay the foundation for understanding disorders of spoken language that may occur in certain deaf persons. Comparisons of the processes of spoken language perception and signed language perception in normal and language-disordered hearing and deaf individuals provide a unique means of determining those aspects of language that are independent of the mode (signed or spoken) of communication. Such findings may be used to develop appropriate rehabilitation strategies, depending upon the nature of the language deficit.

Studies of the acquisition of sign suggest that infants are very good at relating information in one sensory modality with information in another. Deaf infants learning a signed language rely on movement of the hands and arms, as well as processing by the eye. New technology for three-dimensional motion analysis has been developed for the study of signed language perception, and investigations are now under way that will allow one to separate constraints imposed by the transmission modality from more centrally determined factors in the perception of the basic building blocks of language.

Central to the understanding of disorders of spoken and signed language perception in the hearing impaired is an understanding of normal processes. Research advances in the past 10 years have focused primarily on spoken language perception in normal persons and while many advances have been made, scientists are only beginning to understand fully the nature of the spoken and signed language perception process.

For most people, spoken or signed language, or a combination of the two, are the ways to express thoughts and ideas and to communicate with each other. How spoken or signed language perception interacts with syntactic and semantic knowledge in language comprehension is still not understood. The increased availability of precise instrumentation techniques and use of more sophisticated research methods promise to provide a richer understanding of the nature of spoken and signed language perception. Largely through the efforts and cooperation of many different kinds of scientists (speech, language and hearing scientists, engineers, linguists and psychologists) research on this topic is beginning to contribute a multi- and inter-disciplinary perspective to this complex but critical problem.

Language and Language Disorders in Children

The study of language acquisition in normally-developing hearing children has provided an important foundation for research with language-disordered children. Findings on both the course and underlying bases of language development have been reported. It is clear from this work that infants have available at birth, or quickly develop, many of the perceptual, cross-modal (auditory-visual) and conceptual abilities necessary to learn language. Differences among individual children's language learning patterns have been identified, as well as differences in learning according to the type of language being acquired (e.g., morphologically-rich like Italian vs. word-order-dominant like English). Although much research remains to be done, the existing knowledge has greatly facilitated the study of language impairments.

Language disorders among hearing children can be discussed in terms of whether the language difficulties exist in isolation or in association with other problems and whether the factors interfering with language were present from birth or appeared subsequently.

Many children with isolated language problems that appear to be present from birth are given the clinical label of specifically language impaired (SLI). These children show normal hearing, age-appropriate scores on standardized tests of nonverbal intelligence and no overt evidence of neurological damage. Although U.S. prevalence data need to be more firmly established, it is estimated that approximately five percent of preschool children fall into this clinical category.

Although SLI children do not show signs of frank neurological impairment, neuropsychological studies have revealed that these children perform poorly on perceptual and memory tasks, especially those involving the processing of rapid acoustic changes. These findings cast doubt on the presumed isolation of the language difficulties.

Investigations of the language skills of SLI children have focused on syntax, morphology, phonology and semantic relations. These studies have revealed significant limitations in each of these areas. Although each area is acquired in a manner approximating normal development (albeit more slowly), the language profiles across areas often do not match those of younger, normally developing children in that certain areas (for example, morphology) may show an especially serious deficit. Because studies have focused exclusively on SLI children acquiring English, it is not known whether the observed profiles reflect general difficulties with particular grammatical functions or are influenced by the manner in which these properties are marked in English. Several retrospective, follow-up studies of SLI children have suggested that residual problems with language and language related learning problems may be seen through adolescence and into adulthood.

Research in recent years has begun to address the problem of inadequate subject description of SLI children. This work has provided a protocol for selecting prototypic groups of SLI children. Projects devoted to distinguishing among subgroups of SLI children are now under way.

Efforts aimed at the early identification of SLI children are also in progress. It appears that children's expressive vocabulary size, vocabulary comprehension and use of symbolic gestures assist in determining whether late-talking children are at risk for language impairment.

New technologies such as magnetic resonance imaging (MRI) and event related potentials are beginning to be applied to SLI children. Research to date suggests that SLI children show an atypical left-right hemispheric configuration. Genetic studies of SLI children have also been undertaken. The preliminary findings from these studies suggest that SLI children are more likely than normally-developing children to have other members of the family with present or resolved language difficulties.

Research on the phonologic, morphologic and syntactic features of language that are difficult for SLI children, as well as on the perceptual and motor abilities of these children, has continued. In addition, the lexical (vocabulary) and pragmatic (communicative-conversational) abilities of SLI children have received investigative attention.

Prospective longitudinal research on SLI children has begun. The results of these studies indicate long-term deficits in these children. Evidence is accumulating that young SLI children are clearly at risk for later deficits in reading and that SLI and reading-disabled children represent overlapping populations.

For many children with language disorders, limitations in other areas are also evident. Some of these multiple disabilities result from maternal substance abuse in pregnancy, fetal and infant malnutrition, lead poisoning, congenital AIDS and prematurity in the children of adolescent mothers without prenatal care.

In terms of prevalence, mental retardation is the most common disorder associated with inadequate language development. Recent research shows that children with mental retardation can have a variety of language disorders and that mental retardation often offers an inadequate explanation for communication problems in these children. A common genetic form of mental retardation, Down syndrome, has been shown to be associated with greater impairment of expressive than receptive language. Fragile-X, probably the most common single cause of genetic mental retardation in males, affects language meaning and use more than it does the acquisition of phonology and syntax.

Autistic children constitute another group in whom language is but one area of deficiency. Inadequate communication skills are hallmarks and the most common presenting symptoms of autism, but nonlinguistic deficits make separate contributions to its symptomatology. Nonetheless, it is now clear that, while autism is associated with mental retardation in some children, mental retardation is not a defining feature of the disorder.

Other conditions that can complicate the normal acquisition of language relate to the availability of an adequate listening environment early in life. This need is illustrated by three findings. First, there are some data to suggest that chronic otitis media in the developing infant, when accompanied by a mild and intermittent hearing loss, may be predictive of later language impairment. Second, there is evidence that early amplification and auditory training can significantly affect the deaf child's acquisition of spoken language. Third, there is evidence that normal infants and children need a more favorable signal relative to the background noise to perform at the same level as the adult in spoken language perception tasks.

Some language disorders in children are acquired through infections, tumors, stroke or trauma. Strokes in children are estimated to have an annual incidence of 2.52 per 100,000 children. Other causes, such as head trauma are estimated to be as high as 200 per 100,000 per year.

Advances have been made in specifying the relationship among acquired language deficits and the focality or diffuseness of central nervous system (CNS) involvement, lesion laterality and age at lesion onset. Children with focal, unilateral lesions, such as those sustained following vascular episodes, generally have been found to have better long-term language development and recovery than children with lesions involving more diffuse brain structures, such as CNS tumors treated by whole head radiation and chemotherapy, severe closed head injury or epileptic aphasia. Both fluent and nonfluent aphasias may occur in children with acquired brain lesions, and a variety of syntactic and lexical comprehension and production deficits have been described following left hemisphere lesions. Delays in lexical development and in the development of syntactic structures have been documented following early lesions of either the left or right hemisphere. Attempts to relate language sequelae to lesion location within a hemisphere have been equivocal. Prognosis related to age at lesion onset is controversial and confounded by factors such as the diffuse nature of the lesion, concomitant seizure disorders and questionable premorbid status. Studies using electrophysiologic and neuroimaging techniques are beginning to address the nature of hemispheric reorganization following acquired language loss in children.

Language and Language Disorders in Adults

Current best estimates place at nearly one million the number of adults in the United States with acquired disorders of language due to stroke or traumatic brain injury. Additionally, a large proportion of the estimated two million citizens with progressive dementing disease have significant language impairment. Their disabilities range from partial impairment that affects primarily one or two input or output channels to near total and permanent loss of comprehension and production of speech. While many are rendered totally dependent, there is a wide range of possibilities for rehabilitation of communicative power and, in some cases, the return of economic self-sufficiency.

Impairments in the comprehension, production or use of language by adults are encountered in a variety of clinical settings. Acquired language disorders are frequently observed, for example, in patients with stroke, head injury, dementia, brain tumors and CNS infections (including AIDS). Language disorders are also found in adults who have failed to develop normal language because of childhood autism, hearing impairment or other congenital or acquired disorders of brain development. Although deficits of spoken language frequently affect all language modalities, that is, reading, writing and the signed languages of deaf people, dissociations in performance as a function of language modality do occur. Thus, for example, patients with acquired disorders of reading or writing may be essentially normal in spoken language. Lastly, disorders of language, or communication more generally, may be encountered in patients with dysfunction of the nondominant hemisphere. Specific impairments in the interpretation of communicative intent, as well as in the ability to appreciate several alternate meanings of a word, have been demonstrated after stroke involving the right hemisphere.

Research on the ways in which adult language can break down following brain injury necessarily builds upon an understanding of how language comprehension and production are accomplished by normal people. The development of experimental techniques for analyzing language functions and for investigating the neuroanatomic representation of those functions in the brain constitutes an important component of current efforts in this area.

The understanding of the anatomic and physiologic bases of normal and disordered adult language has, in recent times, been facilitated by the application of a variety of experimental techniques. Contemporary computed tomography (CT) and magnetic resonance imaging (MRI) scans offer precise information about lesion size and location heretofore available only at autopsy. These data have, for example, contributed to a better understanding of the anatomic basis of speech initiation and production. Imaging of brain metabolism and blood flow using positron emission tomography (PET), as well as single photon emission computed tomography (SPECT), has contributed substantially to the understanding of the functional anatomy of the language system in normal subjects as well as in patients with brain dysfunction. These studies of dynamic brain activity have also led to a greater appreciation of the important interactions between language and other cognitive operations. Electro-cortical stimulation techniques have also contributed to the understanding of the functional anatomy of the language system. The analysis of the consequences of transient electrically-induced cerebral "lesions" has facilitated the identification of discrete language mechanisms and has engendered better understanding of the individual variability in the cortical representation of language functions. Finally, additional electrophysiologic techniques, such as event-related potentials (ERP) as well as advances in the mathematical modeling and signal processing of electroencephalographic data, have assisted in the understanding of the temporal course and anatomic representation of language processes.

The theories and methods of modern cognitive science have brought about important refinements in understanding the cognitive processes that normally underlie language functions. For example, chronometric investigations of the course of auditory language comprehension have highlighted the complexity of the processes required to integrate aspects of word meanings with elements of sentence structure. These new insights have motivated the development of tests that allow the attribution of specific aphasic symptoms to failure within identifiable components of the language system. These advances have, in turn, provided the groundwork for the development of new approaches to diagnosis and rehabilitation of aphasia and acquired dyslexia.

Several recent findings await further study and fuller exploration. For example, common mechanisms underlying spoken language and the signed language of deaf people have been dramatized by the identification of striking parallels in the effects of brain injury on these two modes of communication. Artificial intelligence computer models of language have offered insights into the processes mediating language; additionally, disruptions or "lesions" of these models permit the simulation of symptoms and promise to provide a means for the testing of hypotheses concerning the basis of particular language deficits. Cross-language comparisons of sentence production and sentence comprehension disorders have begun to distinguish between symptoms that are universal in their form of presentation and those that are specific to the structure of particular languages.

Recent advances in the remediation of language disorders include the demonstration that some profoundly aphasic patients can learn a computerized system for exchanging information by manipulating visual symbols. In fact, computer-assisted assessment and instruction are active areas of current research interest and promise to allow the testing of previously untapped cognitive capacities in severely-impaired patients. Explorations in the pharmacologic treatment for aphasic symptoms have shown promise for the relief of selective disorders, such as impairments of speech initiation, through the use of the dopamine agonist, bromocriptine.

Several more traditional treatment programs have been shown to be efficacious with specific types of aphasic patients. These include language oriented and language stimulation treatment techniques as well as interventions designed to bring about well-defined outcomes such as the elimination of the perseverative intrusions of earlier utterances. Additional intervention strategies currently being tested include treatment protocols targeted directly at theoretically-defined language components that are found to be impaired. A limited number of such studies conducted to date have demonstrated measurable improvement among individual aphasic patients many years following onset of their aphasia. These studies represent a direct application of results gathered previously in cognitive and linguistic studies of aphasia.

Recent accomplishments in the area of adult language and its disorders have built upon advances in neuroanatomic and neurophysiologic diagnostic procedures, as well as on developments in linguistic theory and cognitive science. Assessment and rehabilitation of these deficits continue to rely on the clinical expertise of speech-language pathologists with new participation from the fields of neuropsychology, pharmacology and computer science. This diversity reflects the complex and multifaceted nature of adult language disorders and provides a broad base upon which to develop a research agenda for the future.

Chapter 33

Developmental Speech and Language Disorders: Hope Through Research

Eliza, age 2-1/2, toddles around her nursery school classroom, the straps of her purple overalls slipping off her shoulders. She watches and smiles, and generally she follows directions, but Eliza is silent. The only words she utters are *dog* to describe a wooden plaything and—when it's time to go home—*bus*.

Ben is older, nearly 5, and as sweet-faced as little Eliza. But his only "words"—used sparingly in two-word phrases—are all but unintelligible to a stranger. Ben wants to join in the activities of his class, but he cannot understand his teacher's instructions about putting a beanbag on his head, on his shoe, on his shoulder. He simply holds on to the beanbag and smiles, waiting to imitate the other children's responses.

Eliza and Ben are in a special program for preschoolers with speech and language disorders. Eliza is language disordered and has a brain dysfunction: she is delayed primarily in her ability to translate thoughts into language, even though she understands almost everything that a child her age is expected to. Ben is disordered in both speech and language. His problems involve the neurological motor skills that produce speech, as well as the brain function of understanding language. The treatment he requires is more complex. And if Ben has normal intelligence—which can be determined by specialized testing—then this intelligence is masked by his halting, stumbling phrases.

NIH Publication No. 88-2757. March 1988. Language Milestones chart is adapted from the Portage Guide to Early Education, ©1976, Cooperative Educational Service Agency.

281

What causes speech and language disorders in children like these? How can the problems be treated? Will children who are slow to speak and understand what is said to them also be slow to read, to write, to think logically? Evidence suggests that the answer to the latter question may be yes for some children, but scientists continue to search for causes and effective treatments that will give parents and professionals a basis for hope. Encouraged by the National Institute of Neurological and Communicative Disorders and Stroke (NINCDS), the primary source of Federal support for research on the brain and disorders of speech and language, investigators around the country are developing new techniques for studying normal and disordered speech and language acquisition as well as treatments for speech and language impairments.

Eliza and Ben have a chance of being helped because their problems have been discovered and are being treated early in life. But many questions will remain unanswered for years. The children will be watched closely when they enter school—Ben probably in a special classroom, Eliza perhaps mainstreamed into a regular school—to see whether their speech and language delays show up later in other guises, particularly as reading disabilities. And as they reach adulthood, another question looms: Will they pass their speech and language difficulties on to their own children?

The Scope of the Problem

A child with a language disorder has difficulty understanding language or putting words together to make sense, indicating a problem with brain function. A child with a speech disorder has trouble producing the sounds of language, often resulting from a combination of brain-coordination and neurological motor dysfunction. Either child will lag significantly behind the level of speech and language development expected of a playmate of the same age, environment, and intellectual ability.

Language impairment may show itself in several ways:

- Children may have trouble giving names to objects and using those names to formulate ideas about how the world is organized. For example, they cannot learn that a toy they play with is called <u>car</u>, or that a toy car of another color, or a real car, can also be called <u>car</u>.

282

- They may have trouble learning the rules of grammar. Such children might not learn, for example, how to use prepositions and other small words like in or the.

- They may not use language appropriately for the context; for example, they might respond to a teacher's question by reciting an irrelevant jingle heard on television.

Speech problems seem to be more prevalent than language problems. Both disorders appear to decline as children get older. Speech disorders affect an estimated 10 to 15 percent of preschoolers, and about 6 percent of children in grades 1 through 12. Language disorders affect about 2 to 3 percent of the preschool population and about 1 percent of the school-age population. In all, nearly 6 million children under the age of 18 are speech or language disordered. Two-thirds of them are boys.

It is difficult to be more precise about just how prevalent the problem is, because the definition itself is so unwieldy. How delayed must a child be to qualify as "disordered"? How does one recognize the delay in the first place?

When Is There a Problem?

Experts use phrases such as *developmental language disorder, delayed speech, impaired language, motor disorder,* and *idiopathic* (no known cause) speech and language disorders to describe a variety of speech and language difficulties in children. In this pamphlet, delayed speech or delayed language means a problem that appears in the course of the child's development and for which there is no apparent cause. Eliminated from this discussion are speech or language problems that can be traced to deafness, mental retardation, cerebral palsy, or autism.

Speech-language pathologists generally define children as disordered if they lag significantly behind their age peers in reaching certain speech and language milestones. The significance of this lag is determined by a thorough professional examination. British studies show that the range of normal for early language acquisition is enormous. Normal children speak their first word at anywhere from 6 to 18 months, and combine words into phrases for the first time at anywhere from 10 to 24 months. It takes a skilled practitioner to distinguish between a slow child who will eventually catch up and a child with a true delay.

Speech and language professionals have devised a general outline of what speech sounds should have been acquired by a certain age. A child who is not quite on schedule, of course, is not necessarily delayed or disordered; it may just be that the child's individual timetable is different from most children's.

An understanding of what constitutes normal language development is helpful when parents try to evaluate whether their child is abnormally slow. The most widely accepted speech and language milestones for children age 1 to 7 years are outlined in the charts at the end of this pamphlet.

Language problems are most obvious among 2- to 3-year-olds, whose language skills are usually developing very rapidly. Many of these problems subsequently resolve themselves; others require the aid of therapy.

Among older children, speech and language disorders might emerge in a different guise. A 5- or 6-year-old might have caught up in language and social skills sufficiently to communicate with others, but not sufficiently for good reading or thinking. Such a child could be considered reading- or learning-disabled.

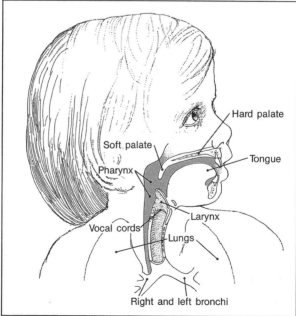

Figure 33.1. The structures of the vocal system.

The Physical Tools of Speech

Speech has four components: articulation, phonation, resonance, and rhythm:

- *Articulation* is the ability to make specific sounds: the g in gum, the b in bear, the s in snake. Articulation is the component most often affected in children with speech disorders of unknown cause.

- *Phonation* is the utterance of vocal sounds—the voice—produced in the larynx or "voice box."

- *Resonance* is the modification of the voice after it leaves the larynx. The voice is modified by the cavities inside the mouth, nose, and pharynx (the throat).

- *Rhythm*, or what scientists call *prosody* involves the rate and timing of speech.

For speech to begin, the brain and the vocal and auditory systems must be in good working order. The human vocal system components are perfectly adapted for speech. Our teeth, for example, are usually evenly spaced and equal in size (unless there are dental problems), and our top and bottom teeth can get close enough to pronounce such sounds as s, f, sh, and th. Our lips have more developed muscles than the lips of other primates, and our relatively small mouths can open and shut rapidly to form sounds such as p and b. The size of our mouth opening can be varied to pronounce a range of vowel sounds.

The location of the larynx is perhaps the most important feature of the human vocal system. In the adult human, the larynx, where the vocal cords are located and voice sounds originate, is located farther down in the throat than is the larynx of any other primate. This extra room allows humans to modulate speech and to pronounce such sounds as the consonants in gut and cut.

The Structures of the Vocal System

Defects in the structure of the lips, palate, or teeth can interfere with a child's ability to make speech sounds correctly. A hole in the palate—the "cleft palate" seen in some newborns—is the most common such problem. A cleft palate can usually be corrected surgically, but even after surgery affected children may have too much nasal resonance and difficulty producing certain speech sounds. Other children with growths in the larynx or vocal cords may have voices with a harsh, husky sound.

The auditory system comprises the three parts of the ear—the outer ear, the middle ear, and the inner ear—and the connections between the inner ear and the auditory center of the brain. The middle ear is prone to infection during childhood because of the angle of the eustachian tube, which connects the middle ear to the throat. When a child has a cold, the short eustachian tube cannot drain excess mucus properly, and the fluid that builds up becomes a breeding ground for bacteria. The resulting condition is called otitis media.

If the auditory system is not in good order and a hearing loss exists as a result of continual ear infections and fluid buildup, the child may mishear adult speech and produce it incorrectly. To avoid this problem, an otolaryngologist, a physician who specializes in ear, nose, and throat disorders, should be consulted at the first sign of a hearing loss. The otolaryngologist may refer the child for testing to an audiologist, an expert on the hearing process.

The Role of the Brain

If scientists were asked to identify the most important feature of the brain that enables humans to speak, they would point to the brain's functional division into left and right hemispheres. This characteristic appears to be related in most people to the brain's asymmetry. Even at birth one can see evidence of this asymmetry: the left hemisphere tends to be larger than the right in most newborns.

Although most complex functions involve both sides of the brain to some extent, certain functions can be traced to one hemisphere or the other. In approximately 90 percent of us, the right hemisphere controls how we see spatial relationships (such as the recognition of faces) and recognize patterns (such as a musical melody). In that same 90 percent of us, the left hemisphere controls how we process sequences of information involving language.

Neuroscientists once thought that a person's handedness showed which side of the brain was dominant for language: right-handed people were thought to derive language skills from the left hemisphere, left-handed people were thought to draw these skills from the right hemisphere. But we now know that the tendency is for most individuals, no matter which hand they prefer, to rely on the left hemisphere for language abilities. In certain situations, however, the right hemisphere can take over language function. In young children, for example, the loss of left-hemisphere language function after certain kinds of brain surgery can be well compensated for by the right hemisphere. But in adolescents and young adults the right hemisphere is less able to take over language or speech production.

The maturing nervous system. The development of the brain's asymmetry is part of the overall maturation of the nervous system which occurs before birth. Scientists believe that sometime in the middle of gestation, nerve cells, or neurons, migrate from germinal zones—areas where cells reproduce—to the regions of the brain in which they will reside. This brain cell migration usually begins at about the 16th week and ends by the 24th week.

Figure 33.2. The axon of a neuron is covered by a myelin sheath, a fatty casing that facilitates the transmission of brain messages.

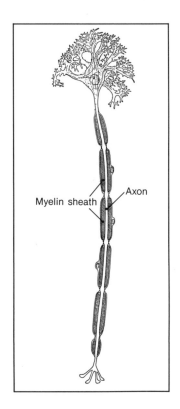

287

If the migration of cells to the brain is incomplete or interrupted by something in the fetus' environment (perhaps an antibody developed by the body in response to a foreign substance), the fetus could die before or shortly after birth. If migration occurs, but with errors, the result could be language delay.

After mid-gestation, and probably through the first decade of life, the neurons of a child's brain begin to mature. As neurons develop, they grow axons: long connecting arms linking one brain cell to another. As neuronal development continues, these axons are covered by a myelin sheath, a fatty casing that protects the axons and helps them transmit messages more efficiently. This myelinization of message pathways in the brain occurs at a rapid rate until about age 2 and continues at a slower pace until puberty. The process is crucial to the child's growing capacity for understanding and expressing language.

The brain's language centers. Two areas in the brain are known to be involved in speech and language. Broca's area, named after the French surgeon Pierre-Paul Broca, is in the left frontal lobe, close to the part of the brain that controls movements of the tongue, larynx, and other structures involved in speech. Broca's area is responsible for translating thoughts into speech.

Wernicke's area, named after the German neurologist Karl Wernicke, is located behind Broca's area, just around the temples. It contributes to the understanding of the spoken and written word, and in most individuals is larger in the left hemisphere than in the right. Wernicke's area is quite close to the auditory cortex, the brain region that controls the input and analysis of sound.

The difference in function of the two language regions is apparent when either area is damaged. Aphasia is the loss of language after a brain injury. An adult aphasic with damage to Broca's area has reduced speech that sounds like a message in a telegram: asked about the weather, he might respond "rainy" or, if pressed, "rainy day." An adult with damage to Wernicke's area may articulate well and form grammatically correct sentences, but provides very little coherent information in his speech. Such a patient might answer a question about the weather by saying, "I think it's not good. I don't like it when it's like that." Many aphasic patients may have other language problems as well.

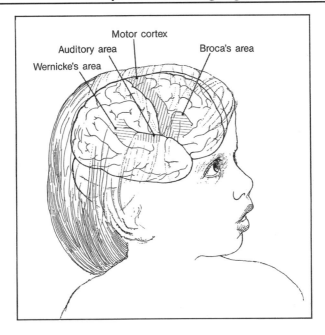

Figure 33.3. The areas of the brain involved in speech and language.

Translating sounds into meaning. Some children may have language difficulty because of a problem with the brain's ability to analyze speech. Research scientists have studied dozens of language-delayed children and found that they are unable to process rapid speechlike signals produced by a computer. But they can be trained to differentiate among sounds if the time between sounds is prolonged.

Scientists now know that soon after birth, babies are able to detect differences between speech sounds. Investigators have found that infants as young as 1 month can detect the minute differences between closely related speech sounds such as <u>p</u>at and <u>b</u>at.

Most children develop a phonological system, an internal sense of how different categories of speech sounds are used, by about age 3. This system differs according to the child's native language. An English-speaking child, for instance, does not have within his phonological system the same <u>s</u> sound as a Spanish-speaking child, a sound that is somewhere between the English <u>s</u> and <u>th</u>, or the gutteral <u>kh</u> sound of a German-speaking child.

Children must first perceive the unique characteristics of a sound in order to be able to repeat it. But many sounds in the English language differ only minutely—and sometimes the differences are a matter of timing. The difference between the initial sounds for the words <u>b</u>in and <u>p</u>in, for example, is a function of something called voice onset time. To utter the <u>b</u> sound, the vocal cords begin to vibrate almost as soon as the speaker releases air by opening the lips. For the <u>p</u> sound, there is a delay of about 20 extra milliseconds between the time the lips first open and the time the vocal cords start vibrating.

Even though these differences are very small, most persons can discriminate between <u>b</u> and <u>p</u>, or <u>d</u> and <u>t</u>, or g and <u>k</u>—consonants distinguishable by short differences in voice onset time. Speech-language pathologists believe that when children consistently fail to make these distinctions, they may have incorrectly established the sounds in their phonological systems.

Think of what happens to an adult trying to learn a foreign language. The adult can generally imitate the sounds of that language after hearing a word about 50 to 100 times, but still does not know the phonology—the range of possible sounds of the language and the rules for their order. Similarly, a child can imitate the sounds his speech pathologist urges him to make, but to him they're like a foreign tongue. A little boy who speaks like Elmer Fudd, the cartoon character who calls Bugs Bunny a "scwewy wabbit," may be capable of making an <u>r</u> sound the way he's told to, but to him the <u>r</u> sound isn't supposed to sound like an <u>r</u>. He thinks it should sound like a <u>w</u>.

Other Influencing Factors

The normal development of speech and language depends largely on the health of the brain and the vocal and auditory systems. But children who are abnormally slow in speech or language acquisition may show no signs of physical problems that could explain the delay. In such cases, certain other factors may be slowing things down.

Ear Infections. Controversy exists about the relationship between chronic otitis media and the rapidity with which a child learns to speak. Most studies investigating the question have found no clear association between otitis media and language disorder, unless a hearing loss is present. The prudent course is to treat ear infections promptly and to be alert to signs of poor hearing—inattentiveness, failure to respond, requests to have words repeated or to have the television volume raised—in a child with frequent otitis media. Treatment may include antibiotic therapy and the insertion of a tube into the middle ear to drain the fluid. Recent NINCDS-supported studies found that decongestant and antihistamine compounds are ineffective for otitis media but that the antibiotic amoxicillin is effective.

Poor models in the home. The role of the environment in language acquisition has never been fully explained. For example, a normal child whose parent suffers from a language problem may reach full language competence despite an environment in which language models are scant. Psycholinguists, who study the psychological and biological roots of language, believe most children have an innate drive to learn the language of the community no matter what the environment.

But children whose brain structures are abnormal, even in quite subtle ways, may be born with a tendency toward language problems, and if their environments are language-deficient they just don't have the inner resources to compensate. In addition, a vicious cycle of silence is all too easy to establish in the home of a language-impaired child. Parents react to the cues their babies give them. If a baby does not respond with sounds and words, the parent is unlikely to know that the baby is indeed ready for conversation. According to one scientist, the communication difficulties of language-impaired children have a direct impact on the parent's efforts to talk to them.

A Collection of Disorders

Speech and language disorders wear many faces. Common speech disorders include:

- *Phonological impairment,* also called misarticulation. Here the child says the sounds wrong, or omits or duplicates certain sounds within a word. The problem may reflect poor neurological motor skills, a learning error, or difficulty in identifying certain speech sounds. Examples of common errors are <u>wabbit</u> for <u>rabbit</u>, <u>thnake</u> for <u>snake,</u> <u>dood</u> for <u>good</u>, and <u>poo</u> for <u>spoon</u>.

  Another phonological impairment is unstressed syllable deletion, in which a child simply skips over a syllable in a long word, as in <u>nana</u> for <u>banana</u> or <u>te-phone</u> for <u>telephone</u>. Many of these misproductions are a part of normal development and are expected in the speech of very young children,

291

but when they persist past the expected age they are considered abnormal and usually indicate brain dysfunction.

- *Verbal dyspraxia.* This term is used by some scientists and clinicians to describe the inability to produce the sequential, rapid, and precise movements required for speech. Nothing is wrong with the child's vocal apparatus, but the child's brain cannot give correct instructions for the motor movements involved in speech. This disorder is characterized by many sound omissions. Some verbally dyspraxic children, for instance, speak only in vowels, making their speech nearly unintelligible. One little boy trying to say "My name is Billy" can only manage "eye a eh ee-ee. " These children also have very slow, halting speech with many false starts before the right sounds are produced. Their speech errors may be similar to those of children with phonological impairment.

- *Dysarthria.* Here muscle control problems affect the speech-making apparatus. Dysarthria most commonly occurs in combination with other nervous system disorders such as cerebral palsy. A dysarthric child cannot control the muscles involved in speaking and eating, so the mouth may be open all the time or the tongue may protrude.

A child with a language problem has difficulty comprehending or using language, and several different types of errors may result. Three of the more common are:

- *Form errors.* These are present when the child cannot understand or use the rules of grammar. A child with this problem might say "We go pool" instead of "We went to the pool. "

Language-disordered children seem to have particular difficulty with complex sentence constructions such as questions and negative forms. Examples of form errors [are listed below showing correct sentences followed by disordered sentences]:

> They won't play with me—They no play with me.
> I can't sing—I no can sing.
> He doesn't have money—He no have money.

When will he come?—When he will come?
What is that?—What that?

- *Content errors.* This language disorder is involved when the semantics, or what the child understands or talks about, is limited or inaccurate. The child may have a limited vocabulary or may fail to understand that the same word—match, for example—can have multiple meanings.

- *Use errors.* This term concerns what linguists call pragmatics, the ability of the child to follow the rules of communication: when to talk, how to request information, how to take turns. A child with a use error might be unable to ask an adult for help, even though he knows that help is needed and the adult can provide it. Autistic children who have difficulty communicating with people may have use errors.

Categorizing Patients

If children with a speech or language problem are to benefit from different treatment approaches now available, they must be accurately subgrouped according to type of impairment. In categorizing speech- and language-impaired children, experts tend to ask two questions. First, is the disorder expressive, receptive, or a mixture of both? Second, is the child simply delayed in speech or language development, or is the child not only delayed but abnormal in speech and language when these skills begin to develop?

Expressive or receptive? Some language-impaired children have primarily expressive (speaking) disorders; others have mainly receptive (understanding) disorders. Most have a combination of both.

Clinicians often encounter children who may be unable to communicate effectively, but nonetheless show signs of understanding others quite well. Consider Becky, a 6-year-old girl seen at a speech clinic. Her conversation with a clinician goes like this:

Clinician: What is your favorite game?
Becky: Doctor.
Clinician: How many can play that game?

Becky: Two four.
Clinician: Two or four?
Becky: Or three.
Clinician: How do you play doctor?
Becky: One has to be doctor.
Clinician: Anything else?
Becky: One operation man.
Clinician: Anything else?
Becky: No.
Clinician: What do you want to be?
Becky: A nurse.
Clinician: Oh, you need a nurse?
Becky: No, you don't.

Becky has an expressive language disorder. Her responses are limited to incomplete sentences that may be inappropriate to the question, and they reveal Becky's inability to use verbs, conjunctions, or any of the subtleties of language. Like some children with expressive language problems, Becky has a good vocabulary, but she has difficulty connecting words. Even though she is 6, she talks like a 2-year-old.

Children with expressive language problems may or may not have articulation problems. But even if their speech is perfectly articulated, communication is impaired because language remains ungrammatical, reduced, babyish.

Paul, who is 7 years old, is Becky's opposite, a child with a receptive language disorder who has difficulty understanding language. Receptive language problems rarely occur alone; usually they are accompanied by at least some degree of expressive language disorder. The condition often is misdiagnosed as attention problems, behavioral problems, or hearing problems. Standardized language tests may reveal, though, that a child with a receptive language disorder is trying to cooperate but simply cannot understand the instructions.

Paul, for instance, cannot point to a picture that best reveals his understanding of single vocabulary words or of grammatical associations between words. When asked to point to a picture of "the ball under the table," Paul might just as readily point to a picture of a ball on the table. When asked to point to the picture of "the boy running after the girl," he might instead choose the one of a girl running after a boy.

Delay or disorder? Scientists have not agreed on whether language-impaired children acquire language normally—but more slowly—than other children or whether they develop language in an abnormal way when they begin to talk and understand. If any consensus has been reached in the past decade, it is that both sides may be right. There may be two quite separate conditions, one in which speech or language is delayed, and another in which speech or language is not only delayed but also incorrect.

In the 1970's, several groups of scientists tackled the problem. Generally, children had been categorized according to certain measures of language development such as the average length of spontaneous sentences. One study found that language-impaired children used simpler grammatical sentences and fewer questions than other children. Another study found that language-impaired children understood the meanings and relationships of words in much the same way that other children did. Language-impaired children seemed to develop their ability to express themselves in the same progression as normal children, but only after they had reached a higher-than-normal level of language comprehension.

The general consensus from research of recent years is: many language-impaired children seem to be merely delayed, but a sizable number also develop language in an abnormal way. The distinction is important, because it can help clinicians recognize that some children should be treated aggressively and others left alone.

A Visit to the Doctor

A child whose parents suspect a speech or language disorder will probably enter the health care system through the pediatrician's office. Before referral to a speech-language pathologist for assessment, the physician will try to determine if there are underlying conditions that might be the indirect cause of the speech or language delay.

A child is likely to be tested to rule out the following conditions:

- *Hearing problems.* Language acquisition is a continual process of hearing, imitating or spontaneously trying a word or phrase, hearing one's own productions, and refining them. Scientists have observed that infants who have impaired hearing from birth tend to be delayed in their instinctive babbling and produce fewer different sounds.

295

A physician faced with a child over 2 years old who does not speak often will refer that child for complete audiological testing. Such tests involve the use of tones delivered through headphones: as soon as the tone is heard, the child responds by raising a finger or performing some other behavior or gesture. Occasionally, children with hearing problems may unintentionally hide their conditions from their parents because they become so adept at using environmental cues—facial expressions, vibrations, and what little hearing they have—to get by. These cues fall short of helping the children learn the complex sounds of language.

- *Mental retardation.* The developmental language disorders described in this pamphlet occur in children of normal or above-normal intelligence. However, language problems are also common among the mentally retarded. Experts estimate that nearly half of all mildly retarded children, 90 percent of severely retarded children, and 100 percent of profoundly retarded children have language disorders of some sort.

  A pediatrician may suspect mental retardation if the delay in achieving speech and language milestones is accompanied by a delay in other mental and physical milestones. Gross neurological motor development—sitting, standing, crawling, and walking—and fine motor development—reaching, grasping, building towers of blocks—are often interpreted as clues to whether a child's mental capacities are normal. If mental retardation is a source of concern, tests are available to see just where a child ranks with his or her age peers in mental and physical areas of development. These tests involve such tasks as having the child imitate an examiner's arrangement of blocks or copy geometric shapes.

- *Autism.* One of the hallmarks of the disorder called autism is the inability of the child to communicate. Autism begins before age 2-1/2 years; it includes particular speech and language problems: total lack of language, a pervasive lack of responsiveness to people, and peculiar speech patterns. The latter include immediate or delayed echoing of another's comments, speaking in metaphors, or reversing pronouns. In addition to having communication problems, autistic children may be resistant to change, may be overly attached to objects, and may have bizarre and unexpected responses to their environments. A child neurologist will ask about the child's behavior to rule out autism.

- *Cerebral palsy.* The muscle control problems characteristic of cerebral palsy can sometimes interfere with speaking. When this happens, children may understand language better than they can speak. They may have trouble expressing themselves because of difficulty moving their lips or tongue.

- *Acquired aphasia.* Children are considered aphasic when the brain injury that causes loss of language occurs after speech and language have begun to develop. Aphasia can occur after severe head trauma or a brain infection. Some acquired aphasia is an unfortunate consequence of surgery, as in those rare cases when children undergoing a heart operation suffer a stroke after blood flow to the brain is blocked.

    Children who suffer damage to the left half of the brain exhibit many of the symptoms that adult aphasics do. Their problems are predominantly expressive but also may be receptive. They may have speech articulation problems or make errors in syntax. They may also speak in reduced, incomplete sentences, just as adults do when there is damage to Broca's area.

    But a child with acquired aphasia is different from an adult aphasic in one important way: the child is better able to recover. Because the brain continues to reorganize itself until adolescence, neurons seem to be capable of compensating for an injury that happens early in life.

- *Other conditions.* A handful of genetic conditions also are characterized by language or speech problems. These include *cri du chat syndrome*, which leads to mental retardation and a tendency to make catlike mewing sounds, and *Tourette syndrome*, a neurological disorder characterized by involuntary sounds such as barking, clicking, and yelping.

A Team of Experts

Once a child has been identified as having a speech or language disorder, most successful diagnosis and treatment involves a team of experts. The audiologist, an expert in the process of hearing, evaluates and assists those with hearing disorders. The audiologist may work in consultation with an otolaryngologist, a physician who specializes in ear, nose, and throat disorders. These two health professionals determine which hearing conditions can be treated—and perhaps corrected—medically or surgically, and which require rehabilitative techniques such as hearing aids or lip reading.

The speech-language pathologist, also called a speech therapist, studies the normal and abnormal processes of speech and language and measures and diagnoses speech and language problems. The pathologist can also enhance early learning of language, teach the correct production of speech and language, and help a child learn to understand words and sentences.

The neurologist is a physician with expertise in the workings of the brain and nervous system. The neurologist may use modern brain imaging techniques to "see" through the skull and detect brain abnormalities in a child with speech or language delay. A range of pencil-and-paper and physical tests have also been devised to help diagnose any underlying brain disorder that might account for the language problem.

The psychologist studies the science of human development and personality, and can administer tests to evaluate the child's cognitive capabilities. Such tests can help determine how the child's language age compares to his or her mental and chronological ages.

The New Therapy

In the 1970's, language-delayed children were taught to repeat sentences in a robotlike fashion. As one NINCDS scientist puts it, "These children could say, 'We went swimming today' perfectly, but they couldn't change it to say the same thing with different words." Today the emphasis in therapy is less on imitation than on grasping the context of language. Children play with toys and are taught to translate their activities into words—a mode of learning that is more meaningful for them and that gives them the tools to construct their own sentences.

For the child whose speech is impaired or delayed, treatment may focus on one sound group at a time, starting with the sounds that babies naturally learn first. Young clients are encouraged to use the sounds in a variety of contexts, to watch the clinician make the sound—even putting their hands on the clinician's throat or mouth while the sound is spoken—and to watch themselves make the sound, putting their hands on their own mouths and watching themselves in a mirror.

The most important and continuous help comes from parents. Guided by speech and language pathologists, parents can do a great deal to improve the language environment in their home.

Parents can learn better ways to respond to their children's utterances so that language skills improve. When a child says, "more milk," a parent may respond several ways. The least helpful are silently to refill the milk glass, or to say, "here milky in cuppy," or some other form of nongrammatical babytalk. But adults are tempted to give such answers with youngsters who never seem to benefit from more sophisticated replies such as, "Do you want more milk?" A better response would be the simple statement, "More milk for Sam."

If the parent peppers responses with what linguists call *expansions*—new words, new sentence constructions, new rules of grammar—the child can eventually learn new bits of language. Expansions introduce new information or help the parent develop the child's words into a grammatically correct sentence.

Ways Adults Can Help a Child Learn Language

- Expand the statement, preserving the child's intent.

  a. Expand the statement using the same noun.
      Child: kitty jump.
      Adult: The kitty is on the chair.
  b. Replace the noun with a pronoun.
      Child: kitty jump.
      Adult: She is jumping.
  c. Expand the statement adding new information.
      Child: kitty jump.
      Adult: The dog is jumping, too.

- Respond by indicating the truth value of the child's utterance, rather than its linguistic accuracy (or inaccuracy).

> *Child:* kitty jump.
> *Adult:* Yes, the kitty is jumping

The Long-Term Outlook

How do speech- and language-impaired children fare in adolescence and adulthood? Most followup studies indicate that speech disorders tend to be outgrown by adolescence, but that difficulties involving language use, production, or understanding can persist into adulthood.

One study from the University of Iowa examined 36 adults, 18 of whom had been diagnosed as speech-disordered and 18 as language-disordered when they were children. Nine of the language-disordered children still had communication and learning difficulties in adulthood, compared to only one in the speech-disordered group.

A Cleveland-based study of 63 preschoolers with speech and language disorders found that 5 years after initial diagnosis, 40 percent of the children still had speech and language problems, and 40 percent had other learning problems such as below-normal achievement in reading and in math. NINCDS-supported scientists at the University of California at San Diego are now conducting a study of 100 language-impaired 4-year-olds to see how they fare up to 5 years after identification of their language problems. Preliminary results suggest that children with only expressive language losses have a lower risk of long-term problems than do children with both expressive and receptive impairments.

The Promise of Research

Scientists are pursuing research leads that promise improved therapy for children with speech and language disorders. Studies of these disorders are supported by NINCDS, other Federal agencies including the National Institute of Mental Health and the National Institute of Child Health and Human Development, and private and medical institutions.

The brain's organization. Studies of cell structure in the brains of dyslexic individuals—otherwise normal people who have extraordinary difficulty learning to read—show that speech and language disorders may be caused by abnormal development of the brain's language centers sometime before or soon after birth.

"From the middle of gestation until about the first or second year, the actual floor plan of the brain is being laid down," says one of the NINCDS grantees who conducted these studies at Boston's Beth Israel Hospital.

Using a technique called cytoarchitectonics, in which the actual structure and arrangement of cells is revealed, the investigators examined the brains of seven adults who had been diagnosed as dyslexic. They found a series of abnormalities in the cerebral cortex. These included _ectopias_, neurons found in the language centers of the brain that seem to have arisen elsewhere and migrated to the wrong area; _dysplasias_, or misshapen neurons; and so-called brain warts, neurons that are nodular in appearance. The brains also failed to show the normal degree of asymmetry.

Other methods are being used to study how the brain may be abnormal in children with speech or language disorders. Some scientists are using brain imaging techniques to try to locate the site of auditory processing in the brains of children with expressive and receptive language impairments. These investigators hope to pinpoint regions where speech sounds are processed and to see how those regions differ between language-impaired and normal children.

The genetic connection. Speech and language problems seem to run in families. This could be accounted for by environmental influences: a home in which language is misused is a home where children develop poor language skills. But most scientists think there may be a large genetic component. Investigators are now studying families with speech and language problems to find out how these disorders are inherited.

Speeding things up. Some language disorders may originate in the abnormally slow rate at which the child's brain is able to process information. To test this theory, scientists are experimenting with ways to train language-impaired children to process speech and language more rapidly. NINCDS grantees at the University of California at San Diego are using computers to teach children to hear the most subtle sound shifts—such as those that differentiate <u>ba</u> from <u>da</u>—by exaggerating those differences. The computer produces and gradually speeds up speech sounds until the children can hear the ba/da distinction at the rate at which it occurs in ordinary conversation.

Some language-delayed children avoid words that are hard to pronounce. In an NINCDS-supported study of word avoidance, scientists at Purdue University are asking both normal and language-delayed children to say the hard-to-pronounce nonsense names assigned to unusual objects and toys. By characterizing the patterns of word avoidance in the two groups, the scientists hope to devise improved treatment methods for the language-delayed children.

As scientists learn more about how the normal brain controls language and initiates speech, they will also discover just what goes wrong in brains when problems arise. After the underlying mechanisms are detected, investigators hope to develop new treatment techniques to help the millions of children whose thoughts and feelings are poorly expressed.

Where to Get Help

A number of private organizations have been set up to help people with speech and language disorders. These organizations distribute educational materials and, in some cases, provide lists of treatment experts. For more information, call or write to the following organizations:

American Speech-Language-Hearing Association
10801 Rockville Pike
Rockville, MD 20852
(301) 897-5700

The Council for Exceptional Children
Division of Children with Communication Disorders
1920 Association Drive
Reston, VA 22091
(703) 620-3660

National Association for Hearing and Speech Action
Suite 1000
6110 Executive Boulevard
Rockville, MD 20852
(301) 897-8682

National Easter Seal Society, Inc.
2023 West Ogden Avenue
Chicago, IL 60612
(312) 243-8400

The Orton Dyslexia Society, Inc.
724 York Road
Towson, MD 21204
(301) 296-0232

Tourette Syndrome Association
42-40 Bell Boulevard
Bayside, NY 11361
(718) 224-2999
(800) 237-0717 (toll free)

NINCDS Information

For more information about the research programs of the NINCDS, contact:

Office of Scientific and Health Reports
National Institute of Deafness and Other Communication Disorders
National Institutes of Health
Bethesda, MD 20892
(301) 496-7243
(301) 402-0252

Language Milestones

[The following list describes the speech behavior a child should have mastered at one to 6 years of age.]

1 Year

- Says 2 to 3 words (may not be clearly pronounced)
- Repeats same syllable 2 to 3 times ("ma, ma, ma")
- Carries out simple direction when accompanied by gestures
- Answers simple questions with nonverbal response
- Imitates voice patterns of others

- Uses single word meaningfully to label object or person

2 Years

- Says 8 to 10 words by age 1-1/2, 10 to 15 words by age 2
- Puts two words together ("more cookie," "where kitty?")
- Points to 12 familiar objects when named
- Names 3 body parts on a doll, self, or another person
- Names 5 family members including pets and self
- Produces animal sound or uses sound for animal's name (cow is "moo-moo")
- Asks for some common food items by name when shown ("milk," "cookie," "cracker")

3 Years

- Produces two-word phrases combining two nouns ("ball chair"), noun and adjective ("my ball"), or noun and verb ("daddy go")
- Uses no or not in speech
- Answers where, who, and what questions
- Carries out a series of two related commands
- Consistently uses ing verb form ("running"), regular plural form ("book/books"), and some irregular past tense forms ("went, " "did," "was")
- Uses is and a in statements ("This is a ball")
- Uses possessive form of nouns ("daddy's")
- Uses some class names ("toy," "animals," "food")

4 Years

- Uses a vocabulary of 200 to 300 words
- Uses is at beginning of questions when appropriate
- Carries out series of two unrelated commands
- Expresses future occurrences with going to, have to, want to
- Changes word order appropriately to ask questions ("Can I?" "Does he?")
- Uses some common irregular plurals ("men," "feet")
- Tells two events in order of occurrence

5 years

- Carries out series of three directions
- Demonstrates understanding of passive sentences ("Girl was hit by boy")
- Uses compound and complex sentences
- Uses contractions can't, don't, won't
- Points out absurdities in picture
- Tells final word in opposite analogies
- Names picture that does not belong in particular class ("one that's not an animal")
- Tells whether two words rhyme

6 Years

- Points to some, many, several
- Tells address and telephone number
- Tells simple jokes
- Tells daily experiences
- Answers why question with an explanation
- Defines words

Chapter 34

Update on Developmental Speech and Language Disorders

The National Institute on Deafness and Other Communication Disorders (NIDCD) has primary responsibility at the National Institutes of Health (NIH) for supporting research on developmental speech and language disorders. The NIDCD, which became one of the institutes of the NIH in October 1988, supports research and research training on normal and disordered processes of hearing, balance, smell, taste, voice, speech, and language. This publication provides an update of current research and recent advances in understanding developmental speech and language disorders.

Language Impairments

Overview. It is estimated that between six and eight million people in the United States have some form of language impairment. A person with a language impairment or disorder has difficulty communicating with others because the ability to understand or produce language is impaired. Understanding spoken words and sentences may be difficult, and the disorder may lead to problems with speaking, reading and writing. Scientists study development of language to understand the nature of the disorders affecting language development and to design teaching or therapeutic strategies to improve the communication process for persons with developmental language disorders._____

This publication, published in December 1991, is an update of the original NIDCD booklet on Developmental Speech and Language Disorders (No. 88-2757).

There are different causes of language disorders in children. Some language disorders are a result of hearing loss, autism, mental retardation, emotional disorders, or neural impairment. However, for a larger number of children, the cause of the disorder is unknown. Scientists use the term specific language impairment (SLI) to describe language disorders of unknown cause. SLI is the type of disorder discussed in this pamphlet update.

Early studies of SLI children found that only a small percentage of these children showed evidence of a neural impairment. However, studies since then have shown that children with SLI may have temporal processing difficulties, in that some perform especially poorly when asked to identify specific sounds when hearing a series of rapid sound changes. Children with SLI also may have problems in coordinating incoming sensations (e.g., sight, sound, touch) with motor activity.

Early studies of children with SLI centered on the features of syntax (sentence structure), morphology (word formation and pronunciation), phonology (the sounds of words), and semantic relations or the meaning of words in a sentence in relation to their location in the sentence. Scientists found that children with SLI had problems in all of these areas. The studies revealed that these children not only develop language more slowly than other children with normal language, but also differently than younger children who are developing language normally. Certain features (e.g., word formation) caused more serious difficulty. Long-term studies of children with language-related learning problems showed that these language problems may continue into adulthood. Young children with language-related learning problems are clearly at risk for later problems in reading.

Recent Advances. Diagnostic techniques, such as magnetic resonance imaging (MRI), are being used to determine if neurogenic disorders might be found in language-impaired children. MRI produces detailed images of the body's inner structures without the use of x-rays.

Genetic studies of SLI children have also been undertaken. The findings from these studies suggest that SLI children are more likely than are normal children to have other family members with language problems. An NIDCD-supported scientist is conducting a genetic study at the University of Iowa to determine factors that contribute to this familial aspect of specific language impairment.

Scientists at the Salk Institute, La Jolla, California, are examining the neurobehavioral development (the brain's impact on behavioral development) in normal children and in language-impaired and reading-disabled (LI/RD) children. They are comparing brain functions during tasks involving sensing, thinking, and language reception and production in normal children and LI/RD children at different ages and different stages of language and thought development. This research will provide an understanding of the best type and timing of intervention for language-impaired individuals.

New studies include comparisons of treatment for children with SLI. Current research includes studies on the lexical (vocabulary) and pragmatic (communicative-conversational) abilities of SLI children. Scientists at Pennsylvania State University are exploring ways to combine imitation training, in which the child imitates the clinician's or teacher's speech, and conversation-based treatment which involves the child in conversation. At an NIDCD-sponsored research study at the University of Washington investigators are looking at the language acquisition process in preschool SLI children to determine whether there are optimum times to begin treatment.

Some of the research priorities of the NIDCD include the integration of speech perception (children's recognition, organization, and interpretation of speech) and speech motor abilities and the relationship of these processes to language acquisition. NIDCD-supported researchers at Purdue University, for example, are examining differences in the processes of speech perception and speech production in normal and SLI children. They are using tests of speech production to determine whether a primary speech motor deficit or a speech motor learning impairment is the cause of language problems in children. These tests will help the scientists determine what extent speech production abilities (i.e., speech motor skills) may be related to how children interpret and produce sentences. Another study by scientists at Indiana University is examining the relationships between speech perception and the more abstract linguistic (language) and cognitive (thinking) processes involved in the understanding of spoken language.

Children with SLI often exhibit difficulties with the way words are used, such as use of past tense and function words, which include articles (i.e., a, an, the) and auxiliary verbs (i.e., be, have, do). A research project is underway at Purdue University to explore the possible bases of these grammatical word limitations and to examine how such limitations may hinder other aspects of these children's language development.

Speech Disorders

Overview. Speech development is a gradual process that requires years of practice. Children spend several years "playing with speech sounds" and imitating the sounds they hear. Most children have mastered all of the speech sounds by six years of age; however, they will continue to refine their speech production for several more years.

By first grade, it is estimated that five percent of children have noticeable speech disorders, the majority of which have no known cause. Although most of these children eventually learn normal speech, about 20 percent will remain speech impaired for the rest of their lives. According to the American Speech-Language-Hearing Association, the major class of speech disorders are articulation disorders of unknown cause. An articulation disorder is an incorrect production of specific speech sounds (e.g., producing a lisp by substituting the /s/ sound for the /th/ sound). These children comprise 40 percent of those seen by school speech clinicians.

Another category of speech disorder is fluency disorders or stuttering. This disorder is characterized by a disruption in the flow of speech. It includes repetitions of speech sounds, hesitations before and during speaking, and/or prolongations of speech sounds. It can be accompanied by evidence of a struggle to speak. The speaker will frequently avoid certain words or phrases and avoid certain difficult speech situations (for example, the telephone). Although stuttering is a type of speech disorder, it is not a developmental speech disorder and is not the focus of this pamphlet.

Recent Advances. NIDCD continues to support research to identify the causes of articulation disorders and to identify factors that may be used in treatment. A research project at Indiana University, for example, is examining whether children perceive distinctions in their own sound productions that are not perceived by other listeners. The researchers will determine if treatment of perceptual knowledge (the listener's interpretation of speech sounds) is as important to learning sounds as treatment of productive knowledge (the process of sound production). It is important to know if some articulation disorders result from a problem in a child's understanding of language messages or a defect in the child's motor system, i.e., the ability to make the movements to produce the sounds. The results of this project will help to identify processes that are essential to learning a sound system. A large research program is being conducted by investigators at the University of Wisconsin to describe, predict, manage, and prevent developmental articulation disorders. Scientists are determining how to predict normal speech following indirect (caregiver-based) and direct (clinician-based) management of speech problems. These findings will have a direct impact on service delivery for preschool children identified as having speech disorders of unknown origin.

As scientists continue to learn more about the underlying causes of speech and language disorders, they will be able to design and develop more appropriate treatment strategies for children with developmental speech and language disorders.

About the NIDCD

The NIDCD conducts and supports research and research training on normal and disordered mechanisms of hearing, balance, smell, taste, voice, speech and language. The NIDCD achieves its mission through a diverse program of research grants for scientists to conduct research at medical centers and universities around the country and through a wide range of research performed in its own laboratories.

The institute also conducts and supports research and research training related to disease prevention and health promotion; addresses special biomedical and behavioral problems associated with people who have communication impairments or disorders; and supports efforts to create devices that substitute for lost and impaired sensory communication function. The NIDCD is committed to understanding how certain diseases or disorders may affect women, men and members of the underrepresented minority populations differently.

The NIDCD has established a national clearinghouse of information and resources. Additional information on developmental speech and language disorders may be obtained from the NIDCD Clearinghouse. Write to:

311

NIDCD Clearinghouse
P.O. Box 37777
Washington, DC 20013-7777

For additional information:

American Speech-Language-Hearing Association
10801 Rockville Pike
Rockville, MD 20852
Voice/TDD (301) 897-5700
Consumer Helpline (800) 638-8255

Central Institute for the Deaf (CID)
818 South Euclid Avenue
St. Louis, MO 63110-1594
(314) 652-3200 voice/TDD

The Council for Exceptional Children
Division of Children with Communication Disorders
1920 Association Drive
Reston, VA 22091
(703) 620-3660

National Rehabilitation Information Center (NARIC)
8455 Colesville Road, Suite 935
Silver Spring, MD 20910
(301) 588-9284 voice/TDD
(800) 34-NARIC

Orton Dyslexia Society
724 York Road
Baltimore, MD 21204
(301) 296-0232
(800) ABCD-123

Chapter 35

Questions and Answers about Articulation Problems

What is articulation?

Articulation is the process by which sounds, syllables, and words are formed when your tongue, jaw, teeth, lips, and palate alter the air stream coming from the vocal folds.

What is an articulation problem?

A person has an articulation problem when he or she produces sounds, syllables, or words incorrectly so that listeners do not understand what is being said or pay more attention to the way the words sound than to what they mean.

Is an articulation problem the same as "baby talk"?

An articulation problem sometimes sounds like baby talk because many very young children do mispronounce sounds, syllables, and words. But words that sound cute when mispronounced by young children interfere with the communication of older children or adults. Older children and adults have so many severe errors that their articulation problems are very different from "baby talk."

What are some types of sound errors?

Most errors fall into one of three categories—omissions, substitutions, or distortions. An example of an omission is "at" for "hat" or "oo" for "shoe." An example of a substitution is the use of "w" for "r," which makes "rabbit" sound like "wabbit," or the substitution of "th" for "s" so that "sun" is pronounced "thun." When the sound is said inaccurately, but sounds something like the intended sound, it is called a distortion.

What causes an articulation problem?

Articulation problems may result from physical handicaps, such as cerebral palsy, cleft palate, or hearing loss, or may be related to other problems in the mouth, such as dental problems. However, most articulation problems occur in the absence of any obvious physical disability. The cause of these so-called functional articulation problems may be faulty learning of speech sounds.

Is an accent an articulation problem?

It can be for some persons. We all have accents—Southern, Eastern, Northern, Western, Chicago, Pittsburgh, Brooklyn, or Boston. An accent may be a problem if it interferes with a person's goals in life.

Can ear problems during infancy have any effect on late sound development?

Children learn their speech sounds by listening to the speech around them. This learning begins very early in life. If children have frequent ear problems during this important listening period, they may fail to learn some speech sounds.

Will a child outgrow a functional articulation problem?

A child's overall speech patten will usually become more understandable as he or she matures, but some children will need direct training to eliminate all articulation errors. The exact speech pattern of the individual child will determine the answer to this question.

Do children learn all sounds at once?

Sounds are learned in an orderly sequence. Some sounds, such as "p," "m," and "b," are learned as early as 3 years of age. Other sounds, like "s," "r," and "l," often are not completely mastered until the early school years.

At what age should a child be producing all sounds correctly?

Children should make all the sounds of English by 8 years of age. Many children learn these sounds much earlier.

How can I help a child pronounce words correctly?

By setting a good example. Don't interrupt or constantly correct the child. Don't let anyone tease or mock (including friends or relatives). Instead, present a good model. Use the misarticulated word correctly with emphasis. If the child says, "That's a big wabbit," you say "Yes, that is a big rabbit. A big white rabbit. Would you like to have a rabbit?"

Can an adult with an articulation problem be helped?

Most articulation problems can be helped regardless of a person's age, but the longer the problem persists, the harder it is to change. Some problems, such as those relating to nerve impulses to the muscles of articulation (dysarthria), are particularly difficult and generally will require a longer period of help than a functional disorder. Other conditions that may influence progress in a child or adult include hearing ability, condition of the oral structures such as the teeth, frequency of help obtained, motivation, intelligence, and cooperation.

Who can help?

Contact a speech-language pathologist if you are concerned about speech. A speech-language pathologist is a professional trained at the master's or doctoral level to evaluate and help the child or adult with an articulation problem as well as other speech and/or language disorders. The speech-language pathologist should be certified by the American Speech-Language-Hearing Association and/or licensed by your state. The speech-language pathologist can advise whether professional help is indicated and how to arrange for assistance. The speech-language pathologist can also give you guidance or provide services to help prevent or eliminate a problem. Early help is especially important for more severe problems.

Is it important to correct an articulation problem?

When you consider the possible impact an articulation problem may have on one's social, emotional, educational, and/or vocational status, the answer becomes obvious. Our speech is an important part of us. The quality of our lives is affected by the adequacy of our speech.

Chapter 36

Facts on Adult Aphasia

What Is Aphasia?

Aphasia is a language disorder that results from damage to the portion of the brain that is dominant for language. For most people, this is the left side of the brain. Aphasia usually occurs suddenly, frequently the result of a stroke or head injury, but it may also develop slowly as in the case of a brain tumor. The disorder may involve aspects of language comprehension and/or expression.

Aphasia treatment strives to improve an individual's ability to communicate. The most effective treatment begins early in the recovery process. Major factors that influence the amount of improvement include the cause of the brain damage, the area of the brain that was damaged, the extent of the brain injury, and the age and health of the patient. Additional factors include motivation, handedness, and educational level.

There are many types of aphasia, however, Broca's aphasia and Wernicke's aphasia are two widely studied aphasic syndromes. Broca's aphasia results from damage to the front portion of the language dominant side of the brain. Wernicke's aphasia results from damage to the back portion of the language dominant side of the brain.

Individuals with Broca's aphasia may speak in short, meaningful sentences. They often omit small words such as "is," "and," and "the."

An unnumbered fact sheet published by the National Institute on Deafness and Other Communication Disorders. September 1994.

Persons with Wernicke's aphasia may speak in long sentences that have no meaning and often add unnecessary words and create new words. Patients with Broca's aphasia are able to comprehend much of the speech of others, but patients with Wernicke's aphasia have notable difficulties understanding speech.

A third type of aphasia, global aphasia, results from damage to a large portion of the language dominant side of the brain. Individuals with global aphasia have major communication difficulties and may be extremely limited in their ability to speak or comprehend language.

Aphasia Research

Language Organization of Deaf Signers

Until recently, little has been known about language organization in the brain of deaf signers. The National Institute on Deafness and Other Communication Disorders (NIDCD) supports research at the Salk Institute, San Diego, California, which has revealed that the left side of the brain is dominant not only for spoken language but for sign language as well. This discovery is particularly interesting since the right side of the brain is dominant for visual and spatial functions. American Sign Language, which is similar in structure to spoken language, is conveyed through hand movements which are visually and spatially oriented. Signers with damage to the right side of the brain had no aphasia for sign language but had difficulty with nonlanguage visual and spatial tasks such as drawing a face. This suggests that, as in those who use spoken language, the right hemisphere in deaf signers develops specialization for nonlanguage visual and spatial functions.

In addition, this research concluded that deaf signers with damage to the left side of the brain demonstrated sign language aphasias similar to the aphasias experienced by those who use spoken language. If the damage was to the front portion of the left side of the brain, the signing would be broken and simplified, much like the broken, effortful speech characteristic of Broca's aphasia. Signers with damage in the back portion of the left side of the brain had fluent signing but poor word selection as well as difficulty understanding the signs of others. This is similar to the word selection and comprehension problems experienced by those with Wernicke's aphasia.

318

A New Look At Aphasia Based On Cross-Language Studies

NIDCD-supported researchers at the University of California at San Diego are studying how damage to specific areas of the brain affects language function across different languages. The characteristics of Broca's and Wernicke's aphasias, for example, may differ across languages primarily because of differences in the languages themselves. At the same time, however, similarities may be found. Results of these cross-language studies suggest that language knowledge is preserved in both Broca's and Wernicke's aphasias but difficulty arises in how the language is accessed and used. This is contrary to the present theory that Broca's and Wernicke's aphasias are primarily disorders of language structure.

A New Way to Select Aphasia Treatment

A number of methods are used to treat aphasia. Health professionals who treat aphasia must select the most effective method of treatment to maximize the aphasic patient's recovery of language function. NIDCD-supported scientists at the Boston University Aphasia Research Center have studied the use of CT scans (computed tomography) to predict the success of one method of treatment, Melodic Intonation Therapy. This form of treatment has been successful for some patients with little or no verbal language following brain injury. The results of this study indicate that information from the CT scan together with results of language assessment by a speech-language pathologist may accurately predict whether this treatment will improve the ability to communicate. Continued research will investigate the use of CT scans, coupled with language tests, to predict the success of other aphasia treatments.

Computers Help Those with Severe Aphasia

Even with therapy, individuals with severe aphasia may have difficulty communicating even the simplest ideas and needs. Scientists at the University of Maryland Medical System in Baltimore have been investigating the use of a nonverbal method of communication for the aphasic patient called computerized visual communication or C-VIC. This method of communication uses pictures on a computer that represent various parts of speech. Seven patients with either severe

Broca's aphasia or global aphasia have recently received training with C-VIC. Six of these patients were able to learn to use the pictures to communicate. The noun pictures were easier for the patients to learn to use than were the verb or action pictures. The information gathered from this research should improve the understanding of the processes underlying language as well as improve the design of speech therapy programs and nonverbal communication systems for individuals with aphasia.

Age and Aphasia

Many professionals who work with aphasic patients believe that it is easier for younger individuals to recover language skills than it is for older individuals. Solid evidence for this concept, however, is lacking. Scientists at the New York University Medical Center in New York City are presently studying how age affects the ability of 90 treated aphasic individuals to relearn language. These individuals range from 50 to 80 years of age and receive comprehensive therapy including speech therapy. It is hoped that the information gained from this study will help select appropriate patients for therapy as well as add to the understanding of how age relates to aphasia.

About the NIDCD

The NIDCD is one of the institutes of the National Institutes of Health (NIH). The NIDCD conducts and supports biomedical and behavioral research and research training on normal and disordered mechanisms of hearing, balance, smell, taste, voice, speech and language.

About the Recent Research Series

This series is intended to inform health professionals, patients, and the public about progress in understanding the normal and disordered processes of human communication through recent advances made by NIDCD-supported scientists in each of the Institute's seven program areas of hearing, balance, smell, taste, voice, speech and language.

For additional information on aphasia, write to:

320

NIDCD Information Clearinghouse

1 Communication Avenue
Bethesda, MD 20892-3456

Chapter 37

Questions and Answers about Adult Aphasia

What is adult aphasia?

Aphasia is the condition in which an individual has difficulty expressing thoughts and understanding what is said or written by others. Aphasia is caused by brain damage, resulting most often from a stroke or direct injury to the head.

What are some of the language problems associated with aphasia?

Persons with aphasia will have difficulty understanding what is said to them and expressing their own thoughts. They will also have reduced ability to read, write, gesture, or use numbers. Speech may be limited to short phrases or single words such as names of objects or actions. Frequently, the smaller words in speech are left out so that the sentence is shortened to "key words" like a telegram. The word order may be incorrect, or the message may be turned around and difficult to understand. Sometimes, sounds and words get changed, for example, calling a table a "chair" or calling a bank teller a "tank beller." Nonsense words like "baba" or "shanna" may even be used. Some people with aphasia may produce speech with obvious effort and misarticulations. The most common characteristic is difficulty in naming. The person with aphasia may know what to do with a toothbrush, for example, but will have forgotten what to call it.

Why does it take a person with aphasia so long to respond?

Persons with aphasia need extra time to understand what is being said to them. They hear the words, but they may not immediately recall the meaning of the word. In some cases, it may sound to the person with aphasia as if the speaker is talking in a foreign language. In addition, they need time to think of the words they want to use.

Once individuals with aphasia think of the word they want to use, will they remember it?

Often they will forget the word once they use it and will have to renew the searching process when they need it again. Their child's name, for example. They may say it several times, but then not be able to recall the name a few minutes later.

Is it typical for individuals with aphasia to swear?

Yes, many times they retain certain automatic responses, such as swearing, counting, naming the days of the week and social responses, such as "fine," "thanks," and "hi." Don't criticize them for swearing. They often won't realize they're saying anything inappropriate.

What other problems can be caused by a stroke or head injury?

Some individuals may have trouble pronouncing words properly. Their speech may be slurred. They may also be more emotional. For example, they may become frustrated more easily, and they may laugh or cry excessively. They may also be confused or forgetful at times.

What are some of the physical problems connected with brain damage?

Aphasia usually is caused by injury to the left side of the brain. When one side of the brain is hurt, the opposite side of the body is affected. Often times persons with aphasia have a weakness of the right arm and leg. Vision may also be affected. In fewer instances, seizures will occur.

What is spontaneous recovery?

As the body recovers from the brain damage on a physical level, some individuals with aphasia will regain former skills, like talking or writing. Improvement may be within days or continue for at least six months, or even longer. This immediate improvement is called spontaneous recovery. Spontaneous recovery seldom produces complete return of function, however.

What help is available for the person with aphasia?

There is help, both for the person with aphasia and for the family who needs to understand aphasia. The speech-language pathologist is the professional who is trained at the master's or doctoral level to evaluate the problem and execute a rehabilitation plan. Although few people can be "cured," most can be helped. Your speech-language pathologist will hold the Certificate of Clinical Competence (CCC) from the American Speech-Language-Hearing Association (ASHA) and/or licensing from your state.

How soon should an individual with aphasia see a speech-language pathologist?

Usually within the first few days following the injury. In addition to providing help for speech and language recovery, the speech-language pathologist can offer hope to the individual and guidance for the family. Often the testing information obtained by the speech-language pathologist will be helpful to the medical staff in caring for the person with aphasia.

Can family and friends help?

Family members and friends are a vital part of the rehabilitation program. The more they understand the problem, the more they can help the recovery of the person with aphasia. The speech-language pathologist will work closely with the family to help them help their loved one.

Chapter 38

Stuttering:
Hope Through Research

*"What dressing will you have on your salad?" the waiter said.
"R-r-r-r-r-ro-ro-roque-roque-I'll have the roque-I think I'd like
to try the ro-ro-ro----Thousand Island."*

Stutterers laugh at that joke, too. For them, however, stuttering
has far more serious consequences than not getting their favorite
salad dressing. The frustration and struggle to get the words out can
embarrass and exhaust both speaker and listener. Some stutterers
avoid the struggle by dodging situations where they have to speak.
Children may say "Don't know," to the teacher—even when they do
know—rather than face laughter and teasing from their classmates.
Other stutterers keep their minds a phrase or two ahead of their
mouths. That way they can pick out problem words and find substi-
tutes. In either case the stutterer suffers the loss of smooth and easy
speech, the spontaneous exchange of feelings and ideas so important
at school or work, among family and friends.

"It is like a sharp mmmmmomentary twist of pain that I eexxsss-
-perience again and again throughout eeeeevery dddddday ah ah of my
life. I ss-ssssssometimes ssssssssssee it as a as a nnnnnail in my shoe
that iiiiiis thththere and p-p-pro-bab-bly always wwww-ww-wi-ll be
there..." says a 36-year-old woman.

Yet there is reason to hope that that woman, and others, particularly younger stutterers, will be able to escape the twist of pain. With

NIH Publication No. 81-2250. May 1981.

therapy—and sometimes without it—many stutterers achieve more normal speech. Studies describing the differences in the way normal and stuttered speech is produced are pointing to new directions in therapy. Spearheading this research is the National Institute of Neurological and Communicative Disorders and Stroke (NINCDS), the leading Federal agency supporting research on speech disorders. The Institute currently supports investigators who are developing new techniques for the study of normal as well as abnormal speech.

Early Warning Signs

Stuttering is a disorder in which the rhythmic flow, or fluency, of speech is disrupted by rapid-fire repetitions of sounds, prolonged vowels, and complete stops—verbal blocks. A stutterer's speech is often uncontrollable—sometimes faster, but usually slower than the average speaking rate. Sometimes, too, the voice changes in pitch, loudness, and inflection.

Observations of young children during the early stages of stuttering have led to a list of warning signs that can help identify a child who is developing a speech problem. Most children use "um's" and "ah's," and will repeat words or syllables as they learn to speak. It is not a serious concern if a child says, "I like to go and and and and play games," unless such repetitions occur often, more than once every 20 words or so.

Repeating whole words is not necessarily a sign of stuttering; however, repeating speech sounds or syllables such as in the song "K-K-K-Katy" is.

Sometimes a stutterer will exhibit tension while prolonging a sound. For example, the 8-year-old who says, "Annnnnnnd---and---thththen I I drank it" with lips trembling at the same time. Children who experience such a stuttering tremor usually become frightened, angry, and frustrated at their inability to speak. A further danger sign is a rise in pitch as the child draws out the syllable.

The appearance of a child or adult experiencing the most severe signs of stuttering is dramatic: As they struggle to get a word out, their whole face may contort, the jaw may jerk, the mouth open, tongue protrude, and eyes roll. Tension can spread through the whole body. A moment of overwhelming struggle occurs during the speech block. The feeling of panic and loss of control is so overwhelming that the stutterer will try to avoid any repetition of the experience in the future. Children may begin to substitute simple words for more troublesome ones; they may giggle before speaking to help get them started, or they may adopt a drawl or other speech mannerism that temporarily displaces the stuttering.

NINCDS is sponsoring a study to analyze the speaking characteristics of young children between 4 and 6 years of age—the time that stuttering most commonly develops. By determining which aspects of speech distinguish those who develop a stuttering problem from those who do not, methods of early detection and improved treatment can be developed.

While the symptoms of stuttering are easy to recognize, the underlying cause remains a mystery. Hippocrates thought that stuttering was due to dryness of the tongue, and he prescribed blistering substances to drain away the black bile responsible. A Roman physician recommended gargling and massages to strengthen a weak tongue. Seventeenth century scientist Francis Bacon suggested hot wine to thaw a "refrigerated" tongue. Too large a tongue was the fault, according to a 19th century Prussian physician, so he snipped pieces off stutterers' tongues. Alexander Melville Bell, father of the telephone inventor, insisted stuttering was simply a bad habit that could be overcome by reeducation.

Some theories today attribute stuttering to problems in the control of the muscles of speech. As recently as the fifties and sixties, however, stuttering was thought to arise from deep-rooted personality problems, and psychotherapy was recommended.

Who Stutters?

Stutterers represent the whole range of personality types, levels of emotional adjustment, and intelligence. Winston Churchill was a stutterer (or stammerer, as the English prefer to say). So were Sir Isaac Newton, King George VI of England, and writer Somerset Maugham.

There are more than 15 million stutterers in the world today and approximately 1 million in the United States alone.

Most stuttering begins after a child has mastered the basics of speech and is starting to talk automatically. One out of 30 children will then undergo a brief period of stuttering, lasting 6 months or so. Boys are four times as likely as girls to be stutterers.

Occasionally stuttering arises in an older child or even in an adult. It may follow an illness or an emotionally shattering event, such as a death in the family. Stuttering may also occur following brain injury, either due to head injury or after a stroke. No matter how the problem begins, stutterers generally experience their worst moments under conditions of stress or emotional tension: ordering in a crowded restaurant, talking over the telephone, speaking in public, asking the boss for a raise.

Stuttering does not develop in a predictable pattern. In children, speech difficulties can disappear for weeks or months only to return in full force. About 80 percent of children with a stuttering problem are able to speak normally by the time they are adults—whether they've had therapy or not. Adult stutterers have also been known to stop stuttering for no apparent reason.

Indeed, all stutterers can speak fluently some of the time. Most can also whisper smoothly, speak in unison, and sing with no hesitations. Country and western singer Mel Tillis is an example of a stutterer with a successful singing career.

Most stutterers also speak easily when they are prevented from hearing their own voices, when talking to pets and small children, or when addressing themselves in the mirror. All these instances of fluency demonstrate that nothing is basically wrong with the stutterer's speech machinery.

If the problem is not in the mouth or the throat, is it in the brain? Stuttering can arise from specific brain damage, but only rarely. In general, stuttering is not associated with any measurable brain abnormality and is not related to intelligence.

The New Research

To find out what is associated with stuttering, investigators are analyzing how speech sounds are normally produced and what goes wrong when a person stutters.

To produce speech, you must shape the sound that is produced as air moves up from the lungs through the throat and into the mouth. Breathing muscles in the chest provide the pressure that drives air up the windpipe across the voice box, or larynx. At the larynx, the air passes between two folds of tissue known as the vocal cords, and sets them vibrating. Like the reeds of oboes, the vibrating cords convert air flow into audible sound.

The shape and amount of tension of the cords determine the pitch of the voice—how high or low it sounds. The further refining of voice into speech sounds depends on the relative shape and position of other parts of the vocal tract: the lips, tongue, jaws, cheeks, and palate. All told, over 100 muscles are involved in speech production.

Because the larynx is the source of sound, scientists are studying it closely, paying particular attention to the muscles that control the vocal cords. One set of muscles pulls the vocal cords apart, opening the airway. Opening allows you to take a deep breath, for example. An opposing set of muscles closes the vocal cords, allowing you to produce voice. The vocal cords are also in a fully closed position when you swallow. That helps prevent food from getting into the airway and causing choking.

Normally the laryngeal muscles work in a coordinated and reciprocal manner: One set of muscles relaxes while an opposing set of muscles contracts. When NINCDS-supported investigators at Haskins Laboratories, New Haven, Conn. studied the behavior of the laryngeal muscles during stuttered speech however, they were astonished to find that both sets of muscles contracted—setting up a virtual tug of war for control of the cords. This striking difference between normal and abnormal muscle behavior can be observed in the same speaker when speaking fluently and when stuttering.

Scientists have also noted excessive muscle activity during stuttering. Not only do both sets of opposing muscles contract during stuttering, but they also contract as hard as they can.

Ingenious techniques have enabled scientists to record the abnormal muscle movements. Investigators can hook wires directly into throat and neck muscles, for example, and pick up the electrical activity associated with muscle movement. They can also observe the movements of the vocal cords directly by using special fiberoptic equipment transmitting light through a flexible narrow tube which is inserted into the subject's nose.

In some cases the inappropriate muscle activity prevents the vocal cords from coming together long enough to make a normal sound. In other cases the vocal cords are so tightly locked no sound at all can emerge: The speaker is totally blocked. Unusually high levels of muscle activity have also been discovered in stutterers' tongue muscles. Whether the extreme muscle contractions cause the failure of coordination of the muscles of speech, or are a reaction to the failure,

331

is not known. Conditions that reduce muscle activity, however, appear to ease stuttering.

The muscle activity associated with partial or complete verbal blocks is not the only aspect of stutterers' speech scientists have analyzed. Both trained and untrained listeners can distinguish the voices of stutterers when speaking fluently from normal speakers. A slower rate of speech and an abnormal rhythm were the cues that identified the stutterers. Such differences may result from the stutterer's habit of planning words ahead to avoid a block and consciously trying to control the speech muscles.

Experiments in several laboratories have shown that stutterers are slower than normal speakers to begin vocalizations (for instance, when they are told to make a sound as soon as a signal goes on). Stutterers are also slower to make transitions from voiced sounds (when the vocal cords vibrate) to unvoiced sounds (when the vocal cords do not vibrate). When a stutterer switches from ordinary speech to some nonstuttering mode, such as choral speaking, the rate of speech also tends to decrease. So some scientists speculate that stutterers have a lower than normal maximum speaking rate. Their everyday speech frequently exceeds that limit, however, and trips them up.

Improved techniques have led to a more detailed description of stuttering and the conclusion by some scientists that what we call stuttering may be more than one condition. Each condition, in turn, may have a different cause. Another conjecture is that stuttering results from the interaction of several factors. For example, a child may inherit a tendency to stutter, but certain environmental conditions may have to be present for stuttering to develop.

Stuttering does seem to run in families, and it affects boys more than girls. NINCDS-supported scientists at Yale University have studied 555 stutterers and more than 2,000 of their close relatives. The results support the idea that a susceptibility to stuttering is inherited, but just how is not clear. Certainly the inheritance pattern does not follow the simple rules that explain how eye color, hair color, or colorblindness is inherited.

To search for a clue to a cause of stuttering—genetic or otherwise—investigators are adopting newly available techniques to investigate brain activity in stutterers. Since the brain is the master regulator and coordinator of all body activity, it is possible that some slight brain dysfunction might disturb the clockwork coordination of the organs of speech. On those occasions when stutterers do speak fluently, the coordination task is usually simplified. Whispering, for example, does not involve vibration of the vocal cords at all.

A subtle brain dysfunction might also affect our ability to hear what we're saying as we say it. Alterations in that hearing "feedback" system or in similar systems monitoring other parts of the speech production machinery, may also be involved in stuttering. Scientists are also just beginning to examine the brain areas that are active during normal and stuttered speech. Important, too, are studies of how the two halves of the brain, the cerebral hemispheres, interact in speech activities.

New Treatments and Old Schools

While research has yet to explain why stuttering occurs, some of the new findings have been applied to therapy:

- *Biofeedback*. One recent approach uses biofeedback techniques to help stutterers relax their throat muscles. The stutterer hears a tone that becomes louder with increased muscle tension, and he or she is instructed to quiet the tone. Usually when the person succeeds in reducing the tension of the throat muscles, he or she is able to speak without stuttering.

- *Larynx control*. Some treatment programs emphasize modifying sound production at the larynx itself. Stutterers are taught to speak with lower levels of laryngeal activity, slower rates of vocal cord opening and closing, and loose rather than tight vocal cord closure. The resultant voice is somewhat lower, softer, smoother, and slower than average speech. To evaluate this technique, as well as other approaches to stuttering therapy, long-term studies will be necessary.

- *Regulating speech rate*. Some patients are taught to slow their overall speech rate. Devices used in such training include ear receivers that play back the speaker's words with a few seconds' delay (delayed auditory feedback). Sometimes a slow "pacing" tone is presented to one ear to provide a rhythm for the stutterer to follow in pronouncing syllables. Although both devices reduce stuttering, they often result in monotonous speech. However, for some patients monotonous but fluent speech may be better than severe stuttering.

333

In general, therapists employing the new techniques in treating stuttering belong to one of two traditional schools: One school believes that stutterers and nonstutterers fall into two distinct groups and that no adult stutterer can be completely cured. Therapists of that conviction teach their clients to stutter easily. Stutterers learn to reduce the tension and struggle so that they do not become completely blocked in speech. Once a person gains confidence in the skill to stutter easily, the frequency of stuttering often drops dramatically. Because normal speakers do stutter occasionally, recipients of the "stutter easy" therapy can learn to speak without noticeable hesitations.

Charles Van Riper, the leading proponent of that approach and a stutterer himself, says, "Stuttering is not the world's worst of all curses...about 99.9 percent of the problem is in the way you respond to the thing!"

The other major school of therapy believes that any stutterer can be taught to be completely fluent. Therapists use methods such as breath control and soft, gentle attacks on words to create fluent speech with no stuttering. Preventing relapses of stuttering once fluency is reached is the most difficult problem with this approach.

A variety of training devices are used by both groups to allow a stutterer to experience fluent speech. A metronome can repress stuttering by setting a slower than normal rate for speech. A relatively new instrument called a masker prevents the stutterer from hearing his or her own voice during a conversation. The portable model consists of earphones and a microphone that rests on the throat near the larynx. Whenever the wearer speaks, the device makes a humming noise in the earphones so the wearer cannot hear his or her words. The device is successful in preventing stuttering even in difficult situations, and some stutterers have found that by using it they eventually learn to speak more fluently unassisted.

The Hope for Children

Therapists from both schools agree that the development of stuttering in young children is reversible. Treatment often includes the parents as well as the child. Parents are cautioned to listen to the content of the child's speech rather than to how he or she speaks. They are encouraged to be patient, and make speech enjoyable by playing word games and by reading or telling stories. The parents themselves are taught to speak slowly, quietly, and calmly, attacking their words gently. Overall, parents are advised to create pleasant and rewarding situations in which the child can communicate, and to reduce stress in the child's life that can disrupt fluency.

Therapists from both schools also agree that motivation is a key to success. The stutterer who feels frustrated and deprived of normal participation in speech is ripe for therapy. Usually it is best for the stutterer to specify exactly what he or she wants to change rather than just express a vague desire to stop stuttering. Results are more likely to be satisfactory if individuals decide that they most want to reduce their physiological problems, for example, or change their speaking pattern, or lower anxiety.

Where to Go for Treatment

In some places in the world anyone can hang out a shingle as a speech therapist. But in the United States, more than 20 states have laws governing the credentials of speech therapists, who also are called speech-language pathologists. The American Speech-Language-Hearing Association, through its standards board, certifies or accredits individual practitioners, educational programs and service agencies. Approximately 24,000 speech pathologists work in U.S. schools, hospitals, clinics, private practices and health departments. Selection of a licensed or certified speech therapist does not guarantee an expert on stuttering therapy, but the therapist should be able to refer the stutterer to an appropriate practitioner.

Evaluating the treatments available for stuttering is a particularly frustrating problem. For one thing, a fraction of stutterers improve with little or no treatment. For another, investigators must follow their subjects for years to see whether any improvement is long lasting. Over a period of 5 to 10 years, therapy techniques continue to evolve. So by the time the results of therapy are evaluated, newer methods may have supplanted those being evaluated.

From another standpoint, the very fact that new techniques are developing and older ones are undergoing revision or refinement is encouraging. Stutterers who quit trying to improve their speech years ago should be advised to try again.

To make a decision about treatment or to exchange ideas and opinions, it may be helpful to join one of the self-help groups for persons who stutter. These groups discuss the problems stutterers face in their daily lives, as well as developments in stuttering research and

335

therapy. They also help stutterers to understand how other people react to them. The National Council of Adult Stutterers and the National Stuttering Project may be able to refer a stutterer to a nearby group.

If you have a friend who stutters or if you come into contact with stutterers, there are ways to ease the embarrassment and frustration. First, try to be patient, though you have other demands on your time. Second, try to maintain eye contact, even when the stutterer looks away during a stuttering block. Finally, never fill in words for the person who stutters. That reinforces a feeling of time pressure and takes away the triumph of finally saying the difficult word.

One scientist who works on stuttering calls it the most fascinating and most frustrating communicative disorder. After years of research the feeling persists that the missing pieces of the stuttering puzzle are close at hand. Rather than having a simple cause—thick tongue or black bile or weak breath control—stuttering may be so complex that scientists will unravel the wonders of normal speech as they search for effective treatment.

For Additional Information:

American Speech-Language-Hearing Association
10801 Rockville Pike
Rockville, MD 20852
(301) 897-5700

National Council of Adult Stutterers
c/o Speech and Hearing Clinic
Catholic University of America
Washington, D.C. 20064
(202) 635-5556

National Stuttering Project
4438 Park Boulevard
Oakland, CA 94602
(415) 530-1678

National Easter Seal Society, Inc.
2023 W. Ogden Avenue
Chicago, IL 60612
(312) 243-8400

Division for Children with Communication Disorders
The Council for Exceptional Children
1920 Association Drive
Reston, VA 22091
(703) 620-3660

National Association for Hearing and Speech Action
Suite 1000
6110 Executive Boulevard
Rockville, MD 20852
(301) 897-8682

Speech Foundation of America
152 Lombardy Road
Memphis, Tenn. 38111
(901) 452-4995

Three good films on the prevention of stuttering were underwritten by the Speech Foundation of America: Part 1—*Identifying the Danger Signs*, Part II—*Parent Counseling and the Elimination of the Problem*, and Part III—*Ssstuttering and Your Child. Is it you? Is it me?* The films are available for purchase or rent to self-help groups, schools, and other organizations interested in speech disorders. Write to:

Seven Oaks Productions
9145 Sligo Creek Parkway
Silver Spring, Md. 20901

Specific inquiries concerning programs on stuttering may be directed to:

NIDCD
National Institutes of Health
Bethesda, Md. 20205

Chapter 39

Update on Stuttering

The National Institute on Deafness and Other Communication Disorders (NIDCD) has primary responsibility at the National Institutes of Health (NIH) for supporting research on stuttering. The NIDCD, which became one of the institutes of the NIH in October 1988, supports research and research training on normal and disordered processes of hearing, balance, smell, taste, voice, speech, and language. This [publication] provides an update of current research and recent advances in understanding stuttering.

Stuttering is a disorder in which the rhythmic flow, or fluency, of speech is frequently disrupted by repetitions of sounds or syllables. Often, stutterers form prolonged vowel sounds, repeat monosyllabic words like "and" or "if," or sometimes experience complete verbal blocks in which no words are spoken. There are over 15 million stutterers in the world, most of whom began stuttering at a very early age. Stutterers of all ages, however, have overcome their stutter through regulated speech-language therapy.

The cause of stuttering is unknown. Many scientists believe stuttering is associated with the intricate muscles involved in speech and vocal cord regulation. Some investigators suggest that psychological reasons may be responsible. Still others believe that it relates to a

This publication was prepared by: Program Planning and Health Reports Branch National Institute on Deafness and Other Communication Disorders National Institutes of Health, Bethesda, Maryland, August 1991.

complex interaction between stutterers' ability to produce speech and the psycho-social environment they experience while speaking.

Much of the current stuttering research focuses on finding a uniform and reliable method of measurement of fluency. Current measurements of the various types of stuttering along with its severity and frequency are subjective, relying almost entirely on a doctor's or therapist's judgement. In the search for an objective measurement, scientists have investigated many different approaches. Some scientists are studying the pathways of nerves that relay information back and forth from the brain to the muscles involved with speech. Plugging into these pathways, or neural networks, with devices like electrodes that measure the nerves' electrical activity can provide a foundation for measuring the severity of a patient's stuttering.

Other NIDCD scientists are studying heart rates. A changing heart rate of a stutterer can provide clues to muscle activity and emotional reactions as the patient casually converses with a therapist. In other studies, investigators are developing low-cost speech analysis programs for personal computers. These computer programs can be standard systems in speech clinics across the country, providing clinicians a uniform measure of fluency.

Once a uniform method of measurement is developed, speech-language pathologists can more accurately assess their patients' stuttering problems and design better therapy treatments for these patients. Through different forms of therapy, stutterers can learn to relax the muscles inside their throat and mouth or speak in softer tones or slower speeds.

Some scientists are searching for common characteristics or factors involved with stuttering. One current research project is tracing 40 stuttering children, probing their family history. In addition to collecting genetic and social background information, scientists are investigating the children's response times to a particular word or set of instructions. This will test the theory that stutterers respond or react to a given situation at a slower rate than nonstutterers. This does not mean, however, that stutterers are less intelligent; it simply suggests that stutterers may produce and respond to language differently.

Whatever causes stuttering, it is clear that it involves a breakdown in fluent speech formation. Scientists, therefore, are investigating the physiological basis for stuttering to understand what causes the disorder.

But speech formation is one of the most complicated skills that a human can learn. What's more, speech can be affected by emotions like excitement or nervousness, which are sometimes magnified when the stutterers realize that their disrupted speech may be making the listener uncomfortable or impatient. To produce speech, the diaphragm pushes air through the lungs to the vocal folds or voice box in the larynx. As air passes between these folds, the folds vibrate, resonating the airflow as it continues up the throat. Then, over 100 different muscles in the throat, mouth and tongue fine-tune this resonation into intelligible language. In addition, speech is produced only after a complicated cognitive process, tapping into a reservoir of nearly a million words in the English language and organizing this information into proper grammar and usage.

As a result, stuttering is a complex problem involving the brain, the muscles, and the emotional processes—incorporating both the psychological history of the stutterer and how that stutterer reacts emotionally to everyday conversations. A problem with any combination of these can cause or exacerbate stuttering. Scientists, therefore, are investigating all of these processes to explain why stuttering can occur or even worsen. As scientists continue to learn more about the physiological causes of stuttering, they can develop better treatment strategies for patients of all ages to overcome their stuttering problems.

About the NIDCD

The NIDCD conducts and supports research and research training on normal and disordered mechanisms of hearing, balance, smell, taste, voice, speech and language. The NIDCD achieves its mission through a diverse program of research grants for scientists to conduct research at medical centers around the country and a wide range of research performed in its own laboratories.

The institute also conducts and supports research and research training related to disease prevention and health promotion; addresses special biomedical and behavioral problems associated with people who have communication impairments or disorders; and supports efforts to create devices that substitute for lost and impaired sensory communication function. The NIDCD is committed to understanding how certain diseases or disorders may affect women, men, and members of the underrepresented minority populations differently.

341

The NIDCD has established a national clearinghouse of information and resources. Additional information on stuttering may be obtained from the NIDCD Clearinghouse. Write to:

NIDCD Clearinghouse
P.O. Box 37777
Washington, DC 20013-7777

For additional information:

American Speech-Language-Hearing Association
10801 Rockville Pike
Rockville, MD 20852
(301) 897-5700 or (800) 638-TALK

National Stuttering Project
4601 Irving Street
San Francisco, CA 94122-1020
(415) 566-5324

The Council for Exceptional Children
Division for Children With Communication Disorders
1920 Association Drive
Reston, VA 22091-1589
(703) 264-9435

Stuttering Foundation of America
P.O. Box 11749
Memphis, TN 38111 -0749
(901) 452-7343 or (800) 992-9392

Chapter 40

Spasmodic Dysphonia

We have all experienced problems with our voices—times when the voice is hoarse or sound will not come out at all! Colds, allergies, bronchitis, exposure to irritants such as ammonia, or cheering for your favorite sports team can result in a loss of voice. But, people with spasmodic dysphonia, a chronic voice disorder, face the persistent question—"What's wrong with your voice?"

With spasmodic dysphonia, movement of the vocal cords is forced and strained resulting in a jerky, quivery, hoarse, tight, or groaning voice. Vocal interruptions or spasms, periods of no sound (aphonia), and periods when there is near normal voice occur.

At first, symptoms may be mild and occur only occasionally. Later on, they may worsen and become more frequent before they stabilize. Even then, symptoms may be worse when a person is tired or stressed. Or, they may be greatly reduced or even disappear, for example, during singing or laughing.

This uncommon voice disorder affects more women than men and is found to strike people in all walks of life. It typically occurs between the ages of 30 and 50 years but is also seen in children and adolescents. Onset may follow an upper respiratory infection or periods of stress.

Causes

When not used for talking, the vocal cords of people with spasmodic dysphonia are normal in appearance and function. However, when the vocal cords are brought together for talking, their movement is uncontrolled.

Symptoms come from more than one source. Some people appear to have nervous system changes that produce an organic tremor of the vocal cords. Others may have dystonia, another kind of neurologic disorder that creates abnormal muscle tone. In rare cases, people can have spasmodic dysphonia symptoms because of acute or chronic life stress.

Diagnosis

There is no simple test for spasmodic dysphonia. Rather, diagnosis is based on the presence of the typical signs and symptoms described above and the absence of other conditions that can produce similar problems. The best evaluation involves an interdisciplinary approach and includes a speech-language pathologist to evaluate voice production and voice quality, an otolaryngologist (ear, nose, and throat specialist) to examine the vocal cords and their movement, and a neurologist who looks for signs of neurological problems.

Treatment

At present, there is no cure for spasmodic dysphonia. However, several treatment options do exist for voice improvement.

Repeat injections of small doses of botulinum toxin (Botox) into one or both vocal cords is frequently recommended. Botox weakens the laryngeal muscles and results in a smoother, less effortful voice because of less forceful closing of the vocal cords. Temporary breathiness or difficulty swallowing sometimes occurs for a short time after injection. Treatment by a speech-language pathologist may also be recommended following injections to optimize voice production.

Speech-language pathology services alone are most helpful when symptoms are mild. Clients learn techniques such as relaxation, breath control, maintaining a steady flow of air from the lungs during voice production, and pitch and loudness modifications. Surgical cutting of the recurrent laryngeal nerve to paralyze one vocal cord initially met with good results by reducing the force of vocal cord closure. Surgery was frequently followed by speech-language pathology treatment. Long-term follow-up has shown return of voice symptoms within 6 months to 3 years of surgery in almost two thirds of these patients with a disturbing number who were worse than before surgery.

Psychological or psychiatric counseling is most useful when acceptance of the disorder and learning coping techniques are the desired goals. Career or vocational counseling may also be advised for persons who fear that the disorder threatens their occupation. Participation in local self-help support groups can also promote adjustment to the problem and provide contact with excellent sources of information.

For additional information and referral, you may contact:

American Speech-Language-Hearing Association
10801 Rockville Pike
Rockville, MD 20852
(800) 638-8255
(301) 897-8682

For more information, contact the following organizations:

Dystonia Medical Research Foundation
One East Wacker Drive
Chicago, IL 60601-2098
(312) 755-0198
(312) 321-5710 FAX

National Institute on Deafness & Other Communication Disorders
National Institutes of Health
Bethesda, MD 20892
(301) 496-9365

National Spasmodic Dysphonia Association (NSDA)
P.O. Box 1574
Birmingham, Ml 48009-1574
(810) 646-6885;
(810) 645-9352 FAX

Our Voice
156 Fifth Ave., Suite 1033
New York, NY 10010-7002
(212) 929-4299 or 929-4397
(212) 929-4099 FAX

Chapter 41

Submucous Cleft Palate

What Is a Submucous Cleft Palate?

A submucous cleft palate is one type of cleft palate. The word "palate" refers to the roof of the mouth and the term "cleft" indicates a split in the palate. The palate consists of both a bony portion (hard palate) and a muscular portion (soft palate). At the end of the soft palate, the small finger-like projection of tissue that hangs down is called the "uvula". The term "submucous" refers to the fact that the cleft is covered over by the lining (mucous membrane) of the roof of the mouth. This covering of mucosa makes the cleft difficult to see when looking in the mouth.

A submucous cleft of the soft palate is characterized by a midline deficiency or lack of muscular tissue and incorrect positioning of the muscles. A submucous cleft of the hard palate is defined as a bony defect in the midline or center of the bony palate. This can sometimes be felt as a notch or depression in the bony palate when the palate is palpated with a finger. Often a submucous cleft palate is associated with a bifid or cleft uvula.

Effects of Submucous Cleft Palate

When a submucous cleft is present, the muscles of the soft palate may not function properly and the individual is at risk for speech

This fact sheet was originally published by the Cleft Palate Foundation. Used by permission.

347

problems, middle ear disease, and swallowing difficulties. However, there are some individuals with a submucous cleft who have no apparent problems. Of importance to all persons with the submucous cleft, and their family, is the knowledge that submucous cleft has the same genetic (hereditary) risk as an obvious cleft of the palate.

How Can a Submucous Cleft Palate Be Identified?

The most common reason that a child is evaluated for a submucous cleft palate is abnormal nasal speech. Other symptoms may include persistent middle ear disease and feeding/swallowing difficulties. A submucous cleft palate may be identified by the presence of a bifid uvula; a very thin translucent strip of lining (mucosa) in the middle of the roof of the mouth; and, a notch at the back edge of the hard palate that can be felt by the fingertip. However, in some children, the palate may appear normal on physical examination despite the fact that the child is experiencing speech problems, persistent ear disease, and/or swallowing difficulties. In such cases, special tests are necessary to fully assess the palate. These tests include x-ray examination and nasopharyngoscopy (looking at the palate through a very small tube that is placed in the nose). These evaluations are most commonly done by members of a cleft palate team. If you suspect your child has a submucous cleft, you should contact a local cleft palate team.

Should a Submucous Cleft Be Treated?

The decision to treat a submucous cleft palate depends upon the consequences of the submucous cleft and is not based on the fact that it is present. The most common reason for treating an individual with a submucous cleft of the palate is because of abnormal speech. The speech has a nasal sound because air is lost through the nose. In such cases the child's speech should be evaluated by a speech pathologist who, in consultation with other professionals, can diagnose the cause of the problem. If the palate cannot prevent air from escaping through the nose during speech, called velopharyngeal incompetence or VPI, then surgical repair of the palate will be required. Speech therapy alone cannot correct velopharyngeal incompetence.

Feeding/swallowing problems can sometimes be managed

through the use of special techniques which the feeding consultant on the cleft palate team can suggest.

Ear problems should be treated by the child's regular physician or by an ear, nose, throat specialist. Treatment may include the use of antibiotics and/or surgical insertion of ventilating tubes in the ear drum. Proper management of the child's ears is essential to ensure good hearing and proper speech development.

If the feeding problems and/or chronic middle ear disease persist and are related to abnormal soft palate muscle function, then treatment of the submucous cleft palate is indicated.

What Treatment Is Available for Submucous Cleft Palate?

For individuals with submucous cleft and velopharyngeal incompetence, the most common treatment is surgical. The surgery consists of reconstruction of the abnormal tissues with a palatal repair with or without pharyngeal flap (pharyngoplasty) A primary goal of this surgery is to allow for normal speech production. This surgery is done in a hospital under general anesthesia. Pre- and post-surgical evaluation by members of a cleft palate team should be part of the overall treatment program.

In a limited number of cases, velopharyngeal incompetence associated with a submucous cleft palate can be treated with an appliance that fits in the mouth and attaches to the teeth. This appliance is generally made by a dental specialist (prosthodontist) associated with a cleft palate team. Again, pre- and post-treatment evaluation by the cleft palate team should be part of this treatment program.

How Can a Cleft Palate Team Be Located?

The Cleft Palate Foundation can refer you to local cleft palate teams and to parent support groups They also provide brochures and fact sheets about various aspects of clefting. Please contact the:

Cleft Palate Foundation
1218 Grandview Avenue
Pittsburgh, PA 15211
(800)24-CLEFT
(412)481-1376

Chapter 42

Treatment for Adults with Cleft Lip and Palate

What treatment is available for adults with cleft lip and palate?

Treatments currently available to infants and children with cleft lip and palate are also available to adults with clefts. Although every attempt is made to complete cleft care by the late teens, some ongoing treatment still may be required or some unmet patient need may become apparent in later years. In addition, new approaches for management of clefts become available as time passes. Finally, adults may desire genetic counselling in order to determine the likelihood of having an infant with a cleft.

How can treatment needs be determined?

Evaluation by a Cleft Palate Team can provide the adult with a cleft with information regarding clefting and its management. A Cleft Palate Team consists of a group of specialists with particular expertise in cleft lip and palate. Specialties represented on the team include plastic surgery, ear-nose and throat, hearing, dentistry, speech, oral surgery, nursing, and psychology among others. You can obtain the names of Cleft Teams in your locality by phoning 1-800-24-CLEFT.

This fact sheet was originally published by the Cleft Palate Association. Used by permission.

What are the most frequent concerns of adults with clefts?

Adults, just like younger individuals with clefts, are most concerned about the appearance of their lip and nose, the ability to speak clearly, the quality of their hearing, and the appearance and function of their teeth.

What can be done about the appearance of the lip and nose?

Although the scar of the repaired cleft lip is permanent, it may be possible to improve the quality of that scar. Surgery also can change the shape of the lip, the deformity of the nose, and the obstruction to nasal breathing. Such revision cleft surgery is usually done on an outpatient basis. Specific questions about changing the appearance of the lip or nose should be directed to the surgeon to determine what is surgically possible and what such surgery will require in terms of time, discomfort, and expense.

Is improvement in speech possible for an adult who has a cleft?

Although the most dramatic changes in speech are observed in children following treatment for their clefts, significant improvement also can be achieved in adults with speech problems related to cleft palate. The speech pathologist and other members of the Cleft Team evaluate speech and advise the individual whether or not improvement is possible. This may require renewed speech therapy, an oral speech appliance or even an additional operation. Adults with clefts may also have some hearing impairment. Hearing loss may reduce speech clarity and often makes communication more difficult. Adults should have their ears and hearing checked routinely by an ear-nose-throat (ENT) specialist and an audiologist so that necessary treatment can be recommended.

What treatment is available for adults with abnormalities of teeth and jaws resulting from clefts?

Adults with clefts may have crooked, poorly shaped, or missing teeth. Crooked teeth can be straightened with "braces." Poorly shaped and missing teeth can be restored or replaced with dental bridges or jaw implants. In addition, teeth may not meet properly because of an abnormal jaw relationship. Failure of the teeth and jaws to meet together properly can interfere with chewing, speech, and attractiveness. Surgery can reposition jaws which do not come together properly. The Cleft Team orthodontist, prosthodontist, oral surgeon, and plastic surgeon work together to determine the best treatment plan for each individual patient.

Can something be done to help adults with clefts who feel embarrassed and who lack self confidence?

Psychological counselling, along with the other restorative treatments mentioned above, can help an individual with a cleft feel better about himself or herself. Concerns about appearance, the ability to get along with others, satisfaction with one's job, goals for the future, and the hopes for a loving, and happy family relationship are concerns that may be discussed with members of the Cleft Team, particularly the psychologist and social worker. Interaction with other adults with clefts, through a patient-parent group, also can be beneficial.

Are there sources of financial support for adults when they need and desire treatment?

Funding through Children's Special Health Services (formerly Crippled Children's Services) stops between 18 and 21 years of age depending upon the regulations of each state. Some adults obtain funding for cleft services through their state Division of Vocational Rehabilitation (or State Rehabilitation Services) if a structural problem causes significant difficulties in areas such as speech related to employment. Sometimes standard medical insurance will pay for part of the treatment; however, many claims are rejected due to "preexisting condition" clauses. The social worker on the Cleft Team can assist in finding sources of funding for needed treatment.

Can adults benefit from membership in support groups?

The Cleft Palate Foundation provides referrals to patient/parent support groups throughout the country. Adults with clefts may wish to join such a group to meet other adults with similar concerns. In addition, adults with clefts can provide valuable assistance as role models for younger individuals with clefts and their families. Membership in the patient/parent support group also can provide an opportunity for the adult with a cleft to advocate for better insurance coverage and state and federal programs for others with similar problems.

For further information, contact the:

Cleft Palate Foundation
1218 Grandview Avenue
Pittsburgh, PA 15211
(800)24-CLEFT
(412)481-1376

Chapter 43

Dental Care of a Child with Cleft Lip and Palate

How Does Cleft Lip/Palate Affect the Teeth?

A cleft of the lip, gum (alveolus), and/or palate in the front of the mouth can produce a variety of dental problems. These may involve the number, size, shape, and position of both the baby teeth and the permanent teeth. The teeth most commonly affected by the clefting process are those in the area of the cleft, primarily the lateral incisors. Clefts occur between the cuspid (eye tooth) and the lateral incisor. In some cases the lateral incisor may be entirely absent. In other cases there may be a "twinning" (twin = two) of the lateral incisor so that one is present on each side of the cleft. In still other cases the incisor, or other teeth, may be present but may be poorly formed with an abnormally shaped crown and/or root. Finally, the teeth in the area of the cleft may be displaced, resulting in their erupting into abnormal positions. Occasionally the central incisors on the cleft side may have some of the same problems as the lateral incisor.

What Does This Mean for Future Dental Care?

A child with a cleft lip/palate requires the same regular preventive and restorative care as the child without a cleft. However, since children with clefts may have special problems related to missing,

This fact sheet was originally published by the Cleft Palate Foundation. Used by permission.

malformed, or malpositioned teeth, they require early evaluation by a dentist who is familiar with the needs of the child with a cleft.

Early Dental Care

With proper care, children born with a cleft lip and/or palate can have healthy teeth. This requires proper cleaning, good nutrition, and fluoride treatment. Appropriate cleaning with a small, soft-bristled toothbrush should begin as soon as teeth erupt. Oral hygiene instructions and preventative counseling can be provided by a pediatric dentist or a general dentist. Many dentists recommend that the first dental visit be scheduled at about one year of age or even earlier if there are special dental problems. The early evaluation is usually provided through the Cleft Palate Team. Routine dental care with a local dentist begins at about three years of age. The treatment recommended depends upon many factors. Some children require only preventative care while others will need fillings or removal of a tooth.

Orthodontic Care

The first orthodontic evaluation may be scheduled even before the child has any teeth. The purpose of this visit is to assess facial growth, particularly the growth of the jaws. Later as teeth begin to erupt, the orthodontist will make plans for the child's short and long-term dental needs. For example, if a child's upper teeth do not fit together (occlude) properly with the lower teeth, the orthodontist may suggest an early period of treatment to correct the relationship of the upper jaw to the lower jaw. It is not unusual for this initial period of treatment to be followed by a long rest period when the orthodontist monitors facial growth and dental development. With the eruption of the permanent teeth, the final phase of orthodontics completes alignment of the teeth.

Coordinated Dental-Surgical Care

Coordination of treatment between the surgeon and dental specialist is important since several procedures may be completed during the same anesthesia. Restorations or dental extractions can be scheduled at the same time as other surgery.

Coordination between the surgeon and the orthodontist becomes most important in the management of the bony defect in the upper jaw that may result from the cleft. Reconstruction of the cleft defect may be accomplished with a bone graft performed by the surgeon. The orthodontist may place an appliance on the teeth of the upper jaw to prepare for the bone graft. A retainer is usually placed after the bone graft until full braces are applied.

When the child approaches adolescence the orthodontist and the surgeon again coordinate their efforts if the teeth do not meet properly because the jaws are in abnormal positions. If the tooth relations cannot be made normal by orthodontics alone, a combined approach of both orthodontics and surgical repositioning of the jaws is necessary. Such surgery is usually performed after the pubertal growth spurt is completed.

Prosthodontic Care

The maxillofacial prosthodontist is a dental specialist who makes artificial teeth and dental appliances to improve the appearance of individuals with cleft and to meet their functional requirements for eating and speaking. The prosthodontist may make a dental bridge to replace missing teeth. Oral appliances called "speech bulbs" or "palatal lifts" may help close the nose from the mouth so that speech will sound more normal. The prosthodontist must also coordinate treatment with the surgeon and/or the orthodontist to assure the best possible result. For the child or adult who wears one of these appliances, the care of the teeth holding the appliance is of particular importance.

How Can I Get the Best Care for My Child?

Children with cleft lip and/or palate require the coordinated services of a number of specialists. For this reason many parents seek care for their child at a cleft palate or craniofacial treatment center. At such a center evaluation, treatment planning, and care are provided by an experienced, multidisciplinary team composed of representatives from a variety of dental, medical, and other health care specialties. Even if you do not have such a center locally, the care your child will receive in such a center may be well worth the inconvenience of traveling to another city.

Parent/patient support groups are located throughout the country. You might want to join one to obtain support and practical help from others who share common problems. To obtain a list of cleft palate-craniofacial centers and parent/patient support groups in your region contact the Cleft Palate Foundation:

Cleft Palate Foundation
1218 Grandview Avenue
Pittsburgh, PA 15211
(800)24-CLEFT
(412)481-1376

Chapter 44

Information about Treacher Collins Syndrome (Mandibulofacial Dysostosis)

What is Treacher Collins syndrome?

Treacher Collins syndrome is the name given to a birth defect which may affect the size and shape of the ears, eyelids, cheek bones, and upper and lower jaws. The extent of facial deformity varies from one affected individual to another. A physician named Treacher Collins was the first to describe this birth defect. "Syndrome" refers to the group of deformities which characterizes affected individuals. Another commonly used medical name for this syndrome is "mandibulofacial dysostosis."

What causes it?

This syndrome is caused by an abnormality in the genes. If both parents are normal, that is showing no signs of the syndrome themselves, this abnormality is the result of a change in the genetic material at the time of conception. The exact cause of this change is not known. If one parent is affected, the abnormal gene is then known to have been contributed by that parent.

This fact sheet and other publications on craniofacial anomalies are available from the Cleft Palate Foundation, 1218 Grandview Avenue, Pittsburgh, PA 15211 (800)24-CLEFT. Contact the Foundation for a free list of publications. Used by permission.

Does this mean that this can happen again in my family?

If both parents are normal, the chances of a second child being born with this syndrome are extremely small. However, if one parent is affected, the chances that any pregnancy will result in a child with Treacher Collins is 1 out of 2 (50% risk). For this reason, it is very important that both parents of an affected child be thoroughly examined before any recurrence risks are quoted to them.

If my child, who has Treacher Collins, marries and has children, will all the children have it too?

No. The risk is 50% for each pregnancy.

What are the risks that my other children will transmit this syndrome to their own children?

If your other children are normal (showing no signs of the syndrome), there is no increased risk to their children. If another family member shows any feature of syndrome, the occurrence risk for each pregnancy is 50%.

Will my child be mentally retarded?

There is no evidence that mental retardation is a feature of this syndrome. Hearing loss, however, is present in most affected individuals to some degree. Early diagnosis and treatment of the hearing loss can prevent associated developmental and educational handicaps.

Will my child be deaf?

The term "deaf" applies only to very severe hearing loss in which the nerves for hearing, in the ear or in the brain, do not function properly. The hearing loss in Treacher Collins syndrome is due to abnormalities in the structures of the outer and middle ear which conduct sound to the nerve endings in the inner ear. Thus, the loss in Treacher Collins syndrome is usually termed "conductive" and in the majority of affected children it is not of sufficient severity to be termed "deafness." However any degree of hearing loss may affect the development of speech and language and ability to succeed in school.

What kinds of problems can I expect?

First, Treacher Collins syndrome, like nearly all birth defects, varies in severity from patient to patient. In fact, some cases are so mild that they are never recognized unless they are seen by specialists experienced in making such a diagnosis. In other children, the physical abnormalities of the face and ears are much more obvious and functional problems may develop.

Second, both the oral cavity (mouth) and the air passage (nose and throat) tend to be small in persons who have this syndrome. This may produce problems for the affected infant with breathing and feeding. You should be on the alert for such problems. If your child has difficulty breathing or feeding, or has weight loss or poor weight gain, discuss your observations and concerns with your child's primary care provider or craniofacial center. Some children who have severe breathing difficulties require and operation to improve breathing and/or feeding.

Third, cleft palate is a frequently associated condition with this syndrome. Cleft palate itself sometimes can cause feeding problems and increase the risk of middle ear problems. Your child's primary care provider or cleft palate or craniofacial center can assist you with management of feeding problems.

The next concern after breathing and feeding is hearing. The hearing loss in Treacher Collins syndrome is usually bilateral (meaning that both ears are affected) and, while it is not severe enough to be termed "deafness," it is severe enough to affect the ability to hear the human voice. Hearing levels can and should be measured. Depending upon the results of the testing, your child may be fitted with a hearing aid to restore his/her access to the world of sound. An early childhood program of speech and language therapy may also be recommended.

The fact that a hearing loss is present does not mean that your child will be dependent upon sign language. The great majority of children with this syndrome do learn to talk. However, there are several features of the syndrome, besides hearing loss, which can affect speech and language development. Particularly in the severely affected child, the size and position of various structures inside the mouth (e.g., the relationship of the upper and lower teeth) may affect the ability to learn certain speech sounds meaning that development will be delayed until the cleft is closed and its function restored.

You can facilitate your child's speech and language development by (1) seeking early evaluation by a specialist in hearing (an audiologist) and a specialist in communication development (a speech/language pathologist), and (2) follow their advice with regard to the need for a hearing aid and for early therapy programs. The specialists most prepared to evaluate and manage your child are those who are members of a multidisciplinary craniofacial team.

What about other areas of development: social, educational, etc.?

The facial deformity and need for treatment of Treacher Collins syndrome may create problems in family and social relationships, in school adjustment, and so on. The craniofacial center may have a psychologist or social worker, or the center can refer you to someone for evaluation and counselling if needed. Remember that children with Treacher Collins syndrome, like all other children, are individuals. They vary in social adjustment, academic achievement, and in their ability to cope with adults. The professionals of craniofacial centers try to maximize each child's potential by offering early diagnosis and treatment when indicated.

What kind of treatment is available for my child?

First, as explained above, your child may need a hearing aid and this can be determined in the first few months of life.

Second, an early childhood program for speech and language stimulation may be recommended.

Third, if a cleft palate is present, the craniofacial team will advise you on the optimum timing for surgical closure of the cleft.

Fourth, reconstructive surgery is available to improve the appearance of the face. The craniofacial center will advise you on what to expect from such surgery and on optimum timing. Since not all children area affected to the same degree, both the necessity and the outcome of reconstructive surgery vary from child to child.

What should I be doing for my child now?

Be certain that the diagnosis is correct. Treacher Collins syndrome shares some features with other syndromes, and not all physicians are aware of this. For this reason, you are best advised to locate a craniofacial center where genetic consultation, evaluation, and treatment planning will be provided by an experienced multidisciplinary staff composed of representatives from a variety of medical, dental, and other health care specialties. You may not have such a center in your locality, but the care your child will be more than worth the inconvenience of traveling to another city. Finally, meet other individuals with similar deformities and their families by joining a parent-patient support group.

Where can I obtain referrals?

To obtain a list of craniofacial centers and/or parent-patient support groups in your region, please contact the:

Cleft Palate Foundation
1218 Grandview Avenue
Pittsburgh, PA 15211
(412) 481-1376
(800) 24-CLEFT

Chapter 45

Information about Pierre Robin Sequence

What is Pierre Robin Sequence?

The term Pierre Robin Sequence is given to a birth defect which involves an abnormally small lower jaw (micrognathia) and a tendency for the tongue to "ball up" and fall backward toward the throat (glossoptosis). Robin Sequence patients may or may not have cleft palate, but they do not have a cleft lip. While the current complete name is "Pierre Robin Malformation Sequence,"[2] it has also been known as "Cleft Palate, Micrognathia and Glossoptosis," "Robin Anomalad,"[6] "Pierre Robin Complex,"[5] and as "Pierre Robin Sequence."[1] The condition was first described in 1822 and is named after the French physician who associated the above problem with breathing problems in affected infants.

What causes the condition?

The immediate cause of Robin Sequence seems to be the failure of the lower jaw to develop. During prenatal development the small jaw seems to prevent the tongue from descending into the oral cavity and so the palate may not close completely.[1] This sequencing of events

---

leads to the classification of this condition as a malformation sequence. The exact reason for the failure of development of the lower jaw remains unknown. To date there is no evidence that it is due to abnormalities of genes or chromosomes or to factors such as drugs, x-rays, or maternal diet.

How common is this condition?

Pierre Robin Sequence is an uncommon condition. It occurs no more frequently than once in every 8,000 live births[5] and may occur as infrequently as once in every 30,000 live births.[4] In contrast, cleft lip or palate occurs once in every 700 to 800 live births.

Will future children be affected?

The risk of having another child with this or another similar condition is commonly considered to be within the 1% to 5% range for parents who already have one child with this condition.[2] However, there have not been enough large scale family studies for geneticists to provide exact risk predictions. There are a number of conditions, most commonly Stickler syndrome, that also include features of Robin Sequence. Consequently it is extremely important that the diagnosis of Robin Sequence is confirmed by an experienced medical geneticist, preferably one associated with a multidisciplinary craniofacial team.

What kinds of problems are associated with this condition?

It is important to remember that Pierre Robin Sequence, like most birth defects, varies in severity from child to child. Thus some children may have many more problems than other children with the same diagnosis. Problems in breathing and feeding in early infancy are most common. Parents are advised on how to position the infant in order to minimize problems (i.e., not place the infant on his/her back). For severely affected children, positioning alone may not be sufficient and the pediatrician may recommend specially designed devices to protect the airway and facilitate feeding. Some children who have severe breathing problems require a surgical procedure to ease their breathing.

Other problems include possible congenital heart murmur and eye defects. The pediatrician will also carefully monitor the baby for ear disease. Virtually all babies with clefts of the palate are prone to build-ups of fluid behind the eardrum. If untreated this could lead to mild or moderate (but reversible) loss of hearing. Since this could affect speech and language development, the baby needs to have his/her hearing monitored from early infancy by audiologists who specialize in testing infants and small children.

What should be done to treat the condition?

Fortunately the small mandible (lower jaw), that is so noticeable when the infant is born, grows rapidly during the first year of life. In some children the jaw may grow so rapidly that by the time the child is approximately six years of age, the profile looks normal.[1] Some minor differences in the shape of the jaw do remain, but are not noticeable except on x-rays of the head. Because of this "catch-up" growth, some children do not require surgery on their jaw. The cleft palate, however, needs to be surgically closed. In some children this surgery is delayed to take advantage of growth which may tend to narrow the opening in the palate. Because children with a cleft of the palate are at higher risk for delayed or defective speech development, their speech development should be monitored by a Speech Pathologist during their early years. If speech is not progressing adequately then the child can be enrolled in speech therapy.

Where can children be best treated?

Since children with Pierre Robin Sequence may have problems in a number of areas, parents are well advised to locate a craniofacial center where evaluation and treatment planning will be undertaken by an experienced multidisciplinary staff composed of health care professionals from many different specialties. If such a center is not located in your city or town, it may well be worth the inconvenience to travel to another city for your child's appointments. To obtain a list of the Teams treating Craniofacial Anomalies, contact the:

Cleft Palate Foundation
1218 Grandview Avenue
Pittsburgh, PA 15211
(412) 481-1376
(800)24-CLEFT

References

1. Gorlin, R. J., Pindborg, J. J., and Cohen, M. M. *Syndromes of the Head and Neck.* 2nd Edition. New York: McGraw-Hill Book Company, 1976.

2. Jones, K. L. *Smith's Recognizable Patterns of Human Malformation.* Philadelphia: W. B. Saunders Company, 1988.

3. Pashayan, H. M. and Lewis, M. B. "Clinical Experience with the Robin Sequence." *Cleft Palate Journal* 21: 270-276, 1984.

4. Rubin, A. *Handbook of Congenital Malformations.* Philadelphia: W. B. Saunders Company, 1976.

5. Sheffield, L. J., Reiss, J. A., and Gilding, M. "A Genetic Follow-Up Study of 64 Patients with the Pierre Robin Complex." *American Journal of Medical Genetics* 28: 25-36, 1987.

6. Williams, M. A., Williams, C.A., and Bush, P. G. "The Robin Anomalad (Pierre Robin Syndrome)—A Follow-Up Study." *Archives of Disease in Childhood* 56: 1981.

Chapter 46

Information about Crouzon Syndrome (Craniofacial Dysostosis)

What is Crouzon Syndrome?

Crouzon syndrome, also called craniofacial dysostosis, is one of the large group of birth defects in which there is abnormal fusion (joining between some of the bones) of the skull and of the face. This fusion does not allow the bones to grow normally, affecting the shape of the head, appearance of the face and the relationship of the teeth. Crouzon syndrome is named after Dr. Crouzon who was the first to record a description of a patient with a characteristic group of deformities (syndrome) which were then observed in other individuals.

What causes it?

Crouzon syndrome is caused by an abnormality in the genes. If both parents are normal, that is showing no signs of the syndrome themselves, this abnormality is the result of a change in the genetic material at the time of conception. The exact cause of this change is not known. However, if one parent is affected, the abnormal gene is known to have been contributed by that parent.

This fact sheet and other publications on craniofacial anomalies are available from the Cleft Palate Foundation, 1218 Grandview Avenue, Pittsburgh, PA 15211 (800)24-CLEFT. Contact the Foundation for a free list of publications. Used by permission.

Can this happen again in my family?

If both parents are normal, the chances of a second child being born with Crouzon syndrome are extremely small. However, if one parent is affected, the chances that any pregnancy will result in a child with this syndrome is 1 out of 2 (50% risk). For this reason, it is important for both parents of an affected child to undergo a thorough physical examination before any recurrence risks are quoted to them.

If my child, who has Crouzon syndrome, marries and has children, will all the children have it too?

If your other children are normal (not showing signs of the syndrome), there is no increased risk to the children of the affected child. If another family member has the syndrome, the occurrence risk for each pregnancy will be 50%.

Will my child be retarded?

There is no data to indicate that mental retardation is a regular feature of this syndrome. Development should be evaluated periodically and if any concerns regarding mental function arise, appropriate referral for testing should be made.

What kinds of problems should I expect?

Like most birth defects, Crouzon syndrome varies in severity from patient to patient causing more problems for some than others. For a complete evaluation, optimum treatment planning, and comprehensive services, we advise you to contact a craniofacial center. At such a center, an experienced multidisciplinary staff composed of representatives from different health care specialties will assist you with care as well as in anticipating and meeting problems.

You should watch for any sign of ear disease and hearing loss, since research indicates that individuals with Crouzon syndrome may be quite vulnerable to ear problems. For an infant, the specialists at the craniofacial center can assess hearing in the early months of life. Hearing should be monitored as your child grows.

While many children with Crouzon syndrome develop speech and language normally, some do not. The speech pathologist at the craniofacial center assesses speech and language development at regular intervals and will advise you if therapy is indicated.

Some individuals with Crouzon syndrome have problems with dry eyes, excessive tearing, or muscle balance (strabismus). A screening eye examination by an ophthalmologist (eye doctor) should be obtained and any problems treated as they arise.

The major problem for individuals with Crouzon syndrome is underdevelopment of the upper jaw. This produces facial deformity (bulging eyes and sunken middle third of face) and malocclusion (abnormal relationship between the upper and lower jaws). Dental and plastic surgery specialists monitor facial growth and correct deformities.

The facial deformity and need for treatment of Crouzon syndrome may create problems in family and social relationships, school placement, and so on. The craniofacial center may have a psychologist or social worker, or may refer you to one for evaluation and counselling if needed. Remember that children are individuals. They vary in social adjustment, academic achievement, and in their ability to cope with adults. The professionals at craniofacial centers try to maximize each child's potential by offering early diagnosis and treatment, when indicated.

Other specialties represented on the team vary somewhat from center to center. If your child has needs or problems requiring other specialties, you will be referred to them as needed.

What kind of treatment is available for my child?

The need, extent and timing for treatment of the deformities of Crouzon syndrome depend on how severely the individual is affected and the age. For the infant, surgery may be required to release and reshape the bones of the skull, so that they may grow more normally. Orthodontics, to straighten the teeth in a more normal position, may be done in childhood, the teens or even the adult years. These are complicated operations which are usually performed by specially trained craniofacial surgeons associated with major craniofacial centers.

What should I be doing for my child now?

First, be certain that the diagnosis is correct. Crouzon syndrome resembles several other syndromes, and not all physicians are aware of this. A geneticist can provide the necessary evaluation and information. Second, locate a craniofacial center. you may not have a center in your city but the care your child will receive will be more than worth the inconvenience of traveling to another city. Third, meet other individuals with similar deformities by joining a parent/patient support group.

Where can I obtain referrals?

To obtain a list of craniofacial centers and/or parent/patient support groups in your region please contact the:

Cleft Palate Foundation
1218 Grandview Avenue
Pittsburgh, PA 15211
(412) 481-1376
(800) 24-CLEFT

Chapter 47

Information about Choosing a Cleft Palate or Craniofacial Team

Throughout the United States there are many qualified health professionals caring for children with cleft lip and palate as well as other craniofacial defects. However, because these children frequently require a number of different types of services which need to be provided in a coordinated manner over a period of years, you may want to search for an interdisciplinary team. Such a team can coordinate and implement all or most of these services through one central facility.

When you are selecting a team, here are some points to consider:

1. The Number of Different Specialists Who Actually Participate on the Team

The more extensive the group of specialists who participate on the team, the more likely every aspect of treatment can be considered during the team evaluation. You should ask how many of the following are represented on the team:

- Plastic Surgeon
- Pediatrician

This fact sheet and other publications on craniofacial anomalies are available from the Cleft Palate Foundation, 1218 Grandview Avenue, Pittsburgh, PA 15211. (800)24-CLEFT. Contact the Foundation for a free list of publications. Used by permission.

- Otolaryngologist
- Geneticist/Dysmorphologist
- Audiologist
- Speech Pathologist
- Orthodontist
- Pedodontist
- Prosthodontist
- Oral Surgeon
- Psychologist
- Social Worker
- Nurse

If your child has a craniofacial defect, then the team you choose may also include the following:

- Neurosurgeon
- Ophthalmologist

2. Qualifications of the Individual Members on the Team

You should inquire of all the members of the team are fully trained and appropriately certified in their areas of specialty, as well as licensed. This may become an issue that will also affect insurance coverage.

3. Experience of the Team

In general, the quality of care increases with the amount of experience the team has. You should ask how often the team meets and approximately how many patients are seen at each meeting. You may also want to try to determine how long this group of professionals has been meeting as a team and also how much experience the various individual professionals have had.

4. Location of the Team

The distance of the team from your home may NOT be an important consideration in choosing a team. In general, the team will be seeing your child only periodically throughout his/her growing years.

Usually routine treatment such as general dental care, orthodontics, speech therapy, and pediatric care will be provided by professionals in your own community who will be in regular contact with professionals on the interdisciplinary team. Thus your travel to a team will usually be limited to several trips a year or even once a year. If a larger, more experienced team is available a few hours away, this may be preferable to a less experienced local team.

Affiliation of the Team and Its Members

You may want to ask if the Team is registered with the American Cleft Palate–Craniofacial Association and how many of the individual members of the Team area also members of the American Cleft Palate–Craniofacial Association. Staying current with recent developments in the field is one sign of a conscientious and concerned health care professional. You may also want to determine whether the team has any relationship to an established hospital or to a medical school or university. Facilities for diagnostic studies and treatment frequently are better with such an affiliation.

For a list of cleft palate or craniofacial teams in your state, or for further information, you may contact:

Cleft Palate Foundation
1218 Grandview Avenue
Pittsburgh, PA 15211
(412) 481-1376
(800)24-CLEFT

Chapter 48

Information about Financial Assistance

Financial resources to help pay all or part of the costs of treating a person with a cleft lip and/or palate fall into three general categories: health insurance; federal and state resources; and private and non-profit agencies, foundations, and service organizations. The most important thing to remember is there are many sources of funds available to help you get the care you need.

Health Insurance

Private and Group Health Insurance will usually cover at least a portion of the cost of the treatment of a cleft lip or palate after the deductible is met. Check your health care plan or call the insurance company for specific coverage information. When choosing health insurance policies, check into coverage of not only surgery and medical care but also dental care and services such as hearing testing, speech and language testing and treatment, and psychological testing and/or counselling. If you have reason to think you are not being covered according to your policy, call your State Insurance Board.

This fact sheet and other publications on craniofacial anomalies are available from the Cleft Palate Foundation, 1218 Grandview Avenue, Pittsburgh, PA 15211 (800)24-CLEFT. Contact the Foundation for a free list of publications. Used by permission.

Federal and State Resources

Champus is a program of medical benefits provided by the Federal Government for members and their dependents who are covered in the uniformed services. Persons covered by Champus should contact the Health Benefits administrator at the nearest military installation for more information.

Medicaid (Title XIX of the Social Security Act of 1966) is a federal program assistance program that covers most of the cost of medical care for people with low incomes who require hospital or physician services, or certain laboratory and X-ray procedures.

In some states, services such as treatment for speech or hearing defects may be covered. Application can be made in the county offices of the Social Services, Welfare, or Human Resources Office.

Recently Medicaid was expanded to include a new program entitled Medical Assistance Pregnant Women and Children's Program (MAPWC). This nationwide program was mandated by Federal legislation to provide medical/dental care for pregnant women and for children from birth to six years of age. The financial eligibility requirements for children under six years of age differs from Medicaid requirements and includes children from working families who might otherwise be excluded from Medicaid benefits. The application form is much shorter and simpler than the forms for Medicaid and income limits are higher. Application can be made in the county offices of the Social Services, Welfare, or Human Resources Office.

Children's Special Health Services (formerly called the Crippled Children's Program) provides comprehensive medical care to children under the age of 21 who have congenital or acquired physically handicapping conditions. Specific medical and financial criteria have to be met by the applicant before financial assistance is approved. Applications are available through the Director, Children's Special Health Services of each state. you may contact your State Department of Health for further information or you may receive information from an agency or medical facility in your community that provides these services.

Vocational Rehabilitation Services are designed for persons 16 years of age and older with emotional, mental, physical/medical and/or developmental disabilities that hinder their prospects for employment. Assistance in obtaining local office telephone numbers can be secured by contacting the State Department of Human Resources of the Welfare Office.

The Hill-Burton Act provides funds for indigent care at hospitals where federal monies were used for construction. The hospital admissions office has information on the availability of these funds and the guidelines for eligibility.

Private and Non-Profit Agencies, Foundations, and Service Organizations

The Easter Seal Society, a non-profit organization, serves physically or developmentally disabled children or adults. Although their primary focus is on patients with cerebral palsy and similar neurological conditions, local chapters provide a variety of other services including speech and hearing services. For a description of services in your area, contact your state office or the national office: The National Easter Seal Society at (312) 726-6200.

The March of Dimes Birth Defects Foundation supports programs designed to prevent birth defects and promotes research, professional education, and treatment. Each local chapter determines how their local funds are to be allocated. While chapters are not encouraged to use funds for treatment of individuals, the local chapter may assist families when no other funds are available in meeting the costs of treatment. The local chapters are usually listed in the telephone directory.

The Grottoes of America provide dentistry to the handicapped. The patient must be under 18 years of age to receive assistance from this organization. In addition they must have one of the following conditions: cerebral palsy, muscular dystrophy, mental retardation, or myasthenia gravis. National Headquarters are in Columbus, Ohio and their telephone number is (614) 860-9193.

379

The National Association for the Craniofacially Handicapped (FACES) provides financial assistance for supportive services, i.e., transportation, food, and lodging, to families of individuals who are receiving treatment for craniofacial deformities resulting from birth defects, injuries, or disease. The Foundation office is located in Chattanooga, Tennessee and their telephone number is (615) 266-1632.

Local Service Organizations such as **Lions, Sertoma, Kiwanis** and **Civitan Clubs** sometimes provide emergency one-time financial aid if funds are available. Local churches and church groups, e.g. the Knights of Columbus, Masons, etc., may also serve as resources. Telephone numbers for these organizations can usually be found in the yellow pages of the telephone directory under Clubs, Fraternal Organizations, and Religious Organizations.

Remember to discuss your financial needs with the team coordinator, social worker or other appropriate member of the local cleft palate team. They may be aware of other funding sources not mentioned above.

The Cleft Palate Foundation can refer you to local cleft palate teams and to parent support groups. They can also refer you to insurance advocates in your region and provide you with brochures and fact sheets about various aspects of clefting. Contact the:

Cleft Palate Foundation
1218 Grandview Avenue
Pittsburgh, PA 15211
(412) 481-1376
(800) 24-CLEFT

Part Three

Voice Disorders

Chapter 49

National Strategic Research Plan for Voice Disorders

Overview

Emergence of Voice Science and the Science of Voice Disorders

Voice production (phonation) is the generation and modulation of sound and is a subset of the more global process of speech production. Disorders of voice involve difficulties with pitch, loudness and quality. Voice disorders can be distinguished from articulation disorders, which present difficulties of speech sound production. Many people who have acquired normal speaking skills become communicatively impaired when their vocal apparatus fails. This impairment is important in modern society because there is much demand for effective speech and oral communication.

Additional demands on the voice are made because of negative influences from noise and pollutants in the environment. There are also increasingly larger populations of the aged and hearing-impaired persons and people under psychological and physical stress. Voice production is not the only function of the larynx (voice box). This organ plays a vital role in protecting the tracheobronchial tree, particularly during swallowing.

This document is a portion of the National Strategic Research Plan for Hearing and Hearing Impairment and Voice and Voice Disorders, compiled by the National Institute on Deafness and Other Communication Disorders, a division of the National Institutes of Health.

Within the last decade, the field of voice science has expanded in several ways. A large new knowledge base has been developed on the mechanisms of phonation. Awareness of voice disorders has increased. A clinical delivery system has emerged with improved diagnosis and treatment of individuals with voice impairment, laryngeal pathology and swallowing disorders. These developments have resulted in the need to address research strategies in the voice and speech systems separately.

Interaction of the Voice and Speech Systems and Their Disorders

In the context of communication, voice is an acoustical representation of language. It is a product of laryngeal and upper aerodigestive tract adjustments that act upon and interact with the respiratory airstream to create the physical disturbances we perceive as sounds. The respiratory system, which is an integral part of the voice production system, provides the energy source and must be coordinated with laryngeal valving and upper aerodigestive tract modulation of the respiratory airflow. Vocal tract shaping above the larynx in the hypopharynx, pharynx, nasopharynx, oral cavity and nasal cavities affects the quality of the voice and is also part of the voice-production system. Speech involves adjustments of the pharynx, tongue, velum (palate), lips and jaw, which modify and enhance the sound source. Articulatory valving and obstructions of the airflow can produce major downward modulations on glottal function. This is only one example of the close interaction between the voice and speech systems. Other significant interactions result from the effects of tongue position on the height of the hyoid bone and larynx during speech.

The same upper aerodigestive tract structures involved in voice and speech production are also required to coordinate the activity of swallowing. Therefore, although normal structure and function and diseases and disorders of the voice, speech systems and swallowing can be studied independently, their interrelations also need to be studied.

Background

The larynx is a valve structure between the trachea (wind pipe) and the pharynx. It has a skeleton consisting of several cartilages, the largest of which is attached to the hyoid bone in the upper part of the neck. Muscles covered with mucous membrane form the vocal folds, which are moved apart to open the larynx or are pulled together for closure.

An important role of the larynx is protection and maintenance of the airway. The vocal folds are separated during inspiration, and air passes into the trachea to the lungs. During expiration, movements of the vocal folds participate in the control of the rate of airflow out of the lungs. During swallowing, the larynx is elevated, moves anteriorly and is closed tightly, while the tongue and pharyngeal muscles move food or fluid into the esophagus. During a cough, the vocal folds close while expiratory muscles contract to increase pressure in the lungs. The larynx opens abruptly, air rushes out and mucus or foreign matter is ejected from the tracheobronchial tree. If the larynx is irritated by particulate matter, reflex closure of the vocal folds and coughing occur. These actions prevent life-threatening aspiration pneumonia.

Voice or phonation is generated by airflow from the lungs as the vocal folds are brought close together. The vocal folds vibrate when air is pushed past them with sufficient pressure. The vibration of the folds causes the airflow to become pulsed. This pulsed airflow is then modulated by aerodigestive tract structures (the pharynx, oral cavity and nasal cavities) to produce the sound that is perceived as voice during speech. Without normal vibration of the vocal folds in the larynx, the sound of speech is absent and words can only be mouthed. They cannot be heard or understood by others, either in face-to-face conversation or over the telephone. To produce a whisper, the vocal folds need to be partially separated, and speech can only be understood by persons very close by.

When vocal fold vibration is impaired, sound generation for speech is affected. An absence of one vocal fold may result in voice loss or impairment. Absence of both vocal folds results in a loss of voice or aphonia. This happens when the larynx is removed, as may be required in laryngeal cancer. Growths on one or both of the vocal folds can change the mechanical properties of the tissue, which affect its vibration. Lesions, such as polyps, result in a hoarse voice caused by irregular vocal fold vibration. Other tissue changes, such as nodules, edema or contact ulcers, can also cause a hoarse voice. Papillomatosis, a spreading of wartlike growths on the vocal folds, also interferes with voice production by limiting vocal fold vibration and the intake of air through the larynx to the lungs.

The nerves controlling the functions of the larynx can be impaired as a result of accidents, surgical procedures or viral infections. When the motor nerves on one side are affected, the muscles moving the vocal fold are paralyzed and the vocal folds cannot come close enough to the center of the larynx. In such individuals, there is excessive air loss between the vocal folds during phonation, which results in a breathy voice. When the nerves on both sides of the larynx are affected, the muscles may not separate the vocal folds properly for breathing. This situation may occur in some motor neuron diseases or following operations on or trauma to the neck.

Both unilateral and bilateral laryngeal nerve paralysis can result in aspiration during swallowing, because laryngeal movement is reduced and the larynx does not close.

Loss of laryngeal sensation can also be a problem. A sensory loss alone can result in food or liquid entering the trachea, and aspiration can cause pneumonia.

The complex functions of the upper aerodigestive tract can be severely impaired by diseases of the central nervous system. Both sensory and motor lesions can significantly impair reflex control as well as voluntary control. Brain stem damage is particularly devastating to swallowing function.

Laryngeal movement disorders have only recently been studied systematically. In spasmodic dysphonia, the muscles of the larynx contract abnormally during speech, causing uncontrolled pitch and voice breaks and sometimes affecting swallowing and breathing. Vocal fold tremor, a disorder attributed to rhythmic contractions of the muscles of the larynx, causes the voice to quaver with frequent pitch and voice breaks. Another disorder, laryngospasm, is an uncontrolled closing of the vocal folds which interferes with breathing.

Interpersonal stress and psychological factors can have a profound impact on the upper aerodigestive tract. This is not surprising, as the voice directly expresses emotion, and eating is a frequent focus of psychogenic disorders.

Incidence, Prevalence and Impact on Society

Most of the statistics regarding voice disorders are from studies of school-age children. In these populations, estimates of the incidence of voice disorders range from six to 23 percent. The majority of these children have hoarseness, which has resulted from vocal abuse.

There are no data available on the incidence of voice disorders in the general adult population. However, voice disorders are believed to be more common in older adults. Voice and swallowing problems are very frequent in patients with acquired neurogenic diseases.

The economic impact of voice disorders on our society cannot be accurately assessed. However, voice disorders can have devastating effects on individuals, interfering with speech. Often, individuals are unable to function in work situations. Use of the telephone may be impossible without utilizing a telecommunication device for the deaf (TDD) and some individuals are forced to rely on writing for communication. Careers can be lost or limited because of the onset of a voice disorder.

Impairment of respiration or swallowing can be life threatening. Often, the only available treatment results in a loss of voice. When swallowing is severely affected, nonoral feeding is required and the quality of life is diminished.

Recent Accomplishments and the Current State of Research

Normal Structure and Function

Laryngeal Physiology

The biomechanics of laryngeal behaviors that produce different movement trajectories during respiration, airway closure, swallowing, coughing, singing and speech have been studied. Recently, properties of laryngeal muscles have been found to differ from properties of other muscles. Laryngeal muscles are resistant to fatigue, are able to contract rapidly and are less susceptible to injury. Experimental studies have demonstrated the possibility of reinnervation of the laryngeal muscles after neural injury with and without surgical intervention.

Lifespan Changes

Research has revealed specific anatomical, physiological and biochemical alterations with maturation of the upper aerodigestive system. Laryngeal position and configuration change during development and with aging. Swallowing is also affected by aging. Prolongation in oral transit times and delay in initiating the pharyngeal phase of swallowing have been defined in the elderly. Changes in laryngeal muscle contraction behaviors with maturation have also been reported. As well, the cellular biology of the upper aerodigestive system has been found to change with age.

A series of histochemical, ultrastructural and stereological investigations have been initiated on the aging human larynx and its innervation. Studies on animal models have demonstrated a number of changes in morphologic parameters that are likely to play key roles in the mechanisms underlying age-related laryngeal dysfunction. In addition, studies on the human superior laryngeal nerve have shown a large, selective loss of the smallest nerve fibers. This finding may help to explain the age-related dysfunction of the laryngeal protective mechanism.

The use of organotypic cultures to study epithelial-mesenchymal interactions and enhance epithelial differentiation *in vitro* has been stimulated by advances in dermatology. Application of these techniques to the larynx has provided insight into the plasticity of the adult human laryngeal epithelium. The differentiation pathway into either stratified squamous or ciliated columnar epithelium can be modulated by changing the concentration of retinoic acid in the medium. This understanding raises questions regarding the use of retinoids in chemoprevention of cancer, and it opens potential avenues of research.

Exceptional Behavior

Training of the voice leads to morphological and behavioral changes in the quality and health of the laryngeal tissues. An understanding of these changes can improve the quality and health of the voices of nonprofessionals as well. Voice training has an important impact on vocal function. Singers have greater frequency and intensity ranges and lower airflows. One consequence of these advances in knowledge is to include singers as a special population in descriptive databases.

There is growing evidence that the voices of trained vocalists change less rapidly with age than those of their nonsinging counterparts. Further study may help develop preventive programs for presbylarynx. In addition, singers appear to be better able to compensate for laryngeal deficits. This finding has implications in voice training for patients with vocal disorders.

Animal Models

Studies are under way to document the role of the central nervous system in the control of laryngeal behavior, vocalization and swallowing. Through the recording of electrical potentials from single neurons in awake, vocalizing animals, the function of various structures is now being understood in the context of the behavior of a normal, healthy animal.

Neural activity has been recorded concomitantly with electromyograms of the upper aerodigestive tract to investigate the integrative actions of the larynx and the rest of the respiratory system in behaviors such as vocalization and swallowing.

Sets of neurons in the periaqueductal gray area of the midbrain have been documented to influence the activity of coordinated groups of neurons to the larynx and the rest of the respiratory system during vocalization. Neurons in the nucleus ambiguus are strongly influenced by cells of the midbrain periaqueductal gray area during vocalization and by cells of the nucleus tractus solitarius and reticular formation during swallowing.

Techniques using multiple arrays of neural recording electrodes have been developed for the study of other systems in awake or anesthetized animals. As the software supporting technology develops, these techniques should yield data on large samples of simultaneously recorded cells and lead to an improved understanding of the functions of specific structures.

Knowledge of the interactions between laryngeal sensory and motor systems has recently been advanced by the development of an animal model that can produce phonation even though the animal is completely anesthetized. This preparation affords researchers the opportunity to study the behavior of laryngeal motor neurons, sensory afferents of the larynx and the mechanisms of how phonatory control interacts with protective reflexes and swallowing.

Anatomy and Physiology of Swallowing

The application of electromyography, endoscopy, manometry and combined techniques (such as videofluoroscopy and manometry combined with computer image analysis) has offered new insights into normal and disordered swallowing. In the past five years, there has been recognition that swallowing is not one behavior but a set of behaviors that vary in their temporal and kinematic characteristics. Some of the factors responsible for systematic variation in swallowing have been identified. These include bolus volume, viscosity and voluntary maneuvers. In particular, the potential for volitional control over laryngeal movement, cricopharyngeal opening and airway closure has been delineated.

The physiology of the upper esophageal sphincter has received special attention relative to the mechanisms of opening and variations with bolus volume. The major elements responsible for opening of the upper esophageal sphincter have been defined as: (1) relaxation of the cricopharyngeal muscle; (2) anterior and vertical laryngeal movement, which opens the sphincter; and (3) bolus pressure, which modulates the width of the opening.

Advances in the Diagnosis and Treatment of Voice Disorders

Vocal Fold Neoplasms

The development of improved visualization of the larynx along with video recordings should lead to improved accuracy in the early diagnosis of laryngeal cancer. When such disorders are detected early, the prognosis for cure while maintaining voice function is good.

Patients can now be fitted with prosthetic devices to redirect airflow and allow voice production soon after surgical removal of the larynx for treatment of laryngeal cancer. Previously, such patients had only two alternatives: to learn esophageal speech or to use a mechanical larynx or electrolarynx. Prostheses provide voice for speech with less training and without an external device. Refinements in design of these prostheses should make speech sound more natural.

Recent advances in the understanding of recurrent respiratory papillomatosis should improve management of this disease and hopefully prevention. The viral cause and latency of the infection are better understood. Quite recently, it was shown that a major contribution to the mass of these tumors is derived from a failure of differentiation rather than increased proliferation. Organotypic tissue cultures mirror this abnormality, thus providing a good model for studying potential modulations of the differentiation process. Interferon cannot eliminate the papilloma virus infection, but it may have a potential adjuvant role in managing patients with severe disease.

Photodynamic therapy using agents that are absorbed by the tumor is currently being evaluated for respiratory papillomas and superficial malignancies.

Vocal Fold Lesions and Glottal Insufficiencies

Phonosurgery is a relatively new specialty that requires skill and new instruments for delicate operations on the vocal folds. Surgical techniques are being designed to improve and restore voice by removing benign growths, correcting structural abnormalities and repairing trauma.

Previous common practices such as vocal fold stripping have been found injurious to the voice. Improvements in technique make it easier to restore normal vocal function.

Neurogenic Disorders

Neurogenic Disease. Neurally based laryngeal problems account for a substantial portion of all voice disorders and such disorders are frequently the first signs of neurogenic disease. Recent technological advances have made it possible to view the laryngeal structure and its gross movement patterns, as well as to make fine measurements of moment-to-moment changes in the cycles of vibration. Voice measurement techniques and computational analysis have yielded information delineating voice changes related to the early course of neurogenic diseases. This information may now be used to make earlier identification of some diseases and to allow investigators to have a measure against which to determine the efficacy of treatment.

Laryngeal Paralysis. Unilateral laryngeal paralysis can result in hoarseness and aspiration due to incomplete closure of the glottis. Vocal fold paralysis abolishes abduction and adduction of the vocal folds and alters the configuration of the glottis. The paralyzed vocal fold is shorter than the normal vocal fold and frequently lies at a different level. Compensatory behavior includes hyperadduction of the mobile vocal fold and anterior-posterior compression of the glottis.

Bilateral paralysis is potentially life threatening, because the airway is severely reduced. Established therapy is to perform a tracheotomy, move one vocal fold laterally or excise an arytenoid. Research is being conducted on alternative therapies, such as reinnervation of laryngeal muscles or artificially stimulated laryngeal movement synchronous with breathing.

Many individuals with clinically apparent laryngeal paralysis do not have muscle denervation that can be demonstrated by electromyography. These individuals seem to have partial neural lesions or ineffective neural regeneration. It is now known that recovery from paralysis requires not only regeneration of a sufficient number of motor nerve fibers but also the connection of nerve fibers to appropriate muscle fibers. Synkinesis is the simultaneous contraction of opposing muscles and results from the innervation of muscles by inappropriate nerves. Research into nerve regeneration may elucidate factors that could prevent synkinesis.

Spasmodic Dysphonia. Spasmodic dysphonia is a voice disorder characterized by frequent voice and pitch breaks or a breathy voice. It is a focal dystonia of the larynx. Dysfunction results from involuntary contractions of laryngeal muscles during speech. Surgical division of the nerve to one side of the larynx can diminish the signs and symptoms of adductor spasmodic dysphonia, but the voice is frequently breathy and the long-term results are often not satisfactory.

Several years ago, botulinum toxin was introduced as an experimental treatment. Minute quantities of the toxin are injected into the affected muscles to produce temporary weakness. Recently, a National Institutes of Health consensus development conference judged this approach to be a safe and effective treatment for patients with adductor spasmodic dysphonia. Although it does not cure the disorder, it significantly reduces signs and symptoms, usually for periods of four to six months.

Other Movement Disorders. Movement disorders affecting the larynx, such as false laryngeal asthma or paradoxical movements, have been recognized. Information concerning the effects of these movement disorders on voice and breathing and their remediation is emerging.

Population Considerations. Advances have been made in recognizing that the impact of vocal lesions is population-specific. For example, singers with vocal nodules may compensate sufficiently to mask vocal signs during speech but have difficulties singing. These population differences help explain some discrepancies in the existing literature and underscore the need to look at singers as a special population even when testing for voice disorders.

Gastroesophageal Reflux. Recent studies have elucidated a variety of disorders caused or aggravated by gastroesophageal reflux to the larynx and pharynx. These disorders include contact ulcers, subglottal stenosis, hoarseness, chronic cough, throat clearing and cancer. There is a need to understand more fully the role of acid and alkaline materials in the causes of these disorders.

Technology

There have been advances in computational tools, both hardware and software. Speed, memory, ease of use, cost and compactness have been improved. These developments have affected virtually all aspects of research in the larynx and upper aerodigestive tract.

Analysis and interpretation of signals from electromyographic, electroglottographic, photoglottographic, accelerometric and aerodynamic transducers can now be accomplished with greater accuracy and ease. The use of microprocessors now permits multichannel data acquisition, near real-time quantification and graphic display of complex data. Furthermore, advanced signal processing techniques, in combination with the general availability of digital signal processing boards, have also made it possible to extract interpretative data for scientific and diagnostic purposes in near real time. Improvements in performance and reductions in size and cost have also increased widespread clinical access to the new technologies.

In conjunction with increasing computational capability and transducer design, important progress has been made in imaging and the interactive display of three-dimensional laryngopharyngeal structures. There have been technological advances in videoendoscopy and related digital imaging, magnetic resonance imaging, computed tomography and ultrasound. Advances in available software make it possible to achieve quantitative evaluation of the images. These developments have led to intraoperative applications that improve surgical results. Currently, intraoperative monitoring of vocal fold kinematics, electrical stimulation and acoustic output are being used. Further advances in surgical technologies have included the use of endoscopic, fiberoptic, tunable lasers for treatment of disease of the airway.

Augmentative and alternative communication devices and aids are beginning to include an increased variety of synthesized voices with better voice quality. These improvements include the choice of a more natural female or male voice. Further computational analyses and modeling of the human vocal tract should lead to the development of prosthetic devices with even more natural sounding voices.

Chapter 50

A Vocologist's Guide: Voice and Voice Therapy

Introduction

This booklet was written for two audiences. It provides a quick reference for practitioners who work with voice: speech-language pathologists, singing teachers and voice coaches. Collectively, these practitioners are called vocologists. Additionally, *A Vocologist's Guide: Voice Therapy and Training* is for individuals with voice problems who want to make educated choices about the treatment they receive.

Current approaches to voice management are presented in summarized formats. Seven clinical voice therapy techniques and four popular voice training techniques from the theatre realm are presented. These techniques are representative samplings of those commonly used in speech-language pathology and theatre, although others are available. Throughout this booklet, an attempt was made to use language easily understood by practitioners with varying backgrounds.

One of the primary goals of this booklet is to encourage clinicians to realize all of the beneficial approaches to voice management available to them. Also, a good grasp of the underlying physiology allows the clinician to better understand how the treatment works. References are provided as a means to gain further information and, possibly, promote implementation of new techniques. Finally, presenting the spectrum of voice management techniques helps foster an inter-disciplinary awareness of the ways voice habilitation is approached from different traditions.

The staff of the National Center for Voice and Speech gratefully acknowledges support from the National Institute on Deafness and Other Communication Disorders (Grant number P60 DC00976). We thank Kate DeVore and Dr. Katherine Verdolini for their assistance in researching, writing and editing this booklet, and to Julie Ostrem for publication design. Special thanks to Dr. Florence Blager, Stefanie Countryman, Heather Dove and Mark Leddy for their valuable insights.

Confidential Voice Therapy

Application

Intended for patients with edema-based (traumatic) injuries such as vocal fold nodules and polyps.

Developer

No single person originally developed this technique, which is used widely in speech pathology for treatment of nodules, polyps, and similar conditions. However, it was perhaps originally called "confidential voice therapy" by Dr. Janina Casper, who, together with her colleagues has also provided physiological descriptions of it.

Description

The method involves speaking as quietly as possible, with a somewhat breathy quality, as if speaking confidentially at close range. A typical therapy hierarchy includes limited work at the single sound and word level, and a rapid progression to the conversational level. Most patients seem to handle this quite readily.

Mechanism

There is evidence that vocal fold adduction during phonation is limited with this method, leading to a limitation in vocal fold impact force. This, in turn, limits the potential for laryngeal trauma.

Efficacy Studies

Verdolini and colleagues examined confidential voice therapy and resonant voice therapy (description of technique follows) as two forms of treatment for vocal nodules. There was evidence of benefit from therapy in the sound of the voice, in phonation effort and in the appearance of the larynx for the combined therapy group as compared to the outcome for a control group. More importantly, patients who received confidential voice therapy and resonant voice therapy had about the same likelihood of benefitting from treatment, provided they actually used the therapy technique outside of the clinic (by their report).

References

Colton, R., & Casper, J. (1990). *Understanding Voice Problems: A Physiological Perspective for Diagnosis and Treatment*. Baltimore, MD: Williams & Wilkins.

Verdolini, K., Burke, M.K., Lessac, A., Glaze, L., & Caldwell, E. (in press). A preliminary study on two methods of treatment for laryngeal nodules. *Journal of Voice*.

Resonant Voice Therapy

Application

This method might be used for patients with many different types of voice disorders for which vocal fold adduction level is a critical issue. Examples are patients with nodules who may need a reduction in adduction and patients with paralysis, who may need an increase.

Developers

In theatre, Arthur Lessac has been one of the primary trainers to develop resonant voice techniques. Dr. Morton Cooper has applied his own version of resonant voice therapy to speech pathology, and Dr. Katherine Verdolini has developed Lessac's technique for application to disordered voice (speech pathology).

Description

In all approaches to resonant voice training and therapy, the emphasis is on oral vibratory sensations during phonation, usually on the anterior palate. In the Lessac approach, the consonant "y" (and sometimes, other voiced consonants, especially nasal ones) is used to facilitate the target voicing in initial phases. In Cooper's approach, the response "um-hmm"—as if agreeing—is used as a facilitatory technique. Typical therapy hierarchies progress from simpler to more complex speech materials.

Mechanism

Research evidence suggests that vocal fold adduction during phonation is limited with this method, as compared to "pressed voice". Because of the limited adduction, there should be limited vocal fold impact force thus preventing and reversing traumatic injuries. At the same time, voice output is characteristically strong, such that an optimal tradeoff is produced between voice output (high) and laryngeal trauma (low).

Efficacy Studies

Verdolini and colleagues examined resonant voice therapy and confidential voice therapy (previously described) as two forms of treatment for vocal nodules. Generally, there was evidence of a benefit from therapy in the sound of the voice, in phonatory effort and in the appearance of the larynx, as compared to the results for a control group. More importantly, patients who received confidential voice therapy and resonant voice therapy had about the same likelihood of benefitting from therapy, provided they actually used the therapy technique outside of the clinic (by their report).

References

Cooper,M.(1973). *Modern Techniques of Vocal Rehabilitation.* Springfield, IL: Charles C. Thomas.

Lessac, A. (1967). *The Use and Training of the Human Voice: A Practical Approach to Voice and Speech Dynamics.* New York: Drama Book Specialists. (2nd edition anticipated, 1994, Mayfield Press, Mountain View, CA).

Verdolini, K., Burke, M.K., Lessac, A., Glaze, L., & Caldwell, E. (in press). "A Preliminary Study on Two Methods of Treatment for Laryngeal Nodules." *Journal of Voice.*

Peterson, L., Verdolini, K., Barkmeier, J., & Hoffman, H. (1994). "Comparison of Aerodynamic and Electroglottographic Parameters in Evaluating Clinically Relevant Voice Patterns." *Annals of Otology, Rhinology and Laryngology*, 103 (5), 335346.

Verdolini, K. & Titze, I.R. (in press). "From Laboratory Formulas to Clinical Formulation." *American Journal of Speech-Language Pathology*.

Flow Mode Therapy

Application

This is an approach to optimal voicing in general, which may be used in normal voice training and for voice disorders. The specific disorder populations have not been formally specified, but the approach should be applicable to the same range of disorders as "resonant voice therapy."

Developer

Dr. Johan Sundberg and his colleagues (Dr. Jan Gauffin, for one) have developed and proposed the technique.

Description

Flow mode is described as the voicing mode produced by the largest amplitude vocal fold vibrations possible, with complete vocal fold closure during each cycle. Biofeedback is proposed in the training of flow mode, using inverse filtered airflow signals to reflect vocal fold vibrational patterns. Laryngeally, the method appears remarkably similar to, if not the same as, resonant voice production already discussed.

Mechanism

As for resonant voice, flow mode may limit vocal fold adduction compared to pathogenic phonation modes (pressed voice), while at the same time maximizing voice output.

Efficacy Studies

No formal studies have been conducted on the efficacy of flow mode, as such. However, if flow mode and resonant voice therapy are similar or even equivalent, as they appear to be, the study by Verdolini and colleagues on resonant voice therapy (previously cited in this booklet) may be relevant.

References

Gauffin, J., & Sundberg, J. (1989). "Spectral Correlates of Glottal Voice Source Waveform Characteristics." *Journal of Speech and Hearing Research*, 32, 556-565.

Accent Method

Application

The technique is proposed for patients with a wide range of voice disorders.

Developer

Svend Smith is credited with development of the technique.

Description

The method is fundamentally a rhythmic approach to speech training. Patients are trained to emphasize accented portions of speech, in contrast to unaccented portions, alternating between a sense of tension and relaxation. The specific training hierarchy includes work on physiological abdominal movements to facilitate airflow during phonation. Sound is subsequently superimposed as gentle pulses. Learners are then encouraged to become aware of the abdominal movements and a sense of alternating "release" and contraction. Following these initial training phases, utterances are then produced rhythmically on /hu/. There is an emphasis on whole body movement to avoid developing new tensions. Articulation is also trained. The program continues with nursery rhymes or similar rhythmic material and finally, to conversational speech.

Mechanism

It is proposed that the rhythmic aspect of the method somehow results in rapid and complete vocal fold closure, thus maximizing harmonic output.

Efficacy Studies

Kotby and colleagues assessed patients with mass lesions, functional voice disorders, and vocal fold immobility. According to their study, benefits from the accent method were obtained in patients' complaints about voice, the sound of the voice, and, for patients with nodules, a reduction in lesion size. Some other physiological parameters were also improved. Smith and Thyme reported an increase in the presence and intensity of high harmonics in the voice output, at frequencies below 1000 Hz, which could account for improved intelligibility of speech.

References

Dalhoff, K., & Kitzing, P. (1989). "Voice Therapy According to Smith. Comments on the Accent Method (A.M.) for Treating Voice and Speech Disorders." *Revue de Laryngologie*, 1 10,407-413.

Kotby, M., El-Sady, S., Basiouny, S., Abou-Rass, Y., & Hegazi, M. (1991). "Efficacy of the Accent Method of Voice Therapy." *Journal of Voice*, 5, 316-320.

Smith, S., & Thyme, K. (1976). "Statistic Research on Changes in Speech Due to Pedagogic Treatment (The Accent Method)." *Folia Phoniatrica*, 28, 98-103.

Facilitating Techniques

Application

Many of the 25 facilitating techniques described by Dr. Daniel Boone may be used across a wide range of disorders, particularly where hyperfunction is involved. Some of the techniques apply instead to under-function, as with paralysis.

Developer

Dr. Daniel Boone has systematically described this corpus of techniques, many of them originally described and used by other clinicians.

Description

The 25 techniques include: altering tongue position; changing loudness; chant tallc; chewing (originally described by Froeschels, 1924); digital manipulation of the larynx; ear training (auditory discrimination); elimination of abuse; elimination of hard glottal attack; establishing a new pitch; explanation of problem; (bio)feedback; half-swallow; head positioning; hierarchy analysis; inhalation phonation; masking; open-mouth approach; pitch inflections; placing the voice (resonant voice); pushing approach; relaxation; respiration training; tongue protrusion; yawn-sigh.

The yawn-sigh was specifically described by Boone and McFarlane (1993) as a technique that promotes laryngeal lowering and supraglottal widening.

Mechanism

Because of the many techniques, no single mechanism can explain the effectiveness for all of them. For the yawn-sigh approach, which was specifically evaluated in a research study, it is easy to speculate that vocal fold adduction is limited, thus limiting vocal fold impact force and laryngeal trauma.

Efficacy Studies

One of the facilitating techniques, digital manipulation of the larynx, was assessed in a treatment study by Roy and Leeper. In that study, patients with voice disorders without any known organic basis received a manual laryngeal muscle tension reduction procedure described by Aronson. The sound of the voice and acoustic measures of the voice improved markedly with this therapy, for many or most subjects.

Another of the facilitating techniques that has been studied empirically is the yawn-sigh technique (Boone & McFarlane; Xu & colleagues)

References

Boone, D., & McFarlane, S (1988). *The Voice and Voice Therapy* (4th ed.). Englewood Cliffs, N.J.: Prentice Hall.

Boone, D., & McFarlane, S. (1993). "A Critical View of the Yawn-Sigh as a Voice Therapy Technique." *Journal of Voice*, 7, 75-80.

Aronson, A.E. (1990). *Clinical Voice Disorders* (3rd ed.). New York, N.Y.: Thieme-Stratton.

Roy, N. & Leeper, H.A. (1993). "Effects of the Manual Laryngeal Musculoskeletal Tension Reduction Technique as a Treatment for Functional Voice Disorders: Perceptual and Acoustic Measures." *Journal of Voice*, 7(3), 242-249.

Xu, J.H., Ikeda, Y., & Komiyama, S. (1991). "Biofeedback and the Yawning Breath Pattern in Voice Therapy: A Clinical Trial." *Auris, Nasus, Larynx*. 18 (1) 67-77.

Vocal Function Exercises

Application

These techniques may be used for any voice disorder for which muscular weakness, hyperfunction or imbalances appear to play an important role.

Developer

Most recently, Dr. Joseph Stemple has developed muscle strengthening exercises. Earlier work was reported by Dr. Bertram Briess.

Description

Vocal function exercise techniques target specific muscles identified as weak or hyperactive, or muscle groups as imbalanced. For example, pitch glides and sustained high or low pitches may be used to address pitch and adduction-related muscles and their interplay (Stemple; Briess).

Mechanism

The mechanism by which muscle exercise techniques may address voice physiology are the same as any physical exercise techniques. That is, muscle states themselves should change with repeated targeted use, as should neurocognitive "programs" or patterns of responding.

Efficacy Studies

In one study, subjects who underwent a "vocal function exercise" program for four weeks improved in phonation volume, flow rate, maximum phonation time, and frequency range, as compared with subjects in placebo and control groups, who did not improve (Stemple et. al., in press).

References

Briess, B. (1959). "Voice Therapy—Part I: Identification of Specific Laryngeal Muscle Dysfunction by Voice Testing." *AMA Archives of Otolaryngology*. 66: 375-382.

Briess, B. (1959). "Voice Therapy—Part II: Essential Treatment Phases of Laryngeal Muscle Dysfunction." *AMA Archives of Otolaryngology*. 69: 61-69.

Stemple, J. (1984). *Clinical Voice Pathology: Theory and Management*. Columbus, OH: Charles E. Merrill.

Stemple, J., Lee, L., D'Amico, B., & Pickup, B. (in press). "Efficacy of Vocal Function Exercises ad a Method of Improving Voice Production." *Jounal of Voice*.

Sabol, J., Lee, L., & Stemple, J. (in press). "The Value of Vocal Function Exercises in the Practice Regimen of Singers." *Journal of Voice*.

Lee Silverman Voice Treatment

Application

The Lee Silverman Voice Treatment is applicable for patients with motor speech disorders, such as Parkinson's disease. The primary assumption is that vocal folds do not adduct completely and increased adduction will improve vocal loudness and increased phonatory effort will improve overall speech production.

Developer

Dr. Lorraine Ramig and her colleagues have been the primary clinicians to develop this technique.

Description

Patients are trained to increase phonatory effort and adduction and carry over this behavior by using "loud" speech. The therapy program has been developed in considerable detail. Generally four essential elements of the program are: the exclusive focus on phonation; the program is intensive (therapy is provided four times a week for four weeks); the program is cognitively simple for the learner—it emphasizes a single parameter ("think loud"); and therapy fundamentally involves a "recalibration" of the patient's sense of phonatory effort and loudness. When the patient reports he/she is "too loud", the voice is considered within normal limits.

More specifically, vocal fold closure is promoted by initiating voice with maximally prolonged vowels while pushing with the hands, and performing repeated pitch glides. Therapy progresses from these simpler tasks to more complex speech drills.

Mechanism

Loud voice production should improve vocal fold adduction (typically impaired in Parkinson disease by vocal fold bowing and by hypokinesia), and pitch glides should improve pitch variability in speech, which is generally limited in persons with Parkinson disease. Other effects are also anticipated as a "by-product". In particular, speech articulation generally improves in clarity. Cognitively, the approach is streamlined for the patient, by focusing on a simple parameter (loud) that holistically generates a series of benefits.

Efficacy Studies

Studies about the effectiveness of LSVT have been conducted by Ramig and colleagues. In the primary study to date, the following effects were noted: (a) perceptual ratings indicated an improvement in loudness, pitch variability, and intelligibility of speech; (b) acoustic measures indicated an improvement in pitch variability during speech and a change in speech pitch towards the norm for males; (c) more isolated speech testing indicated an improvement in maximum vowel duration and in absolute pitch range; (d) forced vital capacity remained constant Studies support maintenance without additional treatment 6-12 months post-treatment.

References

Countryman, S. & Ramig, L. (1993). "Effects of Intensive Voice Therapy on Speech Deficits Associated with Bilateral Thalamotomy in Parkinson's Disease: A Case Study." *Journal of Medical Speech Pathology*, 1(4), 233-249.

Ramig, L.O., Bonitati, C., Lemke, J., & Horii, Y. (in press). "The Efficacy of Voice Therapy for Patients with Parkinson's Disease." *Journal of Medical Speech Pathology*.

Ramig, L.O. (1994). "Speech Therapy for Parkinson's Disease." In Koller, W. and Paulgon, G. (Eds.), *Therapy of Parkinson's Disease*. New York: Marcel Dekker.

Ramig, L.(1992). "The Role of Phonation in Speech Intelligibility: A Review and Preliminary Data from Patients with Parkinson's Disease." In Kent, R.(Ed.) *Intelligibility in Speech Disorders: Theory. Measurement and Management*. Amsterdam: J. Benjamin.

Smith, M., Ramig, L., Dromey, C., Perez, K., & Samandari, R. (in press). "Intensive Voice Treatment in Parkinson's Disease: Laryngostroboscopic Findings." *Journal of Voice*.

Chapter 51

Speaking After Laryngectomy

Laryngectomy, surgical removal of the larynx (voice box) usually due to cancer, can be a life-saving procedure. But, it also removes the vocal cords, the sound source for speech. Therefore, a new sound source must be used:

- esophageal speech
- esophageal speech using a voice prosthesis
- an artificial larynx.

Esophageal Speech

With standard esophageal speech, air is taken in through the mouth, trapped in the throat, and then released. As the air is released, it makes the upper parts of the throat/esophagus vibrate and produce sound. This sound is shaped into words in the same way it was before surgery: with the lips, tongue, teeth, and other mouth parts.

Esophageal speech can be a convenient, efficient, and natural means of communication, but it requires considerable practice.

Voice Prosthesis

A voice prosthesis can also be surgically implanted either at the

This article was originally published by the American Speech-Language-Hearing Association in *Let's Talk*, No. 27. Used by permission.

time of original surgery or at a later date. A small opening (fistula) is made in the back wall of the trachea (windpipe) and in the front wall of the esophagus, near the top of the stoma, an opening in the neck through which people with laryngectomy breathe. The prosthesis is then inserted into the fistula through the stoma.

When the stoma is covered and air from the lungs is exhaled, the air passes through the prosthesis and into the esophagus for speech production. Just as with standard esophageal speech, instruction and practice is necessary to learn how to speak clearly. Speech units can be longer, louder, and more variable in pitch than with standard esophageal speech, but not all people who have had a laryngectomy are suitable candidates for a voice prosthesis.

Artificial Larynx

An artificial larynx is an electronic or mechanical instrument that is held against the neck or placed in the mouth. It provides an external source of sound. The parts of the mouth are still used to shape the sound into words.

Esophageal talkers may also use an artificial larynx in certain settings, for example, in urgent or stressful situations, during a cold, or in noisy places. An artificial larynx is also extremely useful while esophageal speech is being learned. The artificial larynx provides an almost immediate means of communication that is more efficient than writing.

Like the other alternatives, successful use of an artificial larynx requires training and practice to improve intelligibility, resonance, and articulation. And some disadvantages still exist. The artificial larynx has a mechanical voice quality, requires the use of one hand to speak, and draws attention to the speaker.

Speech-Language Pathologist

It is a speech-language pathologist who can recommend the best method or methods of communication and then provide appropriate training. In fact, a preoperative visit by a speech-language pathologist helps to answer questions, explain communication options, and assure family members.

For a list of speech-language pathologists or a more detailed fact sheet on laryngectomy, contact the Consumer Affairs Division, American Speech-Language-Hearing Association, 10801 Rockville Pike, Rockville, MD 20852; (800) 638-8255.

Part Four

Other Sensory Communication Disorders Including Balance, Vestibular, Smell, and Taste Disorders

Chapter 52

Balance and the Vestibular System

Overview

The vestibular system maintains our balance and posture, regulates locomotion and other volitional movements and provides a conscious awareness of orientation in space and a visual fixation in motion. Disease, aging, exposure to unusual motion or altered gravitational environments (e.g., aerospace flight) can impair balance. In the United States, over 90 million people have experienced dizziness or a balance problem. For example, there are an estimated 38,000 new cases of Meniere's disease each year, one of many disorders that affects the vestibular system, and dizziness is the most common reason for seeking medical care in the over-75-year age group. A major consequence of vestibular disturbance is diminished capability and desire for purposeful activity. There may also be incapacitating effects on motor task performance and sensorimotor integration. Furthermore, motivation, concentration, memory, food intake and digestion and many other human activities may be adversely affected.

The vestibular receptors located in the labyrinth of the inner ear signal motion and position of the head. Nerve fibers connecting these receptors to the brain provide information about head movements to

This document is a portion of the National Strategic Research Plan for Balance and the Vestibular System and Language and Language Impairments, compiled by the National Institute on Deafness and Other Communication Disorders, a division of the National Institutes of Health.

413

produce vestibular reflexes. Brain circuits integrate vestibular information with other sensory signals from the eyes, skin, muscles and joints to produce a complex set of reflexes that interact to maintain posture and visual fixation in motion. In addition, the signals contribute to an internal representation or picture of body orientation and self motion.

The vestibular system is a complex, highly-interactive set of brain mechanisms capable of continuous adaptations to changes in the body and the environment. Because it has many components, there are many symptoms that indicate its malfunction, which range from mild discomfort to total incapacitation. Although balance is normally an automatic, unconscious process, it is essential for purposeful movement and effective communication.

Understanding how the vestibular system works is a scientific and technical challenge. The fluid-filled receptor end-organs that detect motion and head position are encased in bone and are difficult to access, manipulate and study. The system is complex because it integrates many kinds of sensory information and utilizes a variety of neurochemical transmitters, and its malfunction results in a multitude of symptoms. The complexity of vestibular system function requires an interdisciplinary approach, including rigorous anatomical, physiological, biochemical, molecular biological, pharmacological, behavioral, perceptual and clinical studies. Biological data should be incorporated into mathematical computational models to examine and understand the integrated action of vestibular receptors and brain circuits in maintaining balance, orientation and the visual fixation and postural stability required for locomotion and other volitional movements. The resulting models should be utilized to predict changes that will result from pathologic conditions. Symptoms of these conditions should be evaluated in the context of the model predictions to reach a global understanding of the normal vestibular system and its pathophysiology.

Symptoms

The symptoms of vestibular system dysfunction are varied, reflecting the complexity of functional interconnections of the vestibular system with vision, tendon and joint position sensors, the digestive system and even the psyche (anxiety disorders).

Dysfunction of the vestibular system, particularly the inner ear and its interconnections with the brain, may cause hallucination of movement, variably described with such terms as dizziness, disorientation, vertigo, spinning, floating, rocking, lightheadedness, giddiness, sense of falling, imbalance, unsteadiness, or difficulty walking.

Symptom characteristics and the degree to which the patient is incapacitated depend upon the nature of the disorder. The symptoms may be episodic or continuous and may vary in frequency, severity and rapidity of onset. If there is damage to the system, the location (either in the inner ear or brain) as well as the magnitude of that damage play roles in the generation of symptoms.

Balance system dysfunction, if severe enough, can also provoke responses in the digestive system (nausea, vomiting and diarrhea), circulatory system (pallor, changes in blood pressure and pulse) and skin (perspiration, cold or clammy sensation).

The psychological impact of vestibular symptoms should not be underestimated. The fear of falling, with the chance of physical injury, adversely affects the individual's sense of independence and quality of life, particularly in the elderly. Similarly, the fear of a sudden attack of dizziness with socially-embarrassing ataxia, nausea and vomiting can cause individuals to become withdrawn. Subconscious fear may play a role in agoraphobia and subtle dysfunction of the vestibular system may underlie difficulties in handwriting and reading. Vestibular dysfunction adversely affects the ability to perform the most routine activities, such as taking a shower, housekeeping duties and driving an automobile, and may prevent patients from holding high-risk jobs, e.g., telephone lineman, mechanic and bus driver.

Disorientation, i.e., wrongly perceived tilt or motion of the body relative to the environment, can arise from abnormalities in the vestibular system or result from subjecting the normal vestibular system to an abnormal environment.

Motion sickness is currently regarded as the brain's response to conflicting sensory messages about the body's orientation and state of motion. The sensors involved include the vestibular part of the inner ear, the eyes and body pressure and joint position sensors. Nausea, vomiting and poor concentration are symptoms provoked by "sensory mismatch."

Dizziness comprises a spectrum of disorders ranging from lightheadedness and giddiness to frank vertigo and dysequilibrium.

415

Attempts to determine precisely the true incidence of vertigo/ imbalance stemming from peripheral and central vestibular system dysfunction are foiled by the nature of the disorders and the complexity of the balance control mechanisms. However, it is clear that balance disorders afflict a large proportion of the population, particularly the elderly.

Prevalence and Costs

Recent estimates exist for the prevalence of balance disorders in general, Meniere's disease and benign paroxysmal positional vertigo (BPPV). Examination of hospital statistics by discharge diagnosis shows that for those people under 65 years of age, 185,680 hospital days per year, on average, are provoked by dysequilibrium. In the general population (all ages), 347,000 hospital days are incurred because of "vertiginous syndromes," 202,000 because of "labyrinthitis" and 184,000 because of "labyrinthitis unspecified," with several thousands more accounted for by other balance disorders, e.g., Meniere's disease. The diagnosis of dizziness or dysequilibrium accounted for 221,000 of the primary discharge diagnoses in 1983. In the 45-to-64-year-old group, 1.3% of all visits to internists are related to vertigo or dizziness, affecting a relatively similar percentage of men and women.

Meniere's disease affects 15.3/100,000 individuals per year, resulting in about 38,250 new cases per year in the United States; in contrast, an incidence of 46/100,000 was found in a Scandinavian population, which would translate into 115,000 new cases per year in the United States. The prevalence figures are even more striking with a rate of 218.2/100,000. It is estimated there are 545,000 individuals in the United States with Meniere's disease.

In Japan, BPPV was determined to affect 10.7/100,000 individuals, with a great deal of inter-regional variability. The Japanese study determined that BPPV peaked in incidence in the fifth decade for both men and women, but that women were more commonly affected than men. BPPV occurred about two-thirds as frequently as Meniere's disease. The incidence of Meniere's disease in Japan is 16.0/100,000, very close to the incidence in the United States.

In looking at outpatient visits, 2.9% of visits to internists by the over-65-years-old group are because of dizziness or vertigo; in the over-75-years-old group, 3.8% of visits were for dizziness or vertigo, the number one reason for going to the physician. Seven percent of those in the over-85-years-old group present to the doctor because of dizziness or vertigo. These numbers reflect just the tip of the iceberg: an interview of those elderly at home showed 47% of the men and 60% of the women over the age of 70 complained of dizziness or vertigo.

In 1976, an estimated $500 million was expended just on visits to physicians for dizziness or vertigo. Assuming, conservatively, a 5% rate of inflation, the costs for medical care alone will approximate one billion dollars in 1991. To this figure must be added the cost of diagnostic testing, as well as therapy. The cost of falls, which potentially lead to fractured limbs, hospitalization, surgery, pneumonia and even death, must also be factored in. An estimated 15 to 23% of those over the age of 65 years who fall do so because of dizziness or vertigo.

The psychological toll of balance disorders on their victims is considerable; of those over the age of 65 years, at least 34% believe that dizziness keeps them from doing things they otherwise could do. This is not a happy way to spend one's "golden years."

If one considers military costs, the Army, Navy and the Air Force lose an average of 30 pilots and their aircraft every year to pilot disorientation and subsequent error. This loss of materiel conservatively represents an estimated cost of $300 million per year. In times of strife, cost estimates are increased three- to four-fold. Also, two-thirds of all astronauts experience motion sickness that can severely reduce their effectiveness for the first three days into orbital flight.

Diagnosis and Treatment

Evaluation of vestibular function has improved in the last 15 years due to the development of tests based on modern anatomic and physiologic concepts and the application of technical advancements. For example, studies of individual neurons are providing data upon which models have been developed to understand precisely vestibular, visual and somatosensory inputs involved in gaze stabilization, balance and orientation. Technical advancements in computer hardware have enabled clinicians to control angular and linear acceleration devices. Methods are being developed to measure different reflex functions (e.g., movements of the eyes, body or extremities) with the aid of microcomputers and programs that permit automatic analysis of data with accuracy and ease.

Tests cannot be limited to measurements of only one aspect of the balance system, however. Normal vestibular and balance function is a result of information about head movement and position from the inner ear, visuo-spatial relationships from the visual system and body relationships to the environment from the somatosensory system. Current methods of evaluating patients with vestibular disorders consist of a battery of tests that quantify the vestibulo-ocular reflex (VOR), the visualoculomotor system and postural responses.

Better techniques to quantify vestibular function and its interaction with other systems, in addition to techniques that aid in early diagnosis such as magnetic resonance imaging (MRI) and techniques that permit evaluation of blood flow and metabolic function of the brain, are resulting in improved diagnosis and management of patients with vestibular disorders. Advancements in our understanding of the pathophysiology of vestibular disorders have also contributed to better medical and surgical management. For example, mortality following resection of vestibular tumors has decreased from 50% to less than 1%.

Rehabilitation procedures are being developed that provide an additional approach to treatment for vestibular disorders. Specific vestibular exercise programs facilitate the rate and final level of recovery from vestibular disorders.

A Current View of Vestibular Function

Understanding the Molecular, Cellular and Neural Basis of Peripheral and Central Vestibular Function

Many of the vestibular reflexes serve to stabilize and coordinate movements of the eyes, head and body. These processes are collectively referred to as the vestibular reflex systems.

The vestibular receptor organs transduce the forces associated with head accelerations and changes in head position relative to gravity. The result is excitation of the nerves leading to control centers in the brain, which use these signals to develop a sense of orientation and to activate automatically muscles that subserve movements of the eyes, locomotion and posture.

While the basic receptors and neural structures are genetically determined, the development and fine tuning of vestibular function is a dynamic process that is dependent upon use and interaction with the environment throughout life. There must be an ongoing process of calibrating reflexes in order to adapt to physical changes in the musculoskeletal system during growth and development as well as to compensate for disorders (for example, inner-ear disease or visual loss) and to adapt to changes in the environment (such as an altered gravitational field, as in space). Thus, the proper responses to vestibular information require learning and memory.

Signal Transduction by Vestibular End-Organs

There are five vestibular end-organs. Two of these, the utricular and saccular maculae, transduce linear acceleration forces acting on the head, while the other three, the cristae of the semicircular canals, transduce angular acceleration forces. The five organs are so arranged in the temporal bone that they collectively provide the brain with a three-dimensional reconstruction of the position and motion of the head relative to the Earth.

Each end-organ consists of a sensory epithelium composed of sensory hair cells and supporting cells, innervated by afferent nerve fibers from the vestibular nerve. Hair cells contain ciliary bundles (hairs) that protrude from their apical surfaces and are embedded in gelatinous structures, the otoconial membranes of the maculae and the cupulae of the cristae. These structures couple the forces acting on the head to the cilia resulting in bending of the cilia. Displacement of the ciliary bundles regulates the opening of transduction channels, thought to be located near the ciliary tips. When the channels are opened, an electrical transducer current flows into the hair cell and changes the voltage. The transducer current modulates ionic currents flowing through the basolateral surface of the hair cell. The basolateral currents alter the electrical response of the hair cell. In addition, one of the basolateral currents adjusts the intracellular concentration of calcium ions and thereby regulates the release of as yet unknown chemical neurotransmitters from the hair cell to the afferent fibers contacting (synapsing with) the hair cell. The result is a change in the nerve impulse frequency of the afferent fibers. Even at rest, hair cells continue to release neurotransmitters and thereby cause nerve fibers to have a background or spontaneous activity. Bending the cilia in one direction causes an increase in transmitter release and nerve activity; bending in the opposite direction results in a decrease. In addition to their afferent innervation, the receptor organs are also provided with efferent nerve fibers arising from the brain and contacting hair cells

419

and afferent terminals. By means of this efferent innervation, the brain can regulate ongoing sensory processing by the end-organs, as well as modulate their function on a longer time scale.

The afferent nerve fibers transmit their impulse activity to the vestibular nuclei and to the cerebellum. These structures are extensively interconnected with each other and with other centers in the brain stem and spinal cord that modulate the activity of the muscles of the eyes, head and body.

Reflex Control of Posture and Gaze

Afferent fibers from the semicircular canals and the otolith organs synapse with neurons in the vestibular nuclei of the brain stem, which form the starting point of neural circuits that regulate movements of the eyes, head and body. These movements take the form of reflexes that compensate for perturbations of head or body position.

Postural reflexes result from the integration of vestibular signals with input from visual and somatosensory receptors and other motor-control systems and generate patterns of activation of leg, trunk and neck muscles that stabilize posture and prevent falling. Maintenance of posture depends on the generation of different stabilizing movements depending upon the context in which adjustments must occur. Vestibular contributions to postural control are difficult to isolate from other postural stabilizing responses.

The direction of visual regard is regulated by gaze reflexes, which are better understood than postural reflexes. Such regulation is required to maintain stability of images on the retina, without which visual acuity is severely reduced. One such reflex, the vestibulo-ocular reflex (VOR), causes eye movement equal but opposite to head movement. When the head is rotated to the right, the horizontal semicircular canal in the right ear is activated and that in the left ear inhibited. Reflex circuits transform these changes in canal afferent activity into activation of muscles that move the eyes to the left by the same angle as the head movement so that the eyes remain directed to a fixed point in space as the head moves. In analogous fashion, when the head is displaced linearly upward (e.g. during running), saccular otoliths are stimulated; and by way of reflex pathways projecting to the ocular motor nuclei, the eyes are moved downwards to compensate for the head displacement.

Despite its seeming simplicity, the VOR requires complex and very accurate processing of semicircular canal, visual and otolith signals to generate the required compensatory eye movement. The angular acceleration signal provided by canals must be converted into a change in angular position of the eyes. Because the canals are not exactly aligned with eye muscles, signals from all canals must be combined to produce a spatial transformation from the three dimensional coordinate frame of the canals to that of the eye muscles. These problems become even more complex in the vestibulo-collic reflex, which must control over 30 neck muscles to stabilize the biomechanically complex head-neck system. Remarkably, the brain is able to perform these functions with relatively simple reflex circuits. The key is in having a parallel processing system with a multiplicity of neurons at each stage of the circuit, which gives the system great processing power and flexibility. Such systems can best be understood by computerized modeling techniques that can represent and explore their structure and computational capabilities.

The most direct neural circuits involved in gaze reflexes are three-neuron vestibulo-ocular and vestibulo-collic reflex arcs that interconnect vestibular afferent fibers, relay neurons in the vestibular nuclei and motor neurons that control eye or neck muscles. Each connection between a labyrinthine receptor and a pool of motor neurons involves several classes of relay neurons, each of which collects input from a different set of vestibular and visual or somatosensory receptors and projects to either a few related or many diverse motor pools. These classes of relay neurons may have distinct biophysical and pharmacological properties which allow them to be regulated independently and which may permit discrete therapeutic intervention to restore deficient reflex function once the mechanisms are known. In addition, the brain has a repertoire of more complex processes for regulating gaze which involve predictive switching, like that seen in postural systems. These are implemented by more complex neural circuits and are as yet poorly understood.

Not surprisingly, to remain effective for visual stabilization, VORs must interact with the visual world during head movements. By receiving visual feedback during head movements, VORs may update their response properties to match what is required to maintain visual stability at any particular time and under a variety of circumstances. That is, the VORs exhibit adaptive plasticity. In addition, recent evidence has shown that VOR characteristics are affected by the vergence state and the direction of gaze in space, indicating that the VOR is not an isolated, simple reflex, but has response properties which are determined by integration of inputs from a variety of nervous system mechanisms and sensors other than vestibular ones.

Sensory Integration in Spatial Orientation, Perception and Motion Sickness

Spatial orientation is the relationship of the head and body to the Earth and to the Earth's gravity. The vestibular system and weight sensors provide information about how the body is oriented relative to the Earth, while other senses such as vision define the relationship of elements of the environment to the body. Balance and equilibrium are processes by which persons move and maintain head and body posture. Maintaining orientation and balance requires the integration of information from many sources, especially the ears, eyes, skin, muscles and joints, and the transformation of these signals into coordinated patterns of muscle activity. To maintain balance and equilibrium under a variety of sensory and support surface conditions, combinations of sensory signals and muscle activity patterns must be interpreted appropriately.

Many sensory inputs are required for the production of a coordinated perception of head and body movement in space. The visual system tells the vestibular nuclei whether the reflexes produced by activation of vestibular end-organs provide the amount of gaze compensation that is required. Visual feedback is critical for proper operation of the VOR. This involves portions of the vestibulo cerebellum, which play a role in adjusting the VOR when visual feedback indicates that it is not correctly stabilizing gaze. Disease of the cerebellum can result in faulty VOR calibration, poor gaze compensation during movement and imbalance and disorientation. Because vestibular signals interact with all of the major sensory systems, a large number of disease processes can impair balance and orientation. While it is clear that many brain structures are involved in determining orientation and balance, their precise roles remain to be determined.

The vestibular system operates largely automatically and without conscious awareness. When normal coordination among the senses is disrupted by disease, a disturbing symptom, known as vertigo, occurs. Similarly, passive or unusual motion conditions (ear and air travel, sea voyages and space flight) induce motion sickness, probably due to unusual combinations of signals from various sensors of motion. Mechanisms underlying the symptoms associated with vertigo and motion sickness are not well understood and are major unsolved problems as exemplified by the very high incidence of motion sickness which occurs during pilot training and reports that about two-thirds of the astronauts suffer from space motion sickness.

Gaze mechanisms involve not only eye movements but head movements as well. Frequently vestibular lesions that affect balance and orientation also affect the way the head is moved. This effect can lead to inappropriate stabilization of the head in an attempt to avoid unpleasant dizziness or vertigo, as well as possible dysfunction of the neck muscles and joints, which can also cause a sense of imbalance. Relatively little is known about the clinical effects of vestibular lesions on neck muscle and joint action or the reverse.

Adaptive Changes in Vestibular Function

A remarkable feature of the vestibular system is its potential for adaptive change (plasticity). This adaptive capacity allows the system to compensate for changes that occur during development and aging or as a result of lesions. Most striking is the rebalancing of the system that occurs after loss of one vestibular nerve or labyrinth. The large postural imbalance and uncontrollable drift of the eyes that are seen immediately after a lesion disappear nearly completely over the course of a few weeks, although these signs can return if the system is stressed. To accomplish this recovery, the adaptive system must compensate for the loss of a large amount of ongoing neural activity that would normally come into the vestibular nuclei via the lesioned nerve. Experimental studies are beginning to reveal some of the neural and pharmacologic aspects of the multi factorial process that is involved.

Another example of adaptive vestibular control is the plasticity of the VOR, which is experienced by anyone who is fitted with a new set of prescription spectacles. Because the lenses magnify or reduce the size of the visual scene, images appear unstable when the head is moved: the VOR is still compensating for image motion that would be different without the lenses. This instability resolves in a few hours because the adaptive system changes the "gain" of the VOR and thus adjusts the speed of reflex eye movement appropriately for the new lens system. Experimentally, large changes in gain can be induced by having subjects wear magnifying and reducing lenses and even the direction of the VOR can be altered by appropriate pairing of head and image motion. Thus, in addition to its clinical relevance, this VOR plasticity has become an important model system for understanding the neural basis of motor learning.

The role of the cerebellum in this process is the subject of current controversy. Cerebellar lesions abolish VOR plasticity, but one group of investigators believe that the cerebellum merely generates error signals that induce learning in the brain stem while another group has provided evidence that cerebellar circuits themselves can undergo plastic changes which account for VOR plasticity. This healthy controversy places the vestibular system at the forefront of attempts to understand sensorimotor systems. What is learned about the role of the cerebellum in the VOR will help scientists understand its role in regulating other types of movements.

As humans venture into space, they will be exposed for increasing periods of time to gravito-inertial fields different from those of Earth. Exposure to microgravity results in profound changes in the balance system. Extended exposure might be expected to have consequences on otolith reflexes involved with control of eye and head movements, posture and locomotion since those reflexes have evolved and function in the gravity of Earth. For example, the linear VOR, which depends on accurate information from otoliths, as well as reflexes dependent upon canal/otolith interactions, would be affected by exposure to space. Diminished accuracy of eye movement control during head movement may result. Thus, in space, adaptive vestibular changes can lead to alterations in behavior and performance, as well as to changes in perception of spatial orientation. Such adaptive alterations can in turn produce difficulties when the individual returns to an Earth gravity environment.

Related Topics

The topics of development and aging, neural modeling and neurotransmitters and molecular biology relate to the four areas discussed in each section of this report, e.g., signal transduction by vestibular end-organs; reflex control of posture and gaze; sensory integration in spatial orientation, perception and motion sickness; and adaptive changes in vestibular function.

424

Development and Aging. The major goal of developmental studies of the vestibular system is to enhance the understanding of the cellular and molecular events leading to neuron proliferation, migration, differentiation and synapse formation. These activities are essential for neuron precursors to become vestibular neurons. In contrast, aging studies focus on postmaturational changes that may result in diminished function and/or cell death. Both types of studies are needed to gain a better understanding of how the brain processes vestibular signals and adapts to change.

One of the major challenges confronting developmental neurobiologists is to understand how connectivity and synaptic specificity are achieved. These issues are confounded in the vestibular system by the highly complex central vestibular network that relies on multisensory inputs for its normal activity and is composed of a highly interconnected network of neurons, with less topologic organization than in other sensory systems. However, there are advantages to the developmental approach which begins by looking at neurons and their connections when the basic components of their organization and function are simpler and more readily apparent. Examining progressively-older neurons and their more complex assemblies should result in further insights into how the system works. Studies of aging vestibular systems should enable us to determine whether the decline in vestibular function is a result of preprogramming (i.e., genetic influences) or the inability of the cells to sustain normal functional demands.

Following injury, the response of the adult vestibular system is characterized by a variety of responses which are species- and age-dependent. In lower vertebrates, hair cells in the inner ear and the vestibular nerve neurons have the capacity to regenerate. This capacity has not yet been demonstrated in mammals. Following the sectioning of amphibian axons, vestibular ganglion cells innervating individual receptor organs find their synaptic locus in the vestibular nuclei. The new connections are functionally operative suggesting that their reestablishment and neuromodulatory function must be genetically imprinted. The central nervous system can compensate for deficits in vestibular function, and this capacity is greatest in primates, including man. Vision has been recognized as an important component in the compensation of VORs of primates and other mammals. There is a paucity of information, however, about the cellular and molecular mechanisms of the repair process. Such mechanisms are being recognized in new experimental work.

425

Neural Modeling. Because of the ability to measure precisely ocular motor and, to some extent, postural compensation in response to vestibular stimulation, mathematical modeling of these systems is an important method for relating their reflex behavior to the neural components that determine that behavior. Dynamic system models have contributed to defining the parameters that characterize the vestibular system. For example, the characterization of the dominant behavior of the VOR and certain postural responses in terms of time constants is a direct consequence of approximating the systems as first-order linear systems. Extensions of these concepts have led to defining parameters of VOR behavior in three dimensions and have given rise to model-based studies that relate these parameters to fundamental organizational principles that determine the behavior of the VOR. Computational models and techniques that predict experimentally-obtained, behavioral results and uncover organizational principles that govern vestibular-induced behavior are needed.

Problems concerning integration of information from the vestibular end-organs and reflex pathways, as well as from other sensory systems, are important to study as a component of vestibular research of balance and posture, both in the civilian sector and in aerospace biomedical research. Computer modeling of neural network function is an important and indispensable tool for understanding how ensembles of neurons produce the required integration of information and generation of motor responses.

Theoretical neurocomputing studies also confront this key problem of information processing (sensory fusion) that has been solved by the brain in the vestibular system. The issue of information integration from different sensors is common to biomedical research, aerospace biology and neurocomputing research. Cooperation among fields will optimize success in each. This success can be achieved by identifying or creating research facilities that can integrate such multidisciplinary efforts.

Neurotransmitters and Molecular Biology. Transmission of vestibular signals from the ear to the brain is initiated when hair cells release molecules of neurotransmitters which react with receptors on the membrane of afferent nerve fibers. Several animal models have demonstrated central nervous system control of labyrinthine receptors by efferent fibers transmitting via acetylcholine. However, despite the identification of glutamate, histamine and other agents as potential

426

afferent transmitters, conclusive evidence that any of these compounds serves as a primary neurotransmitter is still lacking.

It is important to characterize the nature of vestibular neurotransmitters and modulators and their interactions. Motor learning and motor control require continuous remodeling (adaptive plasticity) of neuronal connections and neurotransmission in central vestibular pathways. Understanding the molecular biology and pharmacology of those processes is an important future goal.

Understanding Pathophysiology

Our knowledge of the pathophysiology of many human vestibular disorders comes from experimental observations of the anatomy and physiology of the system together with careful clinical observations and pathologic examination of human temporal bones and the central nervous system. The various mechanisms by which abnormal conditions may disturb the normal structure and function of the vestibular system can be categorized as: traumatic, inflammatory, degenerative, metabolic or neoplastic. These mechanisms may affect the end-organ and/or the vestibular nerve and brain as indicated below:

Trauma to the head may produce fractures or concussions which affect the inner ear or brain. Abnormal stimulation of the end-organ may be associated with otic capsule fistulization from bone resorption, change in the density of a cupula (cupulolithiasis) or an excessively long stapedectomy prosthesis.

Inflammatory destruction (labyrinthitis) is caused by bacterial or viral agents and immune disorders.

Degeneration of the end-organ may be produced by trauma, ototoxic antibiotics (aminoglycosides) and other drugs (loop diuretics, cis-platinum), vascular insufficiency (hemorrhages, infarction), hereditary disorders (Alport's syndrome, Waardenburg's syndrome) or surgical destruction (labyrinthectomy).

Metabolic disorders like diabetes mellitus, hypothyroidism, alcoholism or Paget's disease affect the vestibular system. Metabolic alteration (disturbed labyrinthine fluid composition or function) is commonly considered to be the mechanism by which Meniere's disease and serous labyrinthitis affect the vestibular system.

Neoplastic alteration of the nerve fibers near the end-organ may be caused by an intra-labyrinthine schwannoma.

At the vestibular nerve level, *trauma* may be caused by mechanical compression resulting from arachnoid cysts, arterial loops and bone tumors. *Inflammatory change* is recognized as the pathologic alteration produced by viral and bacterial agents (vestibular neuronitis). *Degenerative changes* are associated with demyelinating disorders, such as multiple sclerosis and surgical transection. *Neoplastic alteration* is most commonly produced by benign tumors (vestibular schwannoma) but may also be associated with metastatic malignancies from other organs.

A variety of neurogenic disorders affect balance and different aspects of brain functions related to vestibular function, such as the control of gaze and posture. These include: hereditary and developmental disorders (congenital nystagmus, migraine, Chiari malformation); several familial ataxia syndromes involving different parts of the cerebellum; degenerative disorders (multiple sclerosis, progressive supranuclear palsies); various neoplastic lesions; vascular disorders, particularly of the brain stem and cerebellum (vascular malformation, infarctions and hemorrhages); and autoimmune disorders, including paraneoplastic syndromes.

Recent Accomplishments

Understanding the Molecular, Cellular and Neural Basis of Peripheral and Central Vestibular Function

Signal Transduction by Vestibular End-Organs

Recent technical advances in membrane biophysics have been applied to hair cells with the result that we now have a qualitative understanding of the events that link the bending of sensory hair bundles with the modulation of afferent impulse activity. Detailed studies in a few end-organs have shown how the various steps in the transduction process can be modified so that different hair cells and afferents become selectively tuned to certain aspects of the mechanical stimulus.

Afferent nerve fibers innervating a particular end-organ differ in their response properties. By the anatomic labeling of individual, physiologically characterized fibers, it has been possible to relate this response diversity to the innervation patterns of the afferents, including their location in the sensory epithelium and the types and number of hair cells that they contact.

Information has been obtained about the response of single vestibular afferent fibers to electrical activation of the efferent axons originating in the brain stem. Studies in alert animals have begun to suggest how efferent activity can modulate afferent discharge under physiological conditions. In addition to classical neurotransmitters such as acetylcholine, efferent neurons contain a variety of neuropeptides and transmitters (metenkephalin and calcitonin gene related peptide) that may influence receptor cells and afferent fibers in the end-organs.

Reflex Control of Posture and Gaze

Over the past five years considerable progress has been made in characterizing the sensory-to-motor transformations that occur in postural and gaze stabilizing reflexes:

- The patterns of limb, trunk and neck muscle activation by postural reflexes have been described and the ways in which they vary with context are being explored.

- Descriptions of the dynamic and three-dimensional spatial transformations that occur in vestibulo-ocular and vestibulocollic reflexes have been obtained. The patterns of muscle activation that result have been described and models have been advanced that successfully predict the muscle patterns that are used during the VOR and vestibulo-collic reflex.

- Information has been obtained in humans and non-human primates on VORs and their interactions with vision in response to linear acceleration. Eye movement control has been shown to involve interactions among otolith, visual and vergence mechanisms, and further understanding of such control mechanisms should lead to the rationale for quantitative tools for clinical assessment of otolith function.

- While understanding of the neuronal substrates of postural reflexes is at a rudimentary stage, great progress has been made in discovering the neural connections that mediate the transformations that occur in gaze-stabilizing reflexes.

- The structure and function of vestibulo-ocular relay neurons that form the middle portion of three-neuron VOR arcs have been described in sufficient detail to reveal how convergent labyrinthine inputs to these neurons and their divergent projections to multiple motor pools could contribute to reflex transformations. Neural network models that explore these possibilities in a formal way are beginning to appear.

- Beginnings have also been made in describing the more complex indirect pathways that contribute to the VOR and in determining how both direct and indirect pathways may be regulated by the cerebellum.

- Research has begun to define the biophysics and pharmacology of neurons in vestibular reflex pathways.

Sensory Integration in Spatial Orientation, Perception and Motion Sickness

Originally, vestibular reflexes were conceived as being automatic and not subject to cognitive control. However, recent research has shown that we can use information from vestibular receptors during movement to determine where we started from and how far we have moved. We can also use the imagined location of near and far targets to adjust the magnitude of eye movements that compensate for linear or angular head movements. Thus, cognitive processing of vestibular information is not only important for determining spatial orientation but also for establishing proper control of VORs.

Great strides have been made in understanding the compensatory responses produced by the otolith organs during linear head movements by considering the eye movements that would be necessary to view real or imagined visual targets. Slower or faster eye movements are required depending on whether targets are far or near. These compensatory eye movements even occur when targets are imagined in darkness.

Studies of this nature have revealed that the VOR is not a simple semicircular canal-mediated response. Instead it encompasses a broad range of reflex responses originating from each of the motion sensors in the labyrinth. Inputs from these sensors are directed toward the vestibular nuclei, where they are integrated with information from the visual and somatosensory systems and from proprioceptors to form signals that direct gaze movements and stabilize posture and equilibrium. Cerebellar participation is essential for proper operation of these vestibular reflexes.

Models of the VOR and of vestibular compensatory eye movements have shown that there are at least two components to the reflex. One operates rapidly to produce quick changes in eye position and eye movement in response to head movement. The other has more sluggish characteristics but outlasts impulses of acceleration and is largely responsible for the characteristics of eye movements induced by rotation. This component has recently been shown to be oriented around gravity. Both components are subject to adaptation, and these types of motor learning are controlled by various portions of the vestibulo-cerebellum. Lesions of the cerebellum cause deficits in compensatory movements, as well as disorientation and dysequilibrium. The current theory of motion sickness holds that it is a by-product of the process of adaptation to unusual sensory inputs or motion conditions. It has been demonstrated that subjects have a remarkable ability to adapt to unusual motion conditions, although the process of adaptation is often associated with motion sickness. When adaptation is finally achieved, the vertigo and/or motion sickness disappears.

Adaptive Changes in Vestibular Function

As described above, the vestibular and balance control systems have the remarkable ability to maintain useful function in many novel motion environments and to adapt to abnormal function of one or more of their components. The ability of these systems to adapt systematically sensory, neural and motor components in order to achieve useful compensation must be more thoroughly understood. Advances in vestibular health care, particularly rehabilitation, should be developed from sound scientific concepts. Therefore, the significance of central nervous system phenomena associated with the adaptive process (such as neural sprouting, reactive synaptogenesis and long-term potentiation or depression of synaptic transmission), which are thought to play important roles in adaptive control, must be measured and correlated systematically with behavior. Some accomplishments that have opened exciting new areas of investigation include:

- The essential role of adaptive plasticity in normal function of the vestibular system has been recognized. This system is unusual in that it is not static. It is constantly changing in response to changes in the environment or internal elements (for example, inner-ear or central nervous system diseases).

- Neural pathways that may play a role in adaptive changes have been identified. As indicated above, there are several possible models of the neural basis of VOR plasticity. Information is also beginning to emerge about the neural changes that accompany recovery from unilateral labyrinthectomy.

- The pharmacologic aspects of adaptive changes and their roles in transmitter synthesis as well as the release, number and sensitivity of receptors have been described.

Research from both U.S. and Soviet space flights has shown alterations in eye movement and postural control, as well as in perception of spatial orientation, both during flight and after return to Earth. It appears that the plasticity of vestibular reflexes, for the most part, allows adaptation during short duration missions, but the effects of vestibular system performance after long exposures is unknown. The precise characteristics of adaptive plasticity in this unique environment and the vestibular function involved in readaptation to Earth's gravity after long-duration exposure to space remain unknown. Vestibular and balance system adaptation to altered gravito-inertial environments has not been measured systematically.

Related Topics

Development and Aging. Recent work suggests that a synchrony may exist between structural maturation of the vestibular end-organs and central vestibular nuclei. In recent developmental studies of the vestibular system, classical approaches have been supplemented with molecular biological probes and innovative techniques. For example, connectivity of the vestibuloocular and vestibulospinal pathways has been studied by the application of fluorescent dyes (e.g. Lucifer yellow, carbocyanine) in brain slices and on cultured brain stem and spinal cord preparations; immunocytochemical probes are used to examine the vestibular pathways and the maturation of otolith organs; and brain slice preparations are employed to obtain membrane and synaptic properties of developing vestibular sensory neurons.

From the combination of electron microscopic methods and tract tracing techniques, we are beginning to determine the steps in the assembly of synaptic inputs to the vestibular brain stem nuclei. Specifically, the first synapses formed in the chick's lateral vestibular nucleus are not formed by primary vestibular fibers but appear to be derived from fibers of central origins. It is important to determine the steps in the assembly of various synaptic inputs to vestibular neurons in order to test what role synaptic formation may play in orchestrating developmental events.

The aging vestibular system also shows interesting changes in the structure of sensory and non-sensory components. Senescence has long been associated with increased vestibular dysfunction in older subjects who have more difficulty with vestibular test performance than younger subjects. Animal studies indicate that neural vestibular components in the ear and brain tend to accumulate a so-called aging pigment or lipofuscin. This and related substances, accumulated during the process of aging, may place a burden on the normal functioning of neurons and may diminish their response to functional demands. The characteristics of structural, functional and behavioral modifications of the aging vestibular system need to be studied. We need to determine if diminished efficiency with age is due to irreversible preprogrammed cessation of function or to reversible cellular modifications.

Neural Modeling. In the past decade, there has been increasing interest in mathematical modeling of vestibular systems at the level of the end-organ, neural pathways and reflex behavior. Models are important because they formalize concepts, organize data and predict responses. Modeling reflex behavior by applying control system analysis, as developed and used in electrical engineering, has been augmented by developing mathematical descriptions of the functioning of parallel neural networks. This conceptual advance is important because it shows that it is possible to reproduce neural behavior by layers of interactive adapting elements. The vestibular system is a natural entry point for the use of such models linking biological and theoretical neural network approaches.

It is not sufficient merely to set up neural networks with a multitude of parameters and adapt them to fit arbitrary data. Studies need to be conducted to derive learning algorithms from fundamental principles that are consistent with mathematically formalized, behavioral constraints. Using realistic models of cellular dynamics as derived from pharmacodynamics could also be helpful in uncovering the principles that govern behavioral learning in the vestibular system such as adaptation and habituation.

Neurotransmitters and Molecular Biology. Considerable progress has been made in identifying the neurotransmitters involved in the vestibular system. The field of potential primary hair cell neurotransmitters has been narrowed to glutamate-related excitatory amino acids. The transmitters liberated from the eighth nerve fibers onto brain stem neurons have not yet been specified, but the inhibitory transmitters of the vestibular commissural systems include gammaamino-butyric acid and glycine. Since data from recent studies on other systems indicate that several neurotransmitters may coexist in the same synapse, this possibility should be investigated in the vestibular system.

Advances in Diagnosis

Thoughtful history taking based on a knowledge of the anatomy, physiology and pathology of the vestibular system provides the core of diagnostic information necessary for clinical practice. This information is enhanced by tests which describe the integrity of vestibular reflexes.

Testing—Physical

Advances in modern technology have made the evaluation of vestibular patients a quantitative science. Because the VOR is the best understood vestibular reflex, scientists have taken advantage of the reliability of eye movement measurement to develop a battery of vestibular function tests to study the integrity of the various VORs.

The function of the cristae of the horizontal semicircular canals, sensors for angular acceleration, can be measured with the caloric test by irrigating, under precisely controlled conditions, the external ear canal with water at different temperatures. The resulting eye movements can be accurately and efficiently measured with the aid of small laboratory computers.

Other methods of evaluating semicircular canal function include the use of rotary platforms and measurements of VOR responses to obtain precise information about the relationship between stimuli and reflex eye movements.

The function of the linear acceleration sensors of the ear (the otolithic organs) has been measured by observing ocular reflex responses to stimulation with various devices including the parallel swing. Also, the evaluation of balance has improved greatly with the use of platforms which measure movement of the patient's center of mass with sensitive force transducers whose signals are analyzed by computer.

The contribution of the visual system to orientation is evaluated by measurement of visual oculomotor reflexes, including the use of tests for smooth pursuit function and optokinetic nystagmus. These tests evaluate the ability of patients to follow small visual images (the smooth pursuit system) or the movement of large visual scenery (optokinetic function). The most revealing information is obtained by combining visual with vestibular stimulation as described above. Given the extent of neural pathways subserving vestibulo-ocular and visuo-oculomotor reflexes, information from these tests provide methods to evaluate large areas of the brain. The combination of such tests in the modern vestibular test battery has allowed the identification of the location within inner ear or specific brain regions of vestibular lesions, a quantitative estimate of the magnitude of the deficit and the ability to follow the course of the disease. Useful features of these tests are their non-invasive nature, their ease of administration and minimal discomfort for the patient.

In addition to these standard tests, new tests are being developed in animal studies and being investigated in humans. Several of the new human vestibular tests are designed to evaluate anterior and posterior semicircular canal function (in addition to horizontal canal function) by rotating subjects about different axes to optimize stimulation of the specific canals. A problem associated with attempts to activate vertical canals is the simultaneous stimulation of the otolithic organs and the complexity of measuring the resulting eye movement. New methods, such as video-based monitors, are being developed to deal with the latter problem.

435

Of all the available vestibular tests, only the caloric test allows specific location of a lesion in one of the ears. All other tests using physiologic stimuli represent the response of a multiplicity of nerve centers. In recent years, however, animal experiments have provided information that suggests the possibility of evaluating lesions specifically located in the vestibular nerve. Vestibular-evoked potentials have been obtained from the nerves of the semicircular and otolith organs in several animal species. Responses from direct electrical stimulation of the vestibular nerve also have been obtained in animal and human experiments.

A major deficiency is the lack of tests for otolithic and proprioceptive reflexes. Tests are being developed to evaluate these systems under operational conditions in freely-moving animals and human subjects. There is interest in the evaluation of head and eye interactions in humans with normal and abnormal vestibular function. Also lacking are tests for the quantitative evaluation of the subjective sensation of motion and of dizziness in patients.

Also, there are no tests that allow the physician to assess the possible role of neck muscle or bone lesions in the production of dizziness, vertigo or postural imbalance.

Testing—Laboratory / Radiology

Tests for antibodies to inner-ear antigens have recently been developed and appear to help in the diagnosis of inner ear autoimmune disease.

Fine resolution imaging has improved with the development of better software and technology for both computed tomography (CT) and magnetic resonance (MR) scanning. Improved use of contrast and speed of image acquisition have made it possible to detect smaller lesions and permit dynamic CT/MR scanning to evaluate blood flow in small regions of the central nervous system. The development of techniques for imaging the individual receptors in the labyrinth would improve diagnosis and understanding of the disease process.

Advances in Treatment

Medical Therapy

Advances in basic research have identified probable transmitters and receptor sites in the vestibular periphery and central connections.

These findings have not only led to clinical trials of transmitter agonist and antagonists but have also resulted in the realization that most pharmacologic agents with potential central nervous system activity may interfere with normal vestibular function. For example, long-acting sleeping pills and tranquilizers are now recognized as a major cause of injuries from falling in nursing home patients.

Clinical trials of antihistamines, anticholinergics and phenothiazines with improved experimental design have been conducted, and these agents appear to be helpful in relieving the symptoms of vertigo. Unfortunately, these agents have side effects such as drowsiness and dry mouth and eyes. The reduction of symptoms, presumably related to increased endolymph fluid, with systemic diuretics appears to be helpful, at least in the early stages of Meniere's disease.

Further studies using systemic, transtympanic or intralabyrinthine aminoglycosides show good results in reducing vertiginous attacks in patients with Meniere's disease but have the potential side effects of loss of hearing or severe loss of vestibular function and oscillopsia (a condition in which objects appear to move up and down or from side to side).

The recognition of the relationship between associated disorders such as depression, anxiety attacks and panic attacks and vestibular disorders suggests the need to investigate these disorders as well. Recent advances in the pharmacologic control of these disorders is encouraging.

Surgical Therapy

Surgical treatment strategies in peripheral vestibular disorders may be grouped into ablative and non-ablative protocols. Ablation procedures relieve the balance symptoms by denervating the altered labyrinth without correcting the lesion. These procedures are 90 to 99 percent effective in relieving episodic dizziness provided that the ablation is complete. If hearing is not useful in the unilaterally-diseased ear, labyrinthectomy (transcanal or transmastoid approach), is a short, relatively-safe technique. If there is useful hearing in an unilaterally-affected ear, selective vestibular neurectomy, via a middle cranial fossa (MF) or posterior cranial fossa (PF) approach, is now the accepted procedure. The MF approach is technically more difficult and is associated with a higher incidence (25 percent) of temporary facial nerve weakness than the PF approach. However, it has a higher success rate

(95 to 98 percent) for vertigo control than the PF method (80 to 90 percent) because of the natural separation of the vestibular and auditory nerves in the internal auditory canal. The separation of these two groups of fibers in the posterior fossa section of the eighth nerve is arbitrarily created by the surgeon.

Selective transection of the posterior ampullary (singular) nerve has been successful in more than 90 percent of patients with chronic disabling positional vertigo (cupulolithiasis). Associated sensorineural hearing loss has occurred in fewer than five percent of the cases.

Non-ablative procedures correct the pathologic derangement responsible for altered vestibular function. Several examples of these are: removal of chronic inflammatory tissue (cholesteatoma) from a bony semicircular canal fistula, removal of an excessively long stapedectomy prosthesis, removal of chronic inflammatory tissue from the oval and round windows and repair of a perilymphatic fistula in the oval or round windows caused by direct or indirect trauma.

The efficacy of vessel loop relocation from the intracranial portion of the eighth nerve has been variable and remains undetermined at this time.

Rehabilitation

The use of exercises to improve gaze and postural stability in patients with vestibular disorders has become increasingly popular in the past five years. The exercises are based in part on anecdotal evidence of improved function in patients following exercise intervention. The exercises are also based on the results of animal research demonstrating that visuo-motor experience can increase the rate of recovery following unilateral vestibular loss and that preventing visual inputs or movement can delay the onset of recovery. Research on human subjects is in progress, but the results are not yet known.

Outcome measures of treatment efficacy include many of the standard methods for quantifying balance but are often dependent on subjective reports. A questionnaire that measures the patient's perception of the extent to which the vestibular or balance disorder is handicapping has been developed and validated.

Chapter 53

Dizziness: Hope Through Research

Most of us can remember feeling dizzy—after a roller coaster ride, maybe, or when looking down from a tall building, or when, as children, we would step off a spinning merry-go-round. Even superbly conditioned astronauts have had temporary trouble with dizziness while in space. In these situations, dizziness arises naturally from unusual changes that disrupt our normal feeling of stability.

But dizziness can also be a sign that there is a disturbance or a disease in the system that helps people maintain balance. This system is coordinated by the brain, which reacts to nerve impulses from the ears, the eyes, the neck and limb muscles, and the joints of the arms and legs. If any of these areas fail to function normally or if the brain fails to coordinate the many nerve impulses it receives, a person may feel dizzy. The feeling of dizziness varies from person to person and, to some extent, according to its cause; it can include a feeling of unsteadiness, imbalance, or even spinning.

Disease-related dizziness, whether it takes the form of unsteadiness or spinning, is fairly common in the older population. Today, both older and younger people with serious dizziness problems can be helped by a variety of techniques—from medication to surgery to balancing exercises. Such techniques have been developed and improved by scientists studying dizziness.

Much of today's research on dizziness is supported by the National Institute of Neurological and Communicative Disorders and

NIH Publication No. 86-76.

Stroke (NINCDS). This Institute is a unit of the National Institutes of Health. It is the focal point within the Federal Government for research on the brain and central nervous system, including studies of the senses through which we interact with our surroundings.

With NINCDS support, scientists are searching for better ways to diagnose and treat dizziness, and are investigating the mechanisms that help us maintain our normal sense of balance. These studies, along with basic research on how the ear, the brain, and the nerves work, hold the best hope for relief for dizziness sufferers.

A Delicate Balancing Act

To understand what goes wrong when we feel dizzy, we need to know about the vestibular system by which we keep a sense of balance amid all our daily twisting and turning, starting and stopping, jumping, falling, rolling, and bending.

The vestibular system is located in the inner ear and contains the following structures: vestibular labyrinth, semicircular canals, vestibule, utricle, and saccule. These structures work in tandem with the vestibular areas of the brain to help us maintain balance.

The vestibular labyrinth is located behind the eardrum. The labyrinth's most striking feature is a group of three semicircular canals or tubes that arise from a common base. At the base of the canals is a rounded chamber called the vestibule. The three canals and the vestibule are hollow and contain a fluid called endolymph which moves in response to head movement.

Within the vestibule and the semicircular canals are patches of special nerve cells called hair cells. Hair cells are also found in two fluid-filled sacs, the utricle and saccule, located within the vestibule. These cells are aptly named: rows of thin, flexible, hairlike fibers project from them into the endolymph.

Also located in the inner ear are tiny calcium stones called otoconia. When you move your head or stand up, the hair cells are bent by the weight of the otoconia or movement of the endolymph. The bending of the hair cells transmits an electrical signal about head movement to the brain. This signal travels from the inner ear to the brain along the eighth cranial nerve—the nerve involved in balance and hearing. The brain recognizes the signal as a particular movement of the head and is able to use this information to help maintain balance.

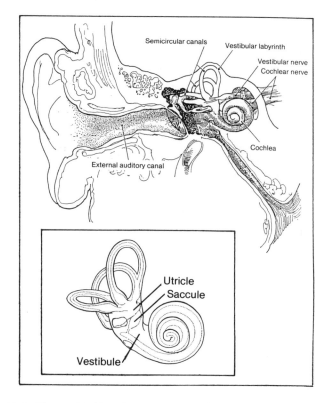

Figure 53.1. *The semicircular canals and vestibule of the inner ear contain a fluid called endolymph that moves in response to head movement.*

The senses are also important in determining balance. Sensory input from the eyes as well as from the muscles and joints is sent to the brain, alerting us that the path we are following bends to the right or that our head is tilted as we bend to pick up a dime. The brain interprets this information—along with cues from the vestibular system—and adjusts the muscles so that balance is maintained.

Dizziness can occur when sensory information is distorted. Some people feel dizzy at great heights, for instance, partly because they cannot focus on nearby objects to stabilize themselves. When one is on the ground, it is normal to sway slightly while standing. A person maintains balance by adjusting the body's position to something close by. But when someone is standing high up, objects are too far away to use to adjust balance. The result can be confusion, insecurity, and dizziness, which is sometimes resolved by sitting down.

441

Some scientists believe that motion sickness, a malady that affects sea, car, and even space travelers, occurs when the brain receives conflicting sensory information about the body's motion and position. For example, when someone reads while riding in a car, the inner ear senses the movement of the vehicle, but the eyes gaze steadily on the book that is not moving. The resulting sensory conflict may lead to the typical symptoms of motion sickness: dizziness, nausea, vomiting, and sweating.

Another form of dizziness occurs when we turn around in a circle quickly several times and then stop suddenly. Turning moves the endolymph. The moving endolymph tells us we are still rotating but our other senses say we've stopped. We feel dizzy.

Diagnosing the Problem

The dizziness one feels after spinning around in a circle usually goes away quickly and does not require a medical evaluation. But when symptoms appear to be caused by an underlying physical problem, the prudent person will see a physician for diagnostic tests. According to a study supported by the National Institute of Neurological and Communicative Disorders and Stroke, a thorough examination can reveal the underlying cause of dizziness in about 90 percent of cases.

A person experiencing dizziness may first go to a general practitioner or family physician; between 5 and 10 percent of initial visits to these physicians involve a complaint of dizziness. The patient may then be referred either to an ear specialist (otologist) or a nervous system specialist (neurologist).

The patient will be asked to describe the exact nature of the dizziness, to give a complete history of its occurrence, and to list any other symptoms or medical problems. Patients give many descriptions of dizziness—depending to some extent on its cause. Common complaints are light-headedness, a feeling of impending faint, a hallucination of movement or motion, or a loss of balance without any strange feelings in the head. Some people also report they have vertigo—a form of dizziness in which one's surroundings appear to be spinning uncontrollably or one feels the sensation of spinning.

The physician will try to determine what components of a patient's nervous system are out of kilter, looking first for changes in blood pressure, heart rhythm, or vision—all of which may contribute to the complaints. Sometimes dizziness is associated with an ear disorder. The patient may have loss of hearing, discomfort from loud sounds, or constant noise in the ear, a disorder known as tinnitus. The physician will also look for other neurological symptoms: difficulty in swallowing or talking, for example, or double vision.

Tests and Scans

After the initial history-taking and physical examination, the physician may deliberately try to make the patient feel dizzy. The patient may be asked to repeat actions or movements that generally cause dizziness: to walk in one direction and then turn quickly in the opposite direction, or to hyperventilate by breathing deeply for 3 minutes.

In another test, the patient sits upright on an examining table. The physician tilts the patient's head back and turns it partway to one side, then gently but quickly pushes the patient backward to a lying down position. The reaction to this procedure varies according to the cause of dizziness. Patients with benign positional vertigo may experience vertigo plus nystagmus: rapid, uncontrollable back-and-forth movements of the eyes.

One widely used procedure, called the caloric test, involves electronic monitoring of the patient's eye movements while one ear at a time is irrigated with warm water or warm air and then with cold water or cold air. This double stimulus causes the endolymph to move in a way similar to that produced by rotation of the head. If the labyrinth is working normally, nystagmus should result. A missing nystagmus reaction is a strong argument that the balance organs are not acting correctly.

NINCDS-supported scientists at The Johns Hopkins University in Baltimore observed that not all patients can tolerate the traditional caloric test. Some become sick when the ear is irrigated with the standard amount of water or air before physicians can measure their eye movements. So the scientists are designing a method of conducting the test more gradually by slowly adjusting the amount of water or air reaching the inner ear. Their goal is to reduce patient discomfort while allowing the test to proceed.

Some patients who cannot tolerate the caloric test are given a rotatory test. In this procedure, the patient sits in a rotating chair, head tilted slightly forward. The chair spins rapidly in one direction, then

443

stops abruptly. Depending on the cause of dizziness, the patient may experience vertigo after this rotation.

In one variation of this test, the chair is placed in a tent of striped cloth. As the chair rotates, electrodes record movements of the patient's eyes in response to the stripes. The physician evaluates these eye movements, a form of nystagmus, to determine if the patient has a disorder of the balance system.

Because disorders of balance are often accompanied by hearing loss, the physician may order a hearing test.

Hearing loss and associated dizziness could also be due to damaged nerve cells in the brain stem, where the hearing and balance nerve relays signals to the brain. To detect a malfunction, the physician may order a kind of computerized brain wave study called a brain stem auditory evoked response test. In this procedure, electrodes are attached to several places on the surface of the patient's scalp and a sound is transmitted to the patient's ear. The electrodes measure the time it takes nerve signals generated by the sound to travel from the ear to the brain stem.

If there is reason to suspect that the dizziness could stem from a tumor or cyst, the patient may undergo a computed tomographic (CT) scan. In a CT scan, x-ray pictures are taken of the brain from several different angles. These images are then combined by a computer to give a detailed view that may reveal the damaging growth.

Sometimes anxiety and emotional upset cause a person to feel dizzy. Certain patients may be asked to take a psychological test, to try to find out whether the dizziness is caused or intensified by emotional stress.

The many tests administered by a physician will usually point to a cause for the patient's dizziness. Disorders responsible for dizziness can be categorized as:

- peripheral vestibular, or those involving a disturbance in the labyrinth.

- central vestibular, or those resulting from a problem in the brain or its connecting nerves.

- systemic, or those originating in nerves or organs outside the head.

Confused Signals

When someone has vertigo but does not experience faintness or difficulty in walking, the cause is probably a peripheral vestibular disorder. In these conditions, nerve cells in the inner ear send confusing information about body movement to the brain.

Ménière's disease. A well-known cause of vertigo is the peripheral vestibular disorder known as Ménière's disease. First identified in 1861 by Prosper Ménière, a French physician, the disease is thought to be caused by too much endolymph in the semicircular canals and vestibule. Some scientists think that the excess endolymph may affect the hair cells so that they do not work correctly. This explanation, however, is still under study.

The vertigo of Ménière's disease comes and goes without an apparent cause; it may be made worse by a change in position and reduced by being still.

In addition to vertigo, patients have hearing loss and tinnitus. Hearing loss is usually restricted at first to one ear and is often severe. Patients sometimes feel "fullness" or discomfort in the ear, and diagnostic testing may show unusual sensitivity to increasingly loud sounds. In 10 to 20 percent of patients, hearing loss and tinnitus eventually occur in the second ear.

Ménière's disease patients may undergo electronystagmography, an electrical recording of the caloric test, to determine if their labyrinth is working normally.

Attacks of Ménière's disease may occur several times a month or year and can last from a few minutes to many hours. Some patients experience a spontaneous disappearance of symptoms while others may have attacks for years.

Treatment of Ménière's disease includes such drugs as meclizine hydrochloride and the tranquilizer diazepam to reduce the feeling of intense motion during vertigo. To control the buildup of endolymph, the patient may also take a diuretic, a drug that reduces fluid production. A low-salt diet—which reduces water retention—is claimed to be an effective treatment of Ménière's disease.

When these measures fail to help, surgery may be considered. In shunt surgery, part of the inner ear is drained to reestablish normal inner ear fluid or endolymph pressure. In another operation, called vestibular nerve section, surgeons expose and cut the vestibular part of the eighth nerve. Both vestibular nerve section and shunt surgery commonly relieve the dizziness of Ménière's disease without affecting hearing.

A more drastic operation, labyrinthectomy, involves total destruction of the inner ear. This procedure is usually successful in eliminating dizziness but causes total loss of hearing in the operated ear—an important consideration since the second ear may one day be affected.

Positional vertigo. People with benign positional vertigo experience vertigo after a position change. Barbara noticed the first sign of this disorder one morning when she got up out of bed. She felt the room spinning. Frightened, she quickly returned to bed and lay down. After about 30 seconds the vertigo passed. Fearing a stroke, Barbara went to the emergency room of a hospital for a medical evaluation, which failed to show a problem. She had no symptoms for several days, then the problem returned. At this point, Barbara was referred to an otoneurologist, a physician who specializes in the ear and related parts of the nervous system.

Like Barbara, most patients with benign positional vertigo are extremely worried about their symptoms. But the patients usually feel less threatened once the disorder is diagnosed.

The cause of benign positional vertigo is not known, although some patients may recall an incident of head injury. The condition can strike at any adult age with attacks occurring periodically throughout a person's life.

In one type of treatment, the patient practices the position that provokes dizziness until the balance system eventually adapts. Rarely, a physician will prescribe medication to prevent attacks.

Vestibular neuronitis. In this common vestibular disorder, the patient has severe vertigo. Jack experienced his first attack of this problem at 2 a.m. when he rolled over in bed and suddenly felt the room spinning violently. He started vomiting but couldn't stand up; finally, he managed to crawl to the bathroom. When he returned to bed, he lay very still—the only way to stop the vertigo. Three days later, he was able to walk without experiencing vertigo, but he still felt unsteady. Gradually, over the next several weeks, Jack's balance improved, but it was a year before he was entirely without symptoms.

Unlike Ménière's disease, vestibular neuronitis is not associated with hearing loss. Patients with vestibular neuronitis first experience an acute attack of severe vertigo lasting for hours or days, just as Jack did, with loss of balance sometimes lasting for weeks or months. About half of those who have a single attack have further episodes over a period of months to years.

The cause of vestibular neuronitis is uncertain. Since the first attack often occurs after a viral illness, some scientists believe the disorder is caused by a viral infection of the nerve.

Other labyrinth problems. Inner ear problems with resulting dizziness can also be caused by certain antibiotics used to fight life-threatening bacterial infections. Probably the best-known agent of this group is streptomycin. Problems usually arise when high doses of these drugs are taken for a long time, but some patients experience symptoms after short treatment with low doses, especially if they have impaired kidneys.

The first symptoms of damage to the inner ear caused by medication are usually hearing loss, tinnitus, or unsteadiness while walking. Stopping the drug can usually halt further damage to the balance mechanism, but this is not always possible: the medicine may have to be continued to treat a life-threatening infection. Patients sometimes adapt to the inner ear damage that may occur after prolonged use of these antibiotics and recover their balance.

Balance can also be affected by a cholesteatoma, a clump of cells from the eardrum that grow into the middle ear and accumulate there. These growths are thought to result from repeated infections such as recurrent otitis media. If unchecked, a cholesteatoma can enlarge and threaten the inner ear. But if the growth is detected early, it can be surgically removed.

Brain and Nerve Damage

The vestibular nerve carries signals from the inner ear to the brain stem. If either the nerve or the brain stem is damaged, information about position and movement may be blocked or incorrectly processed, leading to dizziness. Conditions in which dizziness results from damage to the brain stem or its associated nerves are called central causes of dizziness.

447

Acoustic neuroma. One central cause of dizziness is a tumor called an acoustic neuroma. Although the most common sign of this growth is hearing loss followed by tinnitus, some patients also experience dizziness.

An acoustic neuroma usually occurs in the internal auditory canal, the bony channel through which the vestibular nerve passes as it leaves the inner ear. The growing tumor presses on the nerve, sending false messages about position and movement to the brain.

The hearing nerve running alongside the vestibular nerve can also be compressed by the acoustic neuroma, with resulting tinnitus and hearing loss. Or the tumor may press on other nearby nerves, producing numbness or weakness of the face. If the neuroma is allowed to grow, it will eventually reach the brain and may affect the function of other cranial nerves.

Computed tomography has revolutionized the detection of acoustic neuromas. If an early diagnosis is made, a surgeon can remove the tumor. The patient usually regains balance.

Stroke. Dizziness may be a sign of a "small stroke" or transient ischemic attack (TIA) in the brain stem. TIA's, which result from a temporary lack of blood supply to the brain, may also cause transient numbness, tingling, or weakness in a limb or on one side of the face. Other signs include temporary blindness and difficulty with speech. These symptoms are warning signs: one should see a physician immediately for treatment. If a TIA, is ignored, a major stroke may follow.

Systemic Diseases: Underlying Illness

Dizziness can be a symptom of diseases affecting body parts other than the brain and central nervous system. Systemic conditions like anemia or high blood pressure decrease oxygen supplies to the brain; a physician eliminates the resulting dizziness by treating the underlying systemic illness.

Damaged sensory nerves. We maintain balance by adjusting to information transmitted along sensory nerves from sensors in the eyes, muscles, and joints to the spinal cord or brain. When these sensory nerves are damaged by systemic disease, dizziness may result.

Multiple sensory deficits, a systemic disease, is believed by some physicians to be the chief cause of vaguely described dizziness in the aged population. In this disorder several senses or sensory nerves are damaged. The result: faulty balance.

People with diabetes, which can damage nerves affecting vision and touch, may develop multiple sensory deficits. So can patients with arthritis or cataracts, both of which distort how sensory information reaches the brain. The first step in treating multiple sensory deficits is to eliminate symptoms of specific disorders. Permanent contact lenses can improve vision in cataract patients, for example, and medication or surgery may ease pain and stiffness related to arthritis.

Symptoms of damaged sensory nerves may be relieved by a collar to eliminate extreme head motion, balancing exercises to help compensate for sensory losses, or a cane to aid balance. Some patients are helped by the drug methylphenidate, which can increase awareness of remaining sensations.

Systemic neurological disorders such as multiple sclerosis, Alzheimer's disease, Parkinson's disease, or Creutzfeldt-Jakob disease may also cause dizziness, primarily during walking. However, dizziness is rarely the sole symptom of these nervous system diseases.

Low blood pressure. One common systemic disease causing dizziness is postural or orthostatic hypotension. In this disease, the heart does not move the blood with enough force to supply the brain adequately. Symptoms include sudden feelings of faintness, lightheadedness, or dizziness when standing up quickly.

Because the muscles in aging blood vessels are weak and the arteries inadequate in helping convey blood to the head, older people are particularly susceptible to this condition. Older persons who do not sit or lie down at the first sensation of dizziness may actually lose consciousness.

People who have undetected anemia or those who are taking diuretics to eliminate excess water from their body and reduce high blood pressure are also at risk of developing postural hypotension.

A physician can easily diagnose postural hypotension: the patient's blood pressure is measured before standing abruptly and immediately afterward. Treatment is designed to eliminate dizziness by reducing the patient's blood volume.

A secondary symptom. Dizziness may also be a secondary symptom in many other diseases. Faintness accompanied by occasional loss of consciousness can be due to low blood sugar, especially

449

when the faint feeling persists after the patient lies down.

A common cause of mild dizziness—the kind described as light-headedness—is medicine. A number of major prescription drugs may produce light-headedness as a side effect. Two types of drugs that can cause this problem are sedatives, which are taken to induce sleep, and tranquilizers, which are used to calm anxiety.

When Anxiety Strikes

Tranquilizers may cause a type of dizziness referred to as light-headedness—but so may anxiety. Cynthia is a young woman who becomes light-headed under a variety of stressful circumstances. The light-headedness sometimes is accompanied by heart palpitations and panic. She can produce these symptoms at will by breathing rapidly and deeply for a few minutes.

Cynthia's light-headedness is due to hyperventilation: rapid, prolonged deep breathing or occasional deep sighing that upsets the oxygen and carbon dioxide balance in the blood. The episodes are typically brief and often associated with tingling and numbness in the fingers and around the mouth. Hyperventilation is triggered by anxiety or depression in about 60 percent of dizziness patients.

Once made aware of the source of the symptoms, a patient can avoid hyperventilation or abort attacks by breath-holding or breathing into a paper bag to restore a correct balance of oxygen and carbon dioxide. If hyperventilation is due to anxiety, psychological counseling may be recommended.

Some patients who report dizziness may be suffering from a psychiatric disorder. Generally these persons will say that they experience light-headedness or difficulty concentrating; they may also describe panic states when in crowded places. Tests of such patients reveal that the inner ear is working correctly. Treatment may include counseling.

Demystifying Dizziness through Research

Scientists are working to understand dizziness and its sources among the complex interactions of the labyrinth, the other sense organs, and the brain. The research is offering new insights into the basis of balance, as well as improvements in diagnosis, treatment, and prevention of dizziness.

Innovative surgery. Delicate surgical instruments and operating microscopes have made possible new methods to help patients with dizziness. The symptoms of benign positional vertigo, for example, may be relieved by a microsurgical ear operation called a singular neurectomy in which a tiny portion of the vestibular nerve is divided and cut.

Patients with Ménière's disease may benefit from a microsurgical operation called the cochleosacculotomy. In this procedure, a small curette or wire loop is used to reach into the vestibule of the inner ear and remove the fluid-filled saccule. An investigator at the Massachusetts Eye and Ear Institute in Boston has found that this operation relieves symptoms of vertigo in about 80 percent of patients.

Space biology. Research also promises to help astronauts who suffer from dizziness or space sickness. In one study, a scientist aboard a space shuttle conducted experiments to find out why half the astronauts who have space sickness at the start of a flight overcome this problem before the end of the mission. The investigator, from the Massachusetts Institute of Technology, found that the space traveler's brain no longer relies on the gravity-sensitive inner ear structures for information about position and motion. Instead, the astronaut's brain realizes that the inner ear is sending false information and starts to depend more on the eyes to find out about the body's movements. This finding may enable space biologists to train astronauts before launch to avoid space sickness.

During that same space mission, a German scientist performed experiments that raised questions about the theory behind the caloric test. According to that theory, alternate heating and cooling of the endolymph causes the fluid to form wave-like swirling patterns called convection currents. These currents make the brain think the head is moving. The result is nystagmus.

In space, however, lack of gravity should prevent convection currents from forming, so the eyes were expected to remain still. Instead, they moved just as though the test was being done on Earth in normal gravity. These experiments indicate there is more than one explanation for why the caloric test works: when the endolymph is warmed, the fluid expands and moves the cupula, the top of the cochlear duct. The movement of the cupula cues the brain that the head is moving and the eyes respond.

451

This research helps scientists interpret methods used to test vestibular function. It also promises to increase our understanding of the balance system.

Currently, scientists at the Johnson Space Center in Houston and at the Good Samaritan Hospital in Portland are preparing to study space sickness and vestibular function in a microgravity (near zero gravity) laboratory. The astronauts' vestibular function will be analyzed in a series of experiments, including studies to test whether visual input becomes more important in maintaining balance as weightlessness increases. The scientists anticipate that this research will help all sufferers of motion sickness, not just astronauts.

Improved diagnosis. Back on Earth, improvements are being made in measuring precisely the eye movements of patients undergoing diagnostic tests for dizziness. Investigators at the NINCDS-funded research center at the University of California at Los Angeles have developed a computer-controlled chair in which a patient is shifted into a variety of body positions to stimulate the labyrinth. Eye responses are measured with newly designed computerized instruments. To further stimulate eye movements, a set of computer-generated visual patterns can be moved with the chair or independently of it.

These instruments will extract much information about a patient's ability to integrate information from the eyes and the inner ear, and will help distinguish patients with different disorders of the balance system.

Signaling the brain. To understand dizziness, scientists must find out how stimuli to the labyrinth are translated into information that the brain can use to maintain balance. How, for example, is information from the inner ear sent to the brain and interpreted? Among the scientists studying this question is an NINCDS grantee at the University of Chicago who is looking at the different ways hair cells react to the movement of inner ear fluid. He has identified a characteristic pattern of electrical response in hair cells. The next step is to discover how these messages are interpreted by the nerve cells carrying information to the brain.

Another NINCDS grantee at the University of Minnesota is studying the activity of the brain when it sends balance-preserving signals from the sense organs to the muscles. In one experiment, healthy persons are rotated in the dark at a constant rate. After a few minutes they no longer think they are moving. This is because the inner ear only senses changes in the rate of movement. If the lights are turned on and both the chair and the room rotate at the same constant speed, again the person doesn't sense movement. Both the inner ear and the eyes are fooled into thinking there is no motion.

But the investigator found that if the chair and the room are accelerated, the patient develops what is described as sensory conflict. The acceleration of the chair tells the inner ear that there is movement. But the eyes tell the brain that the body is stationary. How patients react in these conflict situations reveals how the brain puts together various types of sensory information to maintain balance. The results of this and related experiments will help scientists build a mathematical model of the balance system.

Hope for the Future

For those who are healthy, equilibrium is a sense often taken for granted. People can't see their labyrinth, even though it is as much a sense organ as the ears or the eyes. But when it is injured, an ability vital to everyday living is lost.

Scientists already understand a great deal about the labyrinth's function and the way the brain maintains balance. Further research into this complex system should help those who are incapacitated by dizziness when the balance system goes awry.

Voluntary Health Organizations

The following organizations provide information on dizziness or on inner ear diseases that cause dizziness:

Acoustic Neuroma Association
P.O. Box 398
Carlisle, PA 17013
(717) 249-4783

American Academy of Otolaryngology—Head and Neck Surgery
Suite 302
1101 Vermont Avenue, N.W.
Washington, DC 20005
(202) 289-4607

Better Hearing Institute
P.O. Box 1840
Washington, DC 20013
(703) 642-0580
(800) 424-8576 (Toll free)

National Hearing Association
721 Enterprise
Oak Brook, IL 60521
(312) 323-7200

Human Tissue Banks

The study of ear tissue from patients with dizziness and deafness is invaluable in research. Temporal bones willed by people with balance or hearing problems and by people with normal hearing can be used to help research scientists and physicians training to be otolaryngologists. Physicians in training study the basic anatomy of the temporal bone and develop their surgical skills. Scientists use the bones for research on the inner ear and on congenital disorders that cause deafness. Middle ear bones (ossicles) and the eardrum are also used as grafts to surgically correct sound transmission problems of the middle ear.

NINCDS supports four temporal bone banks that supply scientists in every state with tissue from patients who have dizziness or deafness. The donated temporal bone includes the eardrum, the entire middle and inner ear, and the nerve tissues which combine into the brain stem. For information about tissue donation and collection, write to:

National Temporal Bone Bank
Eastern Center
Massachusetts Eye and Ear Infirmary
243 Charles Street
Boston, MA 02114
(617) 523-7900, ext. 2711

National Temporal Bone Bank
Midwestern Center
University of Minnesota
Box 396-Mayo
Minneapolis, MN 55455
(612) 624-5466

National Temporal Bone Bank
Southern Center
Baylor College of Medicine
Neurosensory Center, Room A523
Houston, TX 77030
(713) 790-5470

National Temporal Bone Bank
Western Center
UCLA School of Medicine
31-24 Rehabilitation Center
Los Angeles, CA 90024
(213) 825-4710

Some Useful Definitions

acoustic neuroma: tumor of the vestibular nerve that may press on the hearing nerve causing dizziness and hearing loss.

balance system: complex biological system that enables us to know where our body is in space and to keep the position we want. Proper balance depends on information from the labyrinth in the inner ear, from other senses such as sight and touch, and from muscle movement.

benign positional vertigo: condition in which moving the head to one side or to a certain position brings on vertigo.

brain stem auditory evoked response (BAER): diagnostic test in which electrodes are attached to the surface of the scalp to determine the time it takes inner ear electrical responses to sound to travel from the ear to the brain. The test helps locate the cause of some types of dizziness.

caloric test: diagnostic test in which warm or cold water or air is put into the ear. If a person experiences certain eye movements (nystagmus) after this procedure, the labyrinth is working correctly.

cholesteatoma: a tumorlike accumulation of dead cells in the middle ear. This growth is thought to result from repeated middle ear infections.

computed tomography (CT) scan: radiological examination useful for examining the inside of the ear and head.

diuretic: drug that promotes water loss from the body through the urine. Used to treat hypertension, diuretics may bring on dizziness due to postural hypotension.

dizziness: feeling of physical instability with regard to the outside world.

endolymph: fluid filling part of the labyrinth.

hair cells: specialized nerves found in the semicircular canals and vestibule. Fibers (hairs) sticking out of one end of the hair cells move when the head moves and send information to the brain that is used to maintain balance.

hyperventilation: repetitive deep breathing that reduces the carbon dioxide content of the blood and brings on dizziness. Anxiety may cause hyperventilation and dizziness.

inner ear: contains the organs of hearing and balance.

labyrinth: the organ of balance, which is located in the inner ear. The labyrinth consists of the three semicircular canals and the vestibule.

Ménière's disease: condition that causes vertigo. The disease is believed to be caused by too much endolymph in the labyrinth. Persons with this illness also experience hearing problems and tinnitus.

middle ear: the space immediately behind the eardrum. This part of the ear contains the three bones of hearing: the hammer (malleus), anvil (incus), and stirrup (stapes).

multiple sensory deficits: condition associated with dizziness in which damage to nerves of the eye and arms or legs reduces information about balance to the brain.

neurologist: physician who specializes in disorders of the nervous system.

nystagmus: rapid back-and-forth movements of the eyes. These reflex movements may occur during the caloric test and are used in the diagnosis of balance problems.

orthostatic hypotension: see postural hypotension.

otologist: physician who specializes in diseases of the ear.

peripheral vestibulopathy: vestibular disorder in which the vestibular nerve appears inflamed and paralyzed. Patients may have one or several attacks of vertigo.

postural hypotension (also called orthostatic hypotension): sudden dramatic drop in blood pressure when a person rises from a sitting, kneeling, or lying position. The prime symptom of postural hypotension, which is sometimes due to low blood volume, is dizziness or faintness. The condition can be dangerous in older persons, who may faint and injure themselves.

semicircular canals: three curved hollow tubes in the inner ear that are part of the balance organ, the labyrinth. The canals are joined at their wide ends and are filled with endolymph.

stroke: death of nerve cells due to a loss of blood flow in the brain. A stroke often results in permanent loss of some sensation or muscle activity.

TIA: see transient ischemic attack.

tinnitus: noises or ringing in the ear.

transient ischemic attack (TIA): temporary interruption of blood flow to a part of the brain. Because a TIA may signal the possibility of a stroke, it requires immediate medical attention. During a TIA, a person may feel dizzy, have double vision, or feel tingling in the hands.

vertigo: severe form of dizziness in which one's surroundings appear to be spinning uncontrollably. Extreme cases of vertigo may be accompanied by nausea.

vestibular disorders: diseases of the inner ear that cause dizziness.

vestibular nerve: nerve that carries messages about balance from the labyrinth in the inner ear to the brain.

vestibular neuronitis: another name for peripheral vestibulopathy.

vestibule: part of the labyrinth, located at the base of the semicircular canals. This structure contains the endolymph and patches of hair cells.

Chapter 54

Update on Dizziness

Vestibular System

Special organs called vestibular receptors are located in the inner ear. The vestibular system is responsible for maintaining the body's orientation in space, balance, and posture. The vestibular system also regulates locomotion and other purposeful motions and helps keep objects in visual focus as the body moves.

When balance is impaired, the capability for normal movement is affected. Dizziness and impairment of balance also can affect one's motivation, concentration, and memory. The primary symptoms of vestibular disorders include a sensation of dizziness, spinning or vertigo, falling, imbalance, lightheadedness, disorientation, giddiness, or visual blurring. A person also may experience nausea and vomiting, diarrhea, faintness, changes in heart rate and blood pressure, fear, anxiety, panic attacks, drowsiness, fatigue, depression, impaired memory, and decreased concentration.

Many Americans, age 17 and older, have at some time experienced a dizziness or balance problem. Some groups, especially older people, are particularly at risk for developing balance disorders. In a study of people age 65 to 75, one-third experienced dizziness and imbalance. Other people at risk include those with diseases of the vesti-

This article, published in April 1993, is an update of the original NIDCD booklet on Dizziness.

bular system, such as Meniérè's disease, and those who suffer from motion sickness. Meniérè's disease is a disorder that affects the inner ear and causes periods of vertigo, hearing loss, and tinnitus (roaring or ringing in the ear). Motion sickness is a common cause of dizziness and occurs in healthy people who are exposed to unusual motion conditions as well as to patients with vestibular disorders.

Vestibular function results in specialized reflexes. A reflex is a spontaneous or involuntary reaction or movement. The vestibular reflexes are the body's mechanisms for regulating the position of the eyes and body in relation to changes in head position and motion. A particular reflex called the vestibulo-ocular reflex (VOR) causes the eyes to move in reaction to head motion so it is possible to look steadily at something and keep it in focus when the head moves. When the head is turned to the right, for example, fluid movement in the semicircular canals excites a vestibular receptor in the right ear but inhibits the receptor in the left ear. This sets off a pattern of nerve signals resulting in the eye-stabilizing reflex that allows you to keep your eyes focused on a target while turning your head.

Orientation and Balance

Orientation is knowing the relationship of one's body to the environment. Balance is maintaining the desired body position in the environment. For orientation and balance to be maintained, information from the motion, visual and position receptors located in the ears, eyes, skin, muscles, and joints must be integrated to produce coordinated patterns of muscle activity to maintain balance.

Sometimes the information received from these sensory systems provide conflicting information to the brain. The feeling of continued motion experienced by an individual who steps off a merry-go-round is an example of a sensory conflict situation. When illusions like this are prolonged, motion sickness results.

People with balance or dizziness problems often do not know what is making them feel ill. Physicians may also have difficulty determining the exact cause of their symptoms. This is because the vestibular system is complex, and it interacts with other major systems usually at an unconscious level.

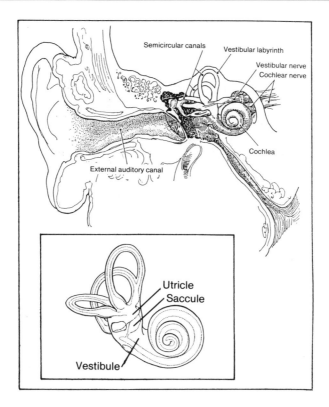

Figure 54.1. *The semicircular canals and vestibule of the inner ear contain a fluid called endolymph that moves in response to head movement.*

Recent Advances

Basic Mechanisms of Vestibular Function

The vestibular system has the remarkable ability to compensate and recover following injury. The system adapts its performance to maintain gaze and postural stability in response to body and environmental changes. Scientists are currently studying how these adaptations are accomplished. They have identified and mathematically modeled some of the features of the neural pathways underlying adaptive changes of the VOR. An understanding of the adaptive capabilities of the vestibular system at the cellular and molecular levels will provide much needed insight into the medical treatment of balance disorders.

461

Diagnosis of Vestibular Disorders

Physicians need to know which structures of the vestibular system cause different symptoms. Disorders may affect one or both ears and can develop gradually or suddenly. The inner ear, the vestibular nerve, the vestibular nuclei or other structures of the vestibular nervous system may be involved. NIDCD-supported scientists have developed new computerized techniques that are helping physicians evaluate balance disorders. Physicians can identify, measure, and localize the source of balance disorders by using the VOR and vestibulospinal reflex evaluation techniques. By precisely measuring the reflexes that stabilize the eyes and body posture under different conditions, scientists can relate these reflex responses to the underlying balance control system.

New computer-controlled rotational chairs and eye movement analysis computer software enable physicians to measure precisely both caloric and rotationally induced vestibular eye movement responses in the clinic. Powerful rotation devices allow physicians to test an expanded range of the VOR. Vestibular responses to rotation in a variety of body positions are being studied at several centers, including the Massachusetts Eye and Ear Infirmary, the Eye and Ear Institute of Pittsburgh, Johns Hopkins University, and the University of California at Los Angeles. A new recording device, called the magnetic search coil system, enables these scientists to measure vertical and "rolling" eye movements as well as horizontal eye movements. Scientists can use this new technology to separate and study eye movements driven by the different vestibular organs of the inner ear.

Other new technology includes imaging techniques, such as magnetic resonance imaging (MRI). Physicians use imaging techniques to identify lesions affecting various parts of brain, cranial nerves, and the inner ear structures. They are also able to screen for blood vessel diseases that cause balance disorders by using MRI and other imaging techniques.

Treatment of Vestibular Disorders

Scientists are developing new treatments for people with vestibular disorders. These treatments include new surgical techniques, drug therapy, and physical therapy.

Because of improved diagnostic tests, physicians can locate small tumors of the vestibular nerve. Often, surgery can be performed before tumors enlarge and compress the brain stem, sparing hearing as well as other important functions. Facial nerve and auditory brain stem response monitoring, as well as improved anesthesia techniques, make these operations safer and reduce the risk of complications. A variety of lasers are also now being used to remove tumors.

Surgeons have developed new operations that have been successful in correcting balance and preserving hearing. For example, surgeons can repair fluid leaks caused by fistulae or ruptures from the inner-ear fluid space to the middle-ear air space to treat dizziness. Surgeons are using new techniques to interrupt the nerve pathways from the inner ear vestibular organs to the brain for treatment of persistent vertigo.

NIDCD-supported scientists at the University of Oklahoma Health Sciences Center are analyzing the chemical changes in the brain that occur when the vestibular system compensates for injury. A description of these chemical changes may help clinical investigators develop drug therapy to help patients recover from vestibular injury. Scientists at Good Samaritan Hospital in Portland, Oregon, are determining the relationships between the recovery of the control of posture and the role of central nervous system compensatory mechanisms.

Scientists at the Johns Hopkins University School of Medicine are studying the effectiveness of certain exercises as a treatment for vertigo caused by degenerative fragments from the inner ear lodged in the receptor region of a posterior semicircular canal. These small fragments make the canal unusually sensitive to changes in the position of the head, causing dizziness. When the head positions of patients in the study were manipulated to dislodge the debris, their dizziness resolved. After treatment, most of the patients in the study had improved enough to return to a normal life. In another study, scientists at the University of Michigan have shown preliminary evidence that suggests that a customized physical exercise program that repeatedly exposes the patient to sensory conflict and provokes vertigo and imbalance is more effective than general exercises for recovery. Such exercises may be a safe and effective alternative to surgery.

Investigators at the Johns Hopkins University School of Medicine have demonstrated the beneficial effects of even brief periods of physical exercise in patients recovering from unilateral vestibular loss. These investigators are studying the effectiveness of patients viewing moving visual scenes and of inducing VOR adaptation with magnifying lenses in the rehabilitation from vestibular disorders. Balance disorders frequently cause falls. According to the National Institute on Aging, falls are the most common cause of fatal injury in older people. In the past, research has focused on the visual-stabilizing reflexes in balance disorders rather than on postural-stabilizing reflexes. Research at the Johns Hopkins University School of Medicine is underway on adaptive strategies of people with balance problems to stabilize posture. Scientists are studying people with and without vestibular disorders to understand these adaptive capabilities. They are comparing the adaptation of the visual reflex with that of the postural reflex. The results of this project will be used to design and assess physical therapy programs.

NIDCD continues to support research concerning the basic mechanisms of balance function, diagnostic procedures, and treatment. The vestibular system is a complex set of inner ear and central nervous system mechanisms that is capable of adapting to changes in the body and the environment. Because of the system's complexity and its interaction with other sensory and motor systems, symptoms are many and varied. As scientists learn more about the vestibular system and its adaptive capabilities, they can develop better diagnostic procedures, medical treatments, surgical techniques, and nonmedical rehabilitative procedures to help patients recover from debilitating disorders of balance.

About the NIDCD

The NIDCD conducts and supports research and research training on normal and disordered mechanisms of hearing, balance, smell, taste, voice, speech, and language. The NIDCD achieves its mission through a diverse program of research grants for scientists to conduct research at medical centers and universities around the country and through a wide range of research performed in its own laboratories.

The institute also conducts and supports research and research training related to disease prevention and health promotion; addresses special biomedical and behavioral problems associated with people who have communication impairments or disorders and supports efforts to create devices that substitute for lost and impaired sensory communication function. The NIDCD is committed to understanding how certain diseases or disorders may affect women, men, and members of underrepresented minority populations differently.

The NIDCD has established a national clearinghouse of information and resources. Additional information on dizziness may be obtained from the NIDCD Clearinghouse. Write to:

NIDCD Clearinghouse
P.O. Box 37777
Washington, DC 20013-7777
or call:
Voice (800) 241-1044
TDD/TT (800) 241-1055

For additional information:

Acoustic Neuroma Association
P.O. Box 12402
Atlanta, GA 30355
Voice (404) 237-8023

American Academy of Otolaryngology—Head and Neck Surgery
One Prince Street
Alexandria, VA 22314
Voice (703) 836-4444
TDD/TT (703) 519-1585

Better Hearing Institute
P.O. Box 1840
Washington, DC 20013
Voice (703) 642-0580
TDD/TT (800) EARWELL

Ear Foundation
2000 Church Street
Box 111
Nashville, TN 37236
Voice or TDD/TT (615) 329-7807
(800) 545-HEAR

Vestibular Disorders Association
P.O. Box 4467
Portland, OR 97208-3079
Voice (503) 229-7705

Center for Hearing and Balance
Johns Hopkins Medical Institutions
550 North Broadway
Baltimore, MD 21205
Voice (410) 955-1078

UCLA Balance and Dizziness Research Program
C 246A RNRC, UCLA School of Medicine
Los Angeles, CA 90024-1769
Voice (310) 825-5910

This publication was prepared by:

NIDCD Clearinghouse
National Institute on Deafness and
Other Communication Disorders
National Institutes of Health
P.O. Box 37777
Washington, D.C.20013-7777
1-800-241-1044 Voice
1-800-241-1055 TDD/TT

Chapter 55

Dizziness and Motion Sickness

What Is Dizziness?

Some people describe a balance problem by saying they feel dizzy, lightheaded, unsteady or giddy. This feeling of imbalance or dysequilibrium, without a sensation of turning or spinning, is sometimes due to an inner ear problem.

What Is Vertigo?

A few people describe their balance problem by using the word vertigo, which comes from the Latin verb "to turn." They often say that they or their surroundings are turning or spinning. Vertigo is frequently due to an inner ear problem.

What is Motion Sickness and Sea Sickness?

Some people experience nausea and even vomiting when riding in an airplane, automobile, or amusement park ride, and this is called *motion sickness*. Many people experience motion sickness when riding on a boat or ship, and this is called *sea sickness* even though it is the same disorder.

A publication of the American Academy of Otolaryngology—Head and Neck Surgery, Inc. One Prince Street, Alexandria, VA 22314. Used by permission.

Motion sickness or sea sickness is usually just a minor annoyance and does not signify any serious medical illness, but some travellers are incapacitated by it, and a few even suffer symptoms for a few days after the trip (the "Mal d'embarquement" syndrome).

The Anatomy of Balance

Dizziness, vertigo and motion sickness all relate to the sense of balance and equilibrium. Researchers in space and aeronautical medicine call this sense *spatial orientation*, because it tells the brain where the body is "in space": what direction it is pointing, what direction it is moving, and if it is turning or standing still.

Your sense of balance is maintained by a complex interaction of the following parts of the nervous system:

1. The inner ears (also called the *labyrinth*), which monitor the directions of motion, such as turning or forward-backward, side-to-side, and up-and-down motions.

2. The eyes, which monitor where the body is in space (i.e. upside down, rightside up, etc.) and also directions of motion.

3. The skin pressure receptors such as the joints and spine, which tell what part of the body is down and touching the ground.

4. The muscle and joint sensory receptors, which tell what parts of the body are moving.

5. The central nervous system (the brain and spinal cord), which process all the bits of information from the four other systems to make some coordinated sense out of it all.

The symptoms of motion sickness and dizziness appear when the central nervous system receives conflicting messages from the other four systems.

For example, suppose you are riding in an airplane during a storm, and your airplane is being tossed about by air turbulence. But your eyes do not detect all this motion because all you see is the inside of the airplane. Then your brain receives messages that do not match up with each other. You might become "air sick."

Or suppose you are sitting in the back seat of a car reading a book. Your inner ears and skin receptors will detect the motion of your travel, but your eyes see only the pages of your book. You could become "car sick."

Or, to use a true medical condition as an example, suppose you suffer inner ear damage on only one side from a head injury or an infection. The *damaged* inner ear does not send the same signals as the *healthy* ear. This gives conflicting signals to the brain about the sensation of rotation, and you could suffer a sense of spinning vertigo, as well as nausea.

What Medical Diseases Cause Dizziness?

1. Circulation: Disorders of blood circulation are among the most common causes of dizziness. If your brain does not get enough blood flow, you feel light headed. Almost everyone has experienced this on occasion when standing up quickly from a lying down position. But some people have light headedness from poor circulation on a frequent or chronic basis. This could be caused by arteriosclerosis or hardening of the arteries, and it is commonly seen in patients who have high blood pressure, diabetes, or high levels of blood fats (cholesterol). It is sometimes seen in patients with inadequate cardiac (heart) function or with anemia.

    Certain drugs also decrease the blood flow to the brain, especially stimulants such as nicotine and caffeine. Excess salt in the diet also leads to poor circulation. Sometimes circulation is impaired by spasms in the arteries caused by emotional stress, anxiety, and tension.

    If the *inner ear* fails to receive enough blood flow, the more specific type of dizziness occurs—that is, vertigo. The inner ear is very sensitive to minor alterations of blood flow, and all of the causes mentioned for poor circulation to the brain also apply specifically to the inner ear.

2. Injury: A skull fracture that damages the inner ear produces a profound and incapacitating vertigo with nausea and hearing loss. The dizziness will last for several weeks, then

slowly improve as the normal (other side) takes over all of the inner ear functions.

3. Infection: Viruses, such as those causing common "cold" or "flu," can attack the inner ear and its nerve connections to the brain. This can result in a severe vertigo, but the hearing is usually spared. However, a bacterial infection such as mastoiditis that extends into the inner ear will completely destroy both the hearing and the equilibrium function of that ear. The severity of dizziness and recovery time will be similar to that described above the skull fracture.

4. Allergy: Some people experience dizziness and/or vertigo attacks when they are exposed to foods or airborne particles (such as dust, molds, pollens, danders, etc.) to which they are allergic.

5. Neurological diseases: A number of diseases of the nerves can affect balance, such as multiple sclerosis, syphilis, tumors, etc. These are uncommon causes, but your physician will think about them during examination.

What Can I Do for Motion Sickness?

1. *Always ride where your eyes will see the same motion that your body and inner ear feel*, e.g., sit in the front seat of the car and look at the distant scenery; go up on the deck of the ship and watch the motion of the horizon; sit by the window of the airplane and look outside. In an airplane choose a seat over the wings where the motion is the least.

2. *Do not read while traveling* if you are subject to motion sickness, and do not sit in a seat facing backwards.

3. *Do not watch or talk to another traveler who is having motion sickness.*

4. *Avoid strong odors and spicy or greasy foods* that do not agree with you (immediately before and during your travel).

Medical research has not yet investigated the effectiveness of popular folk remedies such as "soda crackers and 7 UP® or "cola syrup over ice."

5. *Take one of the varieties of motion sickness medicines* before your travel begins, as recommended by your physician. Some of these medications can be purchased without a prescription (i.e., Dramamine,® Bonnie,® Marezine,® etc.). Stronger medicines such as tranquilizers and nervous system depressants will require a prescription from your physician. Some are used in pill or suppository form; another one (scopolamine) is used as a stick-on patch applied to the skin behind the ear.

Remember: Most cases of dizziness and motion sickness are mild and self-treatable disorders. But severe cases, and those that become progressively worse, deserve the attention and care of a physician with specialized skills in diseases of the ear, nose, throat, equilibrium, and neurological systems.

What Will the Physician Do for My Dizziness?

The doctor will ask you to describe your dizziness, whether it is lightheadedness or a sensation of motion, how long and how often the dizziness has troubled your, how long a dizzy episode lasts, and whether it is associated with hearing loss or nausea and vomiting. You might be asked for circumstances that might bring on a dizzy spell. You will need to answer questions about your general health, any medicines you are taking, head injuries, recent infections, and other questions about your ear and neurological system.

Your physician will examine your ears, nose, and throat and do tests of nerve and balance function. Because the inner ear controls both balance and hearing, disorders of balance often affect hearing, and vice versa. Therefore, your physician will probably recommend hearing tests (audiograms). In some cases the physician might order skull X rays, a CT or MRI scan of your head, or special tests of eye motion after warm or cold water is used to stimulate the inner ear (ENG—electronystagmography). In some cases, blood tests or a cardiology (heart) evaluation might be recommended.

Not every patient will require every test. It will be the physician's judgment (based on each of the findings in each particular patient) that determines which studies are needed. Similarly, the treatments recommended by your physician will depend on the diagnosis.

What Can I Do to Reduce Dizziness?

1. *Avoid rapid changes in position,* especially from lying down to standing up or turning around from one side to the other.

2. *Avoid extremes of head motion* (especially looking up) or rapid head motions (especially turning or twisting).

3. *Eliminate or decrease use of products that impair circulation,* e.g., nicotine, caffeine, and salt.

4. *Minimize your exposure to circumstances that precipitate your dizziness,* such as stress and anxiety or substances to which you are allergic.

5. *Avoid hazardous activities when you are dizzy,* such as driving an automobile or operating dangerous equipment, or climbing a step ladder, etc.

What Is Otolaryngology–Head and Neck Surgery?

Otolaryngology–head and neck surgery is a specialty concerned with the medical and surgical treatment of the ears, nose, throat, and related structures of the head and neck. The specialty encompasses cosmetic facial reconstruction, surgery of benign and malignant tumors of the head and neck, management of patients with loss of hearing and balance, endoscopic examination of air and food passages, and treatment of allergic, sinus, laryngeal, thyroid and esophageal disorders.

To qualify for the American Board of Otolaryngology certification examination, a physician must complete five or more years of post–M.D. (or D.O.) specialty training.

Chapter 56

Acoustic Neuroma

Introduction

The 1991 Consensus Development Conference on Acoustic Neuroma was convened to consider how patients can acquire an accurate diagnosis and to review the best options for management of this disease, including primary therapy, follow-up, and rehabilitation.

We use the term vestibular schwannomas throughout this report because these tumors are composed of Schwann cells and typically involve the vestibular rather than the acoustic division of the 8th cranial nerve. Although benign, because of their location vestibular schwannomas can produce serious morbidity or even death, by compression of vital structures, including the cranial nerves and the brainstem. Advances in microsurgery have dramatically reduced operative mortality and have made tumor removal without additional neurologic deficit a realistic but challenging goal.

An estimated 2,000 to 3,000 new cases of unilateral vestibular schwannoma are diagnosed in the United States each year—an incidence of about 1 per 100,000 per year. The most common presenting symptoms are change in hearing in one ear, tinnitus (noise in the ear), and poor balance. The advent of magnetic resonance imaging (MRI) with gadolinium enhancement has permitted the identification of

Consensus Statement of the NIH Consensus Development Conference, Volume 9, Number 4. December 11-12, 1991.

many very small, previously undetectable tumors. Some studies suggest that the prevalence of vestibular schwannomas at autopsy may be as high as 0.9 percent, but this is quite likely an overestimate. In any event, the vast majority of these tumors are very small and are not recognized clinically. At least 95 percent of diagnosed vestibular schwannomas are unilateral. These tumors are encapsulated, rounded, and usually appear as a single mass. About 5 percent of patients exhibit bilateral schwannomas associated with an inherited syndrome known as neurofibromatosis type 2 (NF2). Population-based data from the United Kingdom suggest that 1 out of every 135,000 individuals carry the gene for NF2.

[The list below] gives criteria that distinguish NF2 from NF1, which is a more common syndrome and rarely associated with vestibular schwannoma.

Distinguishing NF2 from NF1

NF1 may be diagnosed in Caucasians when two or more of the following are present:

- Six or more cafe-au-lait macules whose greatest diameter is more than 5 mm in prepubescent patients and more than 15 mm in postpubescent patients.
- Two or more neurofibromas of any type or one plexiform neurofibroma.
- Freckling in the axillary or inguinal region.
- A distinctive osseous lesion as sphenoid dysplasia or thinning of long-bone cortex, with or without pseudoarthrosis.
- Optic glioma.
- Two or more Lisch nodules (iris hamartomas).
- A parent, sibling, or child with NF1 on the basis of the previous criteria.

NF2 may be diagnosed when one of the following is present:

- Bilateral 8th nerve masses seen by MRI with gadolinium.
- A parent, sibling, or child with NF2 and either unilateral 8th nerve mass or any one of the following:

—neurofibroma
—meningioma
—glioma
—schwannoma
—posterior capsular cataract or opacity at a young age.

What Are Acoustic Neuromas and How Should They Be Classified?

Cytologically, no differences have been found between the vestibular schwannomas of NF2 and those found in sporadic cases. Histologically, however, the tumors in NF2 often appear as grape-like clusters that can infiltrate the fibers of individual nerves and may adumbrate a polyclonal origin. Both unilateral and bilateral tumors vary in their precise location along the vestibular nerve, tending to arise at the border between the central and peripheral segments of the nerve. Why tumors arise at this transition zone is not known, but variation in the site at which a tumor is located can have a major influence on the symptoms it produces.

For clinical management, the most useful classification of vestibular schwannomas is by size, location, and growth rate. However, tumors tend to enlarge unpredictably. Some do not change in size for many years, while others may grow at a rate of up to 20 mm in diameter per year. Currently, the best method to monitor tumor growth is with gadolinium-enhanced MRI. To facilitate the interpretation of clinical studies, both the greatest diameter of the tumor within the posterior fossa and the extent of penetration into the intracanalicular space should be documented.

A second important classification is between familial and sporadic cases. All cases of vestibular schwannomas are thought to result from the functional loss of a tumor-suppressor gene that has been localized to the long arm of chromosome 22. In at least 95 percent of patients, however, the disease is unilateral and the majority of these cases are sporadic, resulting from somatic mutations that are not associated with an increased risk for other tumors either in the individual or in close relatives. About 5 percent of patients exhibit bilateral disease or other features that define NF2. These patients are thought to carry a single germline mutation of the chromosome 22–linked gene and sustain the loss of the remaining normal allele as a somatic event in those cells that give rise to the tumor. Thus, the trait is recessive at the cellular level but exhibits a dominant pattern of genetic transmission in families. Even when a thorough family history is obtained, in about one half of all recognized cases of NF2, no evidence of other affected family members can be found. These patients may represent new germline mutations and are at risk of transmitting the disease to their offspring.

Patients with NF2 who carry new mutations tend to be more severely affected than familial cases, and some recent studies have raised the possibility that in familial cases the onset of symptoms may be earlier and the severity greater when the disease is inherited from the mother. Such effects can arise from genomic imprinting, and although the precise genetic mechanism for this phenomenon is unknown, a growing number of examples of such parental origin effects now have been documented. If confirmed, these findings could have practical implications for the management of families with NF2. Molecular studies on NF2 and on unilateral tumors are at an exciting juncture. The gene for NF2 should soon be identified and may provide molecular explanations for clinical differences among families with NF2 as well as differences in the growth rate among tumors. Further studies on the molecular biology of the gene may suggest treatments for vestibular schwannomas, both in NF2 and in patients with unilateral diseases.

Patients with NF2 may have associated meningiomas and spinal root schwannomas as well as cafe-au-lait spots and peripheral Schwann cell tumors and often develop posterior subcapsular cataracts at an early age. The prevalence of these findings varies greatly among families.

In Whom Should Acoustic Neuroma Be Suspected and Evaluated?

Sporadic Vestibular Schwannoma

The most common symptom, found in up to 90 percent of individuals with vestibular schwannoma, is a progressive, asymmetric, or unilateral sensorineural hearing loss. Approximately 70 percent have a high frequency pattern of loss, while a small number of patients will display either normal hearing or a symmetric hearing loss. A symptom sometimes reported, even in the face of apparently normal hearing, is distorted sound perception, often manifested as difficulty in using the telephone or perceiving instruments to be "off key" in one ear. Although most schwannoma-associated hearing loss is gradual and progressive, approximately 10 percent of patients report sudden loss of hearing. Less commonly reported symptoms in patients with vestibular schwannoma include unilateral or asymmetric tinnitus (ringing in the ears) with or without complaints of dizziness or disequilibrium. These symptoms are generally regarded as "early," but can be seen with both small and large tumors. It should be noted that only a small fraction of patients who suffer any one of the above symptoms will be found to have a vestibular schwannoma.

Other findings, generally regarded as "late" manifestations, are related to compressive effects of tumor mass on neighboring structures. These include headaches, ataxia, cerebellar signs, and compressive cranial neuropathies. The 5th cranial (trigeminal) nerve compression may cause facial pain and/or numbness and corneal insensitivity leading to ulceration. Compression or irritation of the 7th (facial) cranial nerve may result in facial spasm, weakness, or paralysis. Infrequently, involvement of the 6th cranial nerve may cause double vision (diplopia). Compression of the 9th, 10th, or 12th cranial nerves will result in difficulty in swallowing and/or speaking. When the brainstem is sufficiently compressed or distorted by a large tumor, the patient may display nausea, vomiting, or lethargy, leading to coma, respiratory depression, and death. Hydrocephalus and papilledema with increased intracranial pressure also may be seen. With increasing tumor size and severity of symptoms, prompt diagnosis and initiation of treatment become vital.

Bilateral Neurofibromatosis (NF2)

NF2 is a complex syndrome in which many findings in addition to those described above may occur. These include:

- Peripheral or central lenticular cataracts, which may be present even in very young children (80 percent of cases in one series).

- Skin nodules and other lesions that include dermal neurofibromas and cafe-au-lait spots (greater than 60 percent of cases in one series).

- Pain or numbness because of schwannomas of peripheral nerves and/or roots.

- Seizures and other focal neurological symptoms.

- Other findings related to meningiomas, which may be multiple, or to a variety of gliomas (astrocytomas, ependymomas, etc.).

- Similarly affected relatives.

Once the diagnosis of NF2 is made, relatives who are at risk should be screened for the disease. NF2 should also be considered as a diagnostic possibility in patients with unilateral vestibular schwannomas who are under the age of 40.

How Should Patients Be Evaluated?

When vestibular schwannoma is suspected, the evaluation must begin with a thorough clinical and family history. This includes seeking the stigmata of NF2, schwannoma, or other nervous system tumors. The physical examination should focus on the skin and a neurological examination of cranial nerve function. Additional evaluation should include a detailed examination for cataracts and audio-vestibular function.

The initial audiologic evaluation should include pure tone air and bone conduction thresholds, speech reception thresholds, and speech recognition (discrimination) scores. Beyond these tests, two other diagnostic approaches are commonly used. More sophisticated audiological tests such as the determination of acoustic reflex threshold, acoustic reflex decay tests, and brainstem auditory evoked responses (BAER, also termed ABR) may permit assessment of the site of the audiologic lesion. The other approach is gadolinium-enhanced MRI. The decision of which test to use depends on clinical judgement and level of suspicion. These are affected by family pedigree, degree of asymmetry of auditory symptoms brainstem findings, or stigmata of NF2.

The advantages of BAER (ABR) are its ability to measure functional status and its lower cost. Recent experience has shown that the sensitivity of BAER (ABR) is 94 percent and that the specificity is greater than 85 percent for the diagnosis of vestibular schwannoma.

Auditory evoked responses, however, may not be possible in the face of severe hearing loss.

MRI now is regarded as the most definitive study that can be performed, and it is capable of revealing vestibular tumors as small as a few millimeters in diameter. This examination should emphasize thin slice scans in the axial plane with gadolinium enhancement. A negative gadolinium-enhanced MRI is accepted in current practice as effectively excluding the diagnosis of vestibular schwannoma. False positives are rare. A disincentive to the use of MRI as a screening test is its cost.

Vestibular testing is thought to be of less diagnostic value than the audiometric tests listed above, at least in part, because of the compensatory ability of the vestibular system.

Preoperative tests of vestibular function may be important as predictors of postoperative balance and possible hearing preservation at surgery.

Computerized axial tomography (CT) is useful in certain instances for screening purposes, particularly when MRI cannot be obtained. Some surgeons stress the usefulness of CT in preoperative planning.

What Are the Treatment Options for Those With Acoustic Neuroma?

Currently, the ideal treatment for symptomatic patients with vestibular schwannoma is the total excision of the tumor in a single stage with minimal morbidity and mortality and with preservation of neurological function. The other options for management are observation, subtotal removal, and various forms of radiation treatment, including stereotactic radiosurgery. Selection of the appropriate treatment option should be based on the clinical findings and status of the patient.

The question of whether and when to undertake treatment of a vestibular schwannoma is a complex issue. For the majority of patients who present with a symptomatic tumor, expeditious surgery will be the primary treatment modality. Young patients with progressive neurological deficit or evidence of tumor growth clearly are candidates for surgery. However, there are groups of patients for whom conservative approaches, including long-term observation, may be indicated. Elderly patients without severe neurologic symptoms or evidence of tumor growth are one such group. There also is evidence that some patients with unilateral vestibular schwannoma and a subgroup of patients with NF2 may have tumors that fail to progress rapidly, resulting in stable neurologic function for a long time. The use of MRI with contrast enhancement has resulted in the identification of patients with very small, relatively asymptomatic vestibular schwannomas for whom the natural history is still not known. Conservative management may be appropriate for these patients. The risk of neurologic deterioration in conservatively managed patients needs to be recognized and discussed with the patient.

Certain preoperative findings correlate with treatment outcome. When a patient presents with a mild hearing loss and the preoperative ABR recording demonstrates normal results with well formed waves, the prognosis for hearing preservation after surgery is more favorable than when these conditions are not present. Conversely, when MRI shows a tumor that is larger than 2 cm or when the tumor fills the fundus of the internal auditory canal, the likelihood that useful hearing will be preserved is far lower. Expanding our understanding of how these and other preoperative findings correlate with treatment outcome should be a high priority for future research.

Advances in microsurgical technique, anesthesia, and perioperative care have significantly reduced the morbidity and mortality for vestibular schwannoma surgery and now permit total removal in a majority of cases. Excellent results have been reported for three major surgical approaches, each characterized by specific advantages and disadvantages. Hearing preservation should be a goal of surgery when tumor removal can be achieved without compromising the facial nerve. The middle fossa approach provides good extradural exposure for small lesions situated in the internal auditory canal and enables potential hearing preservation, especially for tumors arising from the superior vestibular nerve. This approach is less suitable for larger tumors with intracranial extension. The translabyrinthine approach sacrifices hearing but facilitates ventral exposure of small and large tumors and allows the surgeon to identify and protect the facial nerve. The suboccipital or retrosigmoid approach allows the surgeon to identify the brainstem, cranial nerves, and cerebral vasculature through a wide exposure. In patients with small tumors, this approach facilitates hearing preservation. The approach also is suitable for large tumors. Criteria for the selection of surgical approach should be based on the training, experience, and preference of the surgical team; the status of preoperative hearing; and the location and size of the lesion.

There is a consensus that intraoperative real-time neurologic monitoring improves the surgical management of vestibular schwannoma, including the preservation of facial nerve function and possibly improved hearing preservation by the use of intraoperative auditory brainstem response monitoring. New approaches to monitoring acoustic nerve function may provide more rapid feedback to the surgeon, thus enhancing their usefulness. Intraoperative monitoring of cranial nerves 5, 6, 9, 10, and 11 also has been described, but the full benefits of this monitoring remain to be determined.

In the majority of cases of vestibular schwannoma, the treatment goal is complete removal of the tumor with minimum morbidity and mortality. However, there are clinical situations where the more conservative goal of planned subtotal resection of the tumor may be indicated. Among these are patients requiring decompression in whom recurrence is unlikely because of limited life expectancy, and patients in whom hearing preservation is of importance because of diminished function of the contralateral ear.

The best published surgical outcomes in the treatment of vestibular schwannoma are from medical centers that have highly organized and dedicated teams with a specific interest in these tumors and sufficient continuing experience to develop, refine, and maintain proficiency. Comprehensive surgical treatment of patients with vestibular schwannoma requires collaboration between health care providers from many disciplines, including neuro-otology, otorhinolaryngology, neurosurgery, anesthesiology, radiology, neurology, audiology, nursing, pathology, clinical neurophysiology, plastic surgery, ophthalmology, social service, and rehabilitation medicine, in addition to a strong institutional commitment and support for intensive care in the postoperative period. Teamwork is necessary for both planning and performing the primary surgical procedure and recognizing and managing potential intra- and postoperative complications.

Radiation therapy is a treatment option limited in current practice primarily to patients unable or unwilling to undergo otherwise indicated surgery. The greatest experience to date has been with stereotactic radiosurgery, using multisource Cobalt-60 units for single dose, external gamma ray therapy. Other options include conventional photon beam therapy and particle beam therapy, using either single or fractionated doses. Early reports indicate that retardation of tumor growth is observed in the majority of patients, but long-term follow-up from multiple centers is not yet available to fully assess therapeutic efficacy and complication rates.

Patient follow-up is an important component of management whether the primary treatment is surgery, radiation, or observation. The program for monitoring patients includes obtaining a history of new findings, following the progression of known signs and symptoms, repeated neurologic examination, audiologic assessment, and radiographic imaging. Follow-up intervals may range from every 3 months initially to every 1 to 2 years, depending on the patient's clinical course. The interval between follow-up evaluations may be shorter initially and longer with the passage of time, if there is no evidence of recurrent disease or progression. The duration of patient follow-up may be lifelong, particularly in patients with NF2.

Management of bilateral vestibular schwannomas in patients with NF2 must take into account the risk of hearing impairment in both ears and the disabling consequences of acquired deafness. One side may progress more rapidly and dictate the need and priority of treatment. The previous loss of functional hearing in one ear raises additional management issues for treatment of the tumor on the side with better hearing. More conservative approaches, such as subtotal intracapsular resection or simple observation of the patient's progress, may be indicated.

Rational selection of specific treatment options is impeded by the absence of standardized terminology in the medical literature. In future reports audiometric assessment should be classified according to levels of residual hearing, with specific objective definitions for each level. Such categories might include mild, moderate, severe, and profound hearing loss, as determined by combinations of pure tone averages and speech recognition scores. Imaging of vestibular schwannomas by gadolinium-enhanced magnetic resonance allows tumors to be classified according to volume and tumor location. Specific size categories should be developed to facilitate comparison of patient populations and treatment results. Facial nerve function should be reported according to a standardized grading scale, such as the House-Brackmann classification system. More sophisticated methods of assessing functional speech recognition and facial animation also may be useful in monitoring outcomes and evaluating management options. Patient age groups should also be standardized, with numerical definition of specific age groups. Studies suggest that three or more age groups may be useful.

What Are Possible Adverse Consequences of Treatment and What Are the Management Options for Each?

Both the vestibular schwannoma itself and its management can result in significant morbidity requiring intensive rehabilitative (and sometimes reconstructive) therapy. It is therefore vital that the health care team provide to patients and their families sufficient verbal and written materials so that they have realistic expectations of treatment outcomes. When appropriate, referral to a former patient or peer support/information group can be most helpful.

The most serious perioperative complications occur in the first 72 hours. These include air embolism, intracranial hemorrhage, and stroke. Prompt recognition by the operative team can result in decreased mortality and morbidity. CSF leak and meningitis can occur in a delayed fashion and also require immediate therapy.

Loss of hearing in the operated ear is the most common adverse consequence and can be a serious handicap. These patients have difficulty hearing in even modestly noisy environments and do not have directional hearing. Young children are at an educational disadvantage. There are a number of devices that can be used to allow for partial compensation to make the acoustic signal louder than the background noise or bring sound from the impaired ear to the hearing ear. These devices can be used by both children and adults.

Total loss of hearing occurs in many of the patients with NF2 and in a small number of patients with unilateral tumors who have had hearing loss in the nontumor ear from other causes. These are among the most seriously handicapped of all patients. There are a number of rehabilitation strategies that can be used to restore communication. Many of these are visually based, such as lipreading (speech), use of captions, sign language, etc. Sign language would be more useful if families were also instructed. Patients with visual defects, common in NF2, will have added difficulty in visual communication modes. Tactile systems are somewhat effective for the deaf-blind.

Electroprostheses are being developed and may be of potential benefit in selected patients with postlingual total deafness, secondary to loss of both statoacoustic nerves.

Abnormal vestibular function occurs in almost all patients. Unilateral loss for usual life situations has little morbidity and is compensated rapidly. Vestibular dysfunction becomes significant when it is bilateral or occurs in conjunction with other CNS or sensory impairment. Patients with bilateral vestibular dysfunction are at increased risk for drowning when swimming, diving, or even bathing.

One distressing complication of surgery is disfiguring facial nerve weakness or paralysis, with consequent physical, emotional, psychosocial, and possibly professional dysfunction. Treatment approaches to "reanimation" of the face include surgery (muscle or nerve grafting or rerouting) and physical and occupational therapy (exercise, biofeedback). As yet, none of these can restore normal function and appearance. Strong support from family, friends, the health care team, and patient advocacy/support groups is needed.

When complete closure of the eye is compromised, dryness, irritation, excessive tearing, blurred vision, corneal abrasions, ectropion, entropion, and loss of vision can occur. Surgical reanimation techniques can restore nearly normal function.

Other cranial nerves can be involved, but the particular combination of the 5th and 7th nerves places the cornea at greater risk and must be treated vigorously. The combined involvement of 9th, 10th, and 12th nerves creates difficulty swallowing and places the patient at risk for aspiration.

Headache may be a common and often debilitating complication of surgery. Its intensity can range from moderate to excruciatingly severe, and while most eventually resolve, they can last for months and sometimes years. Evaluation of the true incidence of postoperative headache, its etiology, and possible treatment are needed.

Recurrence can occur in cases where tumors were apparently either totally or partially removed; thus all cases need to be followed by imaging. Those that have recurred may be managed by either reoperation or stereotactic or fractionated radiation. The results are modestly satisfactory for surgery, and marginally satisfactory for fractionated radiation therapy.

Complications of radiation occur late as opposed to the immediate complications of surgery. Stereotactic radiosurgery, a newer modality, has the benefit of a low early complication rate, but unknown long-term complications. The limited data available indicate that there is a high rate of hearing loss within 1 year after therapy. There may be delayed transient dysfunction of the 5th and 7th cranial nerves. Comparison of the complication rate with surgical techniques cannot be done until there are proper long-term data available. If surgery is required after radiation therapy, it may be more difficult and complication prone.

The emotional and interpersonal consequences of vestibular schwannoma on the patient and family must be anticipated. Appropriate and early intervention must be made by a team of professionals and must include advance preparation of the patient and family, emotional support, aggressive physical and rehabilitative therapy, and a carefully coordinated program of follow-up focusing on medical and psychosocial needs. The support team should consist of physicians, audiologists, nurses, social workers, physical and occupational therapists, and behavioral counselors.

Many complications would be deemed far less problematic—certainly less devastating—if patient needs and expectations were addressed preoperatively with precise knowledge of possibilities for their future. The patients should be educated to the degree that they understand the decision they must ultimately make and any potential consequences they will face in accordance with that decision. This may include referral to specialized facilities that deal with their particular problem. Complete and realistic written and audiovisual information should be presented at the time of diagnosis, hospitalization and operation, discharge, and at follow-up. Referral should be made to peer support groups and/or positive former patients early in the process.

Fear of the unknown exacerbates any threatening situation. The more knowledge imparted to patients, the more they participate in a decision, and the better they will be able to live with any possible after effects.

Chapter 57

Facts on Acoustic Neurinoma

An acoustic neurinoma is a benign tumor which may develop on the hearing and balance nerves near the inner ear. The tumor results from an overproduction of Schwann cells—small sheet-like cells that normally wrap around nerve fibers like onion skin and help support the nerves. When growth is abnormally excessive, Schwann cells bunch together, pressing against the hearing and balance nerves, often causing gradual hearing loss, tinnitus or ringing in the ears, and dizziness. If the tumor becomes large, it can interfere with the facial nerve, causing partial paralysis, and eventually press against nearby brain structures, becoming life-threatening.

Early diagnoses of an acoustic neurinoma is key to preventing its serious consequences. Unfortunately, early detection of the tumor is sometimes difficult because the symptoms may be subtle and may not appear in the beginning stages of growth. Also, hearing loss, dizziness, and tinnitus are common symptoms of many middle and inner ear problems. Therefore, once the symptoms appear, a thorough ear examination and hearing test are essential for proper diagnosis. Computerized tomography (CT) scans and magnetic resonance imaging (MRI) are helpful in determining the location and size of a tumor and also in planning its removal.

If an acoustic neurinoma is surgically removed when it is still very small, hearing may be preserved and accompanying symptoms

---

Unnumbered NIDCD Fact Sheet.

may go away. As the tumor grows larger, surgical removal is often more complicated because the tumor may become firmly attached to the nerves that control facial movement, hearing and balance. The removal of tumors attached to hearing, balance or facial nerves can make the patient's symptoms worse because sections of these nerves must also be removed with the tumor.

As an alternative to conventional surgical techniques, radiosurgery may be used to reduce the size or limit the growth of the tumor. Radiosurgery, utilizing carefully focused radiation, is sometimes performed on the elderly, on patients with tumors on both hearing nerves, or on patients with a tumor growing on the nerve of their only hearing ear. If the tumor is not removed, MRI is used to carefully monitor its growth.

There are two types of acoustic neurinomas: unilateral and bilateral. Unilateral acoustic neurinomas affect only one ear and account for approximately 8 percent of all tumors inside the skull. Symptoms may develop at any age, but usually occur between the ages of 30 and 60 years.

Bilateral acoustic neurinomas, which affect both ears, are hereditary. Inherited from one's parents, this tumor results from a genetic disorder known as neurofibromatosis–2 (NF2). Affected individuals have a 50 percent chance of passing this disorder on to their children. Unlike those with a unilateral acoustic neurinoma, individuals with NF2 usually develop symptoms in their teens or early adulthood. Because NF2 patients usually have multiple tumors, the surgical procedure is more complicated than the removal of an unilateral acoustic neurinoma. Further research is needed to determine the best approach in these circumstances.

In addition to tumors arising from the hearing and balance nerves, NF2 patients may develop tumors on other cranial nerves associated with swallowing, speech, eye and facial movement and facial sensation. NF2 patients may also develop tumors within the spinal cord and from the brain's thin covering.

Scientists believe that both types of acoustic neurinoma form following a loss of the function of a gene on chromosome 22. A gene is a small section of DNA responsible for a particular trait like hair color or skin tone. Scientists believe that this particular gene on chromosome 22 suppresses the growth of Schwann cells. When this gene malfunctions, Schwann cells can grow out of control. Scientists also think that this gene may help suppress other types of tumor growth. In NF2 patients. the faulty gene on chromosome 22 is inherited. For individuals with unilateral acoustic neurinoma, however, some scientists hypothesize that this gene somehow loses its ability to function properly as a result of environmental factors.

Once the gene that suppresses Schwann cell growth is "mapped" or located, scientists can begin to develop gene therapy to control the overproduction of these cells in individuals with acoustic neurinoma. Also, learning more about the way genes help suppress acoustic neurinoma may help prevent brain tumors and lead to a treatment for cancer.

Chapter 58

Because You Asked about Ménière's Disease

What is Ménière's disease?

Ménière's disease is an abnormality of the inner ear causing a host of symptoms, including vertigo or severe dizziness, tinnitus or a roaring sound in the ears, fluctuating hearing loss, and the sensation of pressure or pain in the affected ear. The disorder usually affects only one ear and is a common cause of hearing loss. Named after French physician Prosper Ménière who first described the syndrome in 1861, Ménière's disease is now also referred to as endolymphatic hydrops.

What causes Ménière's disease?

The symptoms of Ménière's disease are associated with a change in fluid volume within a portion of the inner ear known as the labyrinth and the membranous labyrinth. The labyrinth has two parts: the bony labyrinth and the membranous labyrinth to balloon or dilate—a condition known as endolymphatic hydrops.

Many experts on Ménière's disease think that a rupture of the membranous labyrinth allows the endolymph to mix with perilymph, another inner ear fluid that occupies the space between the membranous labyrinth and the bony inner ear. This mixing, scientists believe,

NIH Publication No. 95-3403; November 1994.

can cause the symptoms of Ménière's disease. Scientists are investigating several possible causes of the disease, including environmental factors, such as noise pollution and viral infections, as well as biological factors.

What are the symptoms of Ménière's disease?

The symptoms of Ménière's disease occur suddenly and can arise daily or as infrequently as once a year. Vertigo, often the most debilitating symptom of Ménière's disease, forces the sufferer to lie down. Vertigo attacks can lead to severe nausea, vomiting, and sweating and often come with little or no warning.

Some individuals with Ménière's disease have attacks that start with tinnitus, a loss of hearing, or a full feeling of pressure in the affected ear. It is important to remember that all of these symptoms are unpredictable. Typically, the attack is characterized by a combination of vertigo, tinnitus and hearing loss lasting several hours. But people experience these discomforts at varying frequencies, durations, and intensities. Some may feel slight vertigo a few times a year. Others may be occasionally disturbed by intense, uncontrollable tinnitus while sleeping. And other Ménière's disease sufferers may notice a hearing loss and feel unsteady all day long for prolonged periods. Other occasional symptoms of Ménière's disease include headaches, abdominal discomfort and diarrhea. A person's hearing tends to recover between attacks but over time becomes worse.

How is Ménière's disease treated?

There is no cure for Ménière's disease. Medical and behavioral therapy, however, are often helpful in managing its symptoms. Although many operations have been developed to reverse the disease process, their value has been difficult to establish. And, unfortunately, all operations on the ear carry a risk of hearing loss.

The most commonly performed surgical treatment for Ménière's disease is the insertion of a shunt, a tiny silicone tube that is positioned in the inner ear to drain off excess fluid.

In another more reliable operation, a vestibular neurectomy, the vestibular nerve which serves balance is severed so that it no longer sends distorted messages to the brain. But the balance nerve is very close to the hearing and facial nerves. Thus, the risk of affecting the patient's hearing or facial muscle control increases with this type of surgical treatment. Also, older patients often have difficulty recovering from this type of surgery.

A labyrinthectomy, the removal of the membranous labyrinth, is an irreversible procedure that is often successful in eliminating the dizziness associated with Ménière's disease. This procedure, however, results in a total loss of hearing in the operated ear—an important consideration since the second ear may one day be affected. Also, labyrinthectomies themselves may result in other balance problems.

Some physicians recommend a change of diet to help control Ménière's symptoms. Eliminating caffeine, alcohol and salt may relieve the frequency and intensity of the attacks in some people. Eliminating tobacco use and reducing stress levels may lessen the severity of the symptoms. And medications that either control allergies, reduce fluid retention or improve blood circulation in the inner ear may also help.

How is Ménière's disease diagnosed?

Scientists estimate that there are 3 to 5 million people in the United States with Ménière's disease, with nearly 100,000 new cases diagnosed each year. Proper diagnosis of Ménière's disease entails several procedures, including a medical-history interview and a physical examination by a physician; hearing and balance tests; and medical imaging with magnetic resonance imaging (MRI). Accurate measurement and characterization of hearing loss are of critical importance in the diagnosis of Ménière's disease.

Through the use of several types of hearing tests, physicians can characterize hearing loss as being *sensory* arising from the inner ear, or *neural* arising from the hearing nerve. An auditory brain stem response, which measures electrical activity in the hearing nerve and brain stem, is useful in differentiating between these two types of hearing loss. And under certain circumstances, electrocochleography, recording the electrical activity of the inner ear in response to sound, helps confirm the diagnosis.

To test the vestibular or balance system, physicians irrigate the ears with warm and cool water. This flooding of the ears, known as caloric testing, results in nystagmus, rapid eye movements that can help a physician analyze a balance disorder. And because tumor growth can produce symptoms similar to Ménière's disease, magnetic resonance imaging is a useful test to determine whether a tumor is causing the patient's vertigo and hearing loss.

What research is being done?

Scientists are investigating environmental and biological factors that may cause Ménière's disease or induce attack. They are also studying how fluid composition and movement in the labyrinth affect hearing and balance. And by studying hair cells in the inner ear, which are responsible for proper hearing and balance, scientists are learning how the ear converts the mechanical energy of sound waved and motion into nerve impulses. Insights into the mechanisms of Ménière's disease will enable scientists to develop preventative strategies and more effective treatment.

Where can I get more information?

The NIDCD currently supports research on Ménière's disease in medical centers and universities throughout the nation. For more information about Ménière's disease, you can contact:

American Academy of Otolaryngology—Head and Neck Surgery
One Prince Street
Alexandria, VA 22314
Telephone: (703) 836-4444 (519-1585 TTY)

Deafness Research Foundation
9 East 38th Street
New York, NY 10016
Telephone: (212) 684-6556 (684-6559 TTY)
(800) 535-DEAF

Ear Foundation
2000 Church Street, Box 111
Nashville, TN 37236
Telephone: (615) 329-7807 (329-7809 TTY)
(800) 545-HEAR

Vestibular Disorders Association
P.O. Box 4467
Portland, OR 97208-4467
Telephone: (503) 229-7705
(800) 837-8428

Chapter 59

Because You Asked about Smell and Taste Disorders

If you experience a smell or taste problem, it is important to re-member that you are not alone: thousands of other individuals have faced the same situation. More than 200,000 persons visit a physician for a smell or taste problem each year. Many more smell and taste dis-turbances go unreported.

How do smell and taste work?

Smell and taste belong to our chemical sensing system, or the chemosenses. The complicated processes of smelling and tasting begin when tiny molecules released by the substances around us stimulate special cells in the nose, mouth, or throat. These special sensory cells transmit messages through nerves to the brain where specific smells or tastes are identified.

Olfactory or smell nerve cells are stimulated by the odors around us—the fragrance from a gardenia or the smell of bread baking. These nerve cells are found in a small patch of tissue high inside the nose, and they connect directly to the brain.

Gustatory or taste cells react to food and beverages. These sur-face cells in the mouth send taste information to their nerve fibers. The taste cells are clustered in the taste buds of the mouth and throat. Many of the small bumps that can be seen on the tongue contain taste buds.

NIH Publication No. 91-3231; June 1991.

A third chemosensory mechanism, called the common chemical sense, contributes to our senses of smell and taste. In this system, thousands of nerve endings—especially on the moist surfaces of the eyes, nose, mouth, and throat—give rise to sensations like the sting of ammonia, the coolness of menthol, and the irritation of chili peppers.

We can commonly identify four basic taste sensations: sweet, sour, bitter, and salty. In the mouth these tastes, along with texture, temperature, and the sensations from the common chemical sense, combine with odors to produce a perception of flavor. It is flavor that lets us know whether we are eating a pear or an apple. Flavors are recognized mainly through the sense of smell. If you hold your nose while eating chocolate, for example, you will have trouble identifying the chocolate flavor even though you can distinguish the food's sweetness or bitterness. That's because the familiar flavor of chocolate is sensed largely by the odor. So is the well-known flavor of coffee.

What are smell and taste disorders?

The most common chemosensory complaints are a loss of the sense of smell and the sense of taste. Testing may demonstrate a reduced ability to detect odors (*hyposmia*) or to taste sweet, sour, bitter, or salty substances (*hypogeusia*). Some people can detect no odors (*anosmia*) or no tastes (*ageusia*).

In other disorders of the chemical senses, the system may misread and distort an odor, a taste, or a flavor. Or a person may detect a foul odor or taste from a substance that is normally pleasant smelling or tasting.

Overall, smell disorders are more common than taste disorders. They rarely occur together.

What causes smell and taste disorders?

Some people are born with chemosensory disorders, but most develop them after an injury or illness. Upper respiratory infections are blamed for some chemosensory losses, and injuries to the head can also cause smell or taste problems.

Chemosensory disorders may result from polyps in the nasal cavities, sinus infections, hormonal disturbances, or dental problems. Loss of smell and taste also can be caused by exposure to certain chemicals such as insecticides and by some medicines.

Many patients who receive radiation therapy for cancers of the head and neck develop chemosensory disturbances.

How are smell and taste disturbances diagnosed?

The extent of a chemosensory disorder can be determined by measuring the lowest concentration of a chemical that a person can detect or recognize. A patient may also be asked to compare the smells or tastes of different chemicals or to note how the intensities of smells or tastes grow when a chemical's concentration is increased.

Scientists have developed an easily administered "scratch and sniff" test to evaluate the sense of smell. A person scratches pieces of paper treated to release different odors, sniffs them, and tries to identify each odor from a list of possibilities.

In taste testing, the patient responds to different chemical concentrations: this may involve a simple "sip, spit, and rinse" test, or chemicals may be applied directly to specific areas of the tongue.

Are smell and taste disorders serious?

A person with faulty chemosenses is deprived of an early warning system that most of us take for granted. Smell and taste alert us to fires, poisonous fumes, leaking gas, and spoiled food and beverages. Smell and taste losses can also lead to depression.

Abnormalities in smell and taste functions frequently accompany and even signal the existence of several diseases or unhealthy conditions, including obesity, diabetes, hypertension, malnutrition, and some degenerative diseases of the nervous system such as Parkinson's disease, Alzheimer's disease and Korsakoff's psychosis.

Can smell and taste disorders be treated?

If a certain medication is the cause of a smell or taste disorder, stopping or changing the medicine may help eliminate the problem. Some patients, notably those with respiratory infections or allergies, regain their smell or taste upon the resolution of their illness. In many cases, nasal obstructions such as polyps can be removed surgically to restore airflow to the nose. Often the correction of a general medical problem can also correct the loss of smell and taste. Occasionally, recovery of the chemosenses occurs spontaneously.

497

What research is being done?

The National Institute on Deafness and Other Communication Disorders (NIDCD), one of the institutes of the National Institutes of Health, supports basic and clinical investigations of chemosensory disorders at institutions across the nation. Some of these studies are conducted at several chemosensory research centers, where scientists work together to unravel the secrets of smell and taste disorders.

Remarkable progress has been made in establishing the nature of changes that occur in the chemical senses with age. It is now known that age takes a much greater toll on smell than on taste. Scientists have found that the sense of smell begins to decline after age 60. Women at all ages are generally more accurate than men in identifying odors. Smoking can adversely affect the ability to identify odors in both men and women.

Although certain medications can cause chemosensory problems, others notably antiallergy drugs seem to improve the senses of smell and taste. Scientists are working to find medicines similar to antiallergy drugs that can be used to treat patients with chemosensory losses.

Smell and taste cells are the only sensory cells that are regularly replaced throughout the life span. Scientists are examining this phenomenon which may provide ways to replace these and other damaged sensory and nerve cells. NIDCD's research program goals for chemosensory sciences include:

- promotion of the regeneration of sensory and nerve cells
- appreciating the effects of the environment on smell and taste (such as gasoline fumes, chemicals, and extremes of relative humidity and temperature)
- prevention of the effects of aging
- prevention of the access of infectious agents and toxins to the bruin through the olfactory nerve
- development of new diagnostic tests
- understanding associations between chemosensory disorders and altered food intake in aging as well as in various chronic illnesses
- improved methods of treatment and rehabilitation strategies

What can I do to help myself?

Proper diagnosis by a trained professional, such as an otolaryngologist-head and neck surgeon, is important. These physicians specialize in disorders of the head and neck, especially those related to the ear, nose and throat. Diagnosis may lead to treatment of an underlying cause of the disturbance. Many types of smell and taste disorders are curable, and for those that are not, counseling is available to help patients cope with a disorder.

The NIDCD supports research studies at several centers specializing in developing a better understanding of the chemical senses in health and disease:

Richard L. Doty, Ph.D.
University of Pennsylvania Smell and Taste
Research Center
Hospital of the University of Pennsylvania
3400 Spruce Street
Philadelphia, PA 19104-4283
(215) 662-6580

Marion E. Frank, Ph.D.
Taste and Smell Center
Connecticut Chemosensory Clinical Research
Center
University of Connecticut Health Center
Farmington, CT 06032
(203) 679-2459

Maxwell M. Mozell, Ph.D.
SUNY Health Sciences Center at Syracuse
Clinical Olfactory Research Center
766 Irving Avenue
Syracuse, NY 1 3210
(315) 464-4538

Gary Beauchamp, Ph.D.
Monell Chemical Senses Center
3500 Market Street
Philadelphia, PA 19104
(215) 898-6666

Thomas E. Finger, Ph.D.
Rocky Mountain Taste and Smell Center, Box 111
University of Colorado Health Sciences Center
4200 East 9th Avenue
Denver, C0 80262
(303) 270-7464

About the NIDCD

The National Institute on Deafness and Other Communication Disorders (NIDCD) is one of the institutes of the National Institutes of Health. The NIDCD conducts and supports research and research training on normal mechanisms and well as diseases and disorders of hearing, balance, smell, taste, voice, speech and language. The NIDCD achieves its mission through a wide range of research performed in its own laboratories, a program of research grants, individual and institutional research training awards, career development awards, center grants, and contracts to public and private research institutions and organizations.

The Institute also conducts and supports research and research training related to disease prevention and health promotion; addresses special biomedical and behavioral problems associated with people who have communication impairments or disorders; and supports efforts to create devices which substitute for lost and impaired sensory and communication function.

The NIDCD is committed to understanding how certain diseases or disorders may affect women, men, or members of underrepresented minority populations differently.

The NIDCD has a national clearinghouse for information and resources. Additional on smell and taste may be obtained from the NIDCD Clearinghouse. Write to:

NIDCD Clearinghouse
P. O. Box 37777
Washington, DC 20013-7777

Index

Index

A page number in *italics* indicates an illustration.

A

ABC-TV News, live-captioned 37
ABR *see* brain stem auditory evoked response (BAER)
accent, as articulation problem 314
acoupedic method 32
acoustic energy 6
acoustic immittance audiometry, in infants and young children 57
Acoustic Neuroma Association 465
acoustic neuroma (vestibular schwannoma) 473-85, 487-89
  and acquired sensorineural hearing loss 10
  audiological testing for 478-79
  bilateral 488
    see also neurofibromatosis type 2
  classification of 475-76
  defined 455
  diagnosis of 487
  dizziness with 448
  evaluation for 476-79
  psychological aspects of 485
  radiation therapy for 481-82
    complications of 484

acoustic neuroma, continued
  radiosurgery for 488
  recurrence of 484
  sporadic 476-77
    nerve compression in 477
  surgical removal of 480-81, 487-88
  symptoms of 473-74, 487
  treatment of, complications of 483-85
  types of 488
acoustic trauma, defined 112
acquired immunodeficiency syndrome (AIDS), and acquired sensorineural hearing loss 10
acute otitis media (AOM) 71-91
  see also ear infection(s); middle ear disease; otitis media
  defined 69, 75
  polyethelene tubes for 86-87
  recurrent *75*, *76*
    frequently 78-79, *80*
  resistant 79
  treatment of 84-85
  unresponsive 76-78, *77*
ADARA (American Deafness and Rehabilitation Association) 35
adult(s)
  aphasia of 317-21
  with articulation problems 315
  with cleft lip and palate 351-54

503

O

OAE *see* otoacoustic emissions (OAE)
occlusion
of child with cleft lip and palate 356
and Crouzon syndrome (craniofacial dysostosis) 371
Occupational Safety and Health Administration (OSHA), on hearing protection devices 135
occupations
of deaf people 34
noise of 109-10
older people *see* aging people
olfactory (smell) nerve cells 495
OME *see* otitis media, with effusion (OME)
omissions 314
open-set speech recognition 220
optokinetic nystagmus, testing for 435
oral appliances
for clefts 357
for submucous cleft palate 349
oral communication 31-32
oral hygiene *see under* dental care
oral language acquisition in children, impact of cochlear implant on 236-37
organ of Corti (hearing organ) 5
organizations, of and for deaf people 34-36
orientation
and balance 460
sense of 418
orthodontics, for child with cleft lip and palate 356-57
orthostatic (postural) hypotension 457
and dizziness 449
Orton Dyslexia Society 303, 312
oscillopsia 437
OSHA (Occupational Safety and Health Administration), on hearing protection devices 135
ossicles (middle ear bones), donation of for research 454
Osteogenesis imperfecta, gene mapping of 18
otitis media 11-13
acute 71-91
see also acute otitis media (AOM)

otitis media, continued
causes hearing loss in children 3-4, 11-12
research in 19-21
in children 59-62, 63-64
chronic
affects development in speech and language 290-91
defined 69
defined 63, 67, 69
effect of on speech and language development 64, 65, 68, 69
with effusion (OME) 79-81, *82*
defined 75
evaluation of effusions of 73-75
as incidental 81-83
as persistent 79-81, *82*
natural history of 86
polyethelene tubes for 85, 86-87
treatment of 84-85
facts about 67-70
hearing loss in 64, 65
NICD facts about 67-70
occurence of how common 63-64
with perforation 207
questions and answers about 63-66
recurrent
defined 69
see also under acute otitis media
research in 19-21
serous, defined 69
severe, management of 71-91
signs and symptoms of 65, 68, 69
vaccine development for 20
see also acute otitis media (AOM); ear infection(s); middle ear disease
otoacoustic emissions (OAE) 6
defined 6
in infants and young children 58
screening for in infants 52
source of 6
otoconia 440
otolaryngologist 180
defined 69
and speech and language disorders 298
otolaryngology–head and neck surgery defined 206, 209, 472